A Colour Atlas of Surface Anatomy

Reprinted 1989

Copyright © K.M. Backhouse, R.T. Hutchings, 1986
Published by Wolfe Medical Publications Ltd, 1986
Printed by Royal Smeets Offset b.v., Weert, Netherlands
ISBN 0 7234 0801 7
Reprinted 1990

For a full list of anatomy atlases, plus
forthcoming titles and details of our medical,
surgical, dental and veterinary atlases, please
write to Wolfe Medical Publications Ltd,
Brook House, 2-16 Torrinton Place, London WC1E 7LT.

Designer: Iain Wolfe

A Colour Atlas of

Surface Anatomy

clinical and applied

Kenneth M. Backhouse

O.B.E., V.R.D., M.B,B.S., M.R.C.S.
Reader Emeritus in Applied Anatomy, University
of London. Clinical Anatomist, Institute of
Laryngology and Otology and the Royal National
Throat, Nose and Ear Hospital, London. Lecturer
in Anatomy and Orthopaedics, Royal Ballet School,
London. Formerly Reader in Applied Anatomy,
Hunterian Professor, Arris and Gale Lecturer and
Examiner in Anatomy for Primary F.R.C.S. and
F.D.S., Royal College of Surgeons of England.

Ralph T. Hutchings

Freelance Photographer. Formerly Chief Medical
Laboratory Scientific Officer, Royal College of
Surgeons of England.

Wolfe Medical Publications Ltd

Acknowledgements

We would like to thank our models for providing the physical substance for this book, and Professor Robert McMinn for kindly allowing us to use some of the subsurface photographs from his 'Colour Atlas of Human Anatomy'.

Reprinted 1989

Copyright © K.M. Backhouse, R.T. Hutchings, 1986
Published by Wolfe Medical Publications Ltd, 1986
Printed by Royal Smeets Offset b.v., Weert, Netherlands
ISBN 0 7234 0801 7

For a full list of anatomy atlases, plus forthcoming titles and details of our medical, surgical, dental and veterinary atlases, please write to Wolfe Medical Publications Ltd, Brook House, 2-16 Torrinton Place, London WC1E 7LT.

Designer: Iain Wolfe

Contents

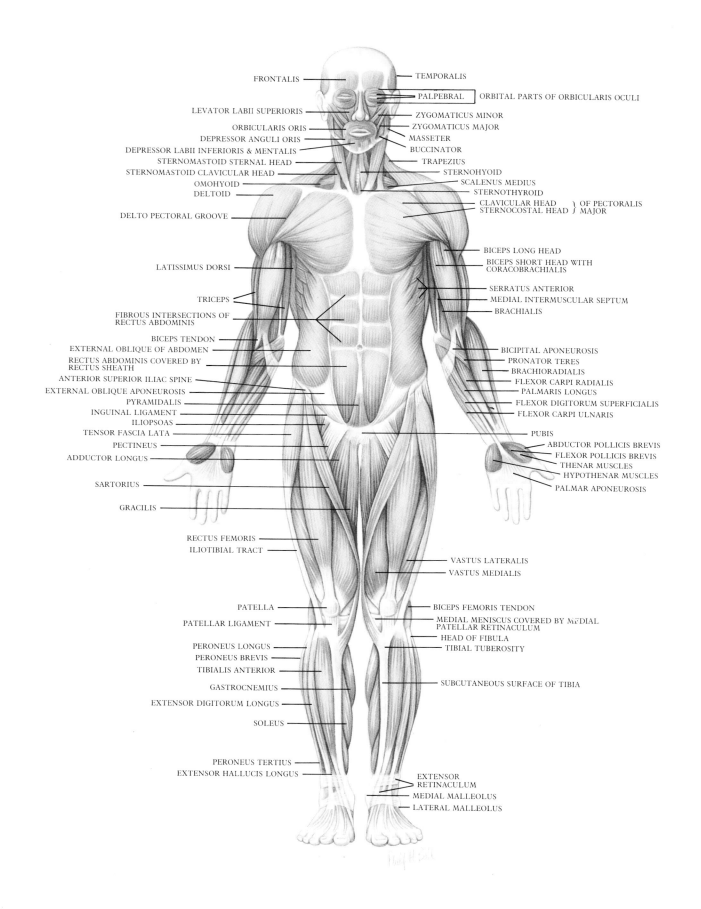

FRONTALIS — TEMPORALIS

PALPEBRAL | ORBITAL PARTS OF ORBICULARIS OCULI

LEVATOR LABII SUPERIORIS — ZYGOMATICUS MINOR

ORBICULARIS ORIS — ZYGOMATICUS MAJOR

DEPRESSOR ANGULI ORIS — MASSETER

DEPRESSOR LABII INFERIORIS & MENTALIS — BUCCINATOR

STERNOMASTOID STERNAL HEAD — TRAPEZIUS

STERNOMASTOID CLAVICULAR HEAD — STERNOHYOID

OMOHYOID — SCALENUS MEDIUS

DELTOID — STERNOTHYROID

CLAVICULAR HEAD | OF PECTORALIS
STERNOCOSTAL HEAD | MAJOR

DELTO PECTORAL GROOVE

BICEPS LONG HEAD

BICEPS SHORT HEAD WITH
CORACOBRACHIALIS

LATISSIMUS DORSI — SERRATUS ANTERIOR

MEDIAL INTERMUSCULAR SEPTUM

TRICEPS — BRACHIALIS

FIBROUS INTERSECTIONS OF
RECTUS ABDOMINIS

BICEPS TENDON

EXTERNAL OBLIQUE OF ABDOMEN — BICIPITAL APONEUROSIS

RECTUS ABDOMINIS COVERED BY
RECTUS SHEATH — PRONATOR TERES

BRACHIORADIALIS

ANTERIOR SUPERIOR ILIAC SPINE — FLEXOR CARPI RADIALIS

EXTERNAL OBLIQUE APONEUROSIS — PALMARIS LONGUS

PYRAMIDALIS — FLEXOR DIGITORUM SUPERFICIALIS

INGUINAL LIGAMENT — FLEXOR CARPI ULNARIS

ILIOPSOAS

TENSOR FASCIA LATA — PUBIS

PECTINEUS — ABDUCTOR POLLICIS BREVIS

ADDUCTOR LONGUS — FLEXOR POLLICIS BREVIS

THENAR MUSCLES

HYPOTHENAR MUSCLES

SARTORIUS — PALMAR APONEUROSIS

GRACILIS

RECTUS FEMORIS

ILIOTIBIAL TRACT

VASTUS LATERALIS

VASTUS MEDIALIS

PATELLA — BICEPS FEMORIS TENDON

PATELLAR LIGAMENT — MEDIAL MENISCUS COVERED BY MEDIAL
PATELLAR RETINACULUM

HEAD OF FIBULA

PERONEUS LONGUS — TIBIAL TUBEROSITY

PERONEUS BREVIS

TIBIALIS ANTERIOR

GASTROCNEMIUS — SUBCUTANEOUS SURFACE OF TIBIA

EXTENSOR DIGITORUM LONGUS

SOLEUS

PERONEUS TERTIUS

EXTENSOR HALLUCIS LONGUS

EXTENSOR
RETINACULUM

MEDIAL MALLEOLUS

LATERAL MALLEOLUS

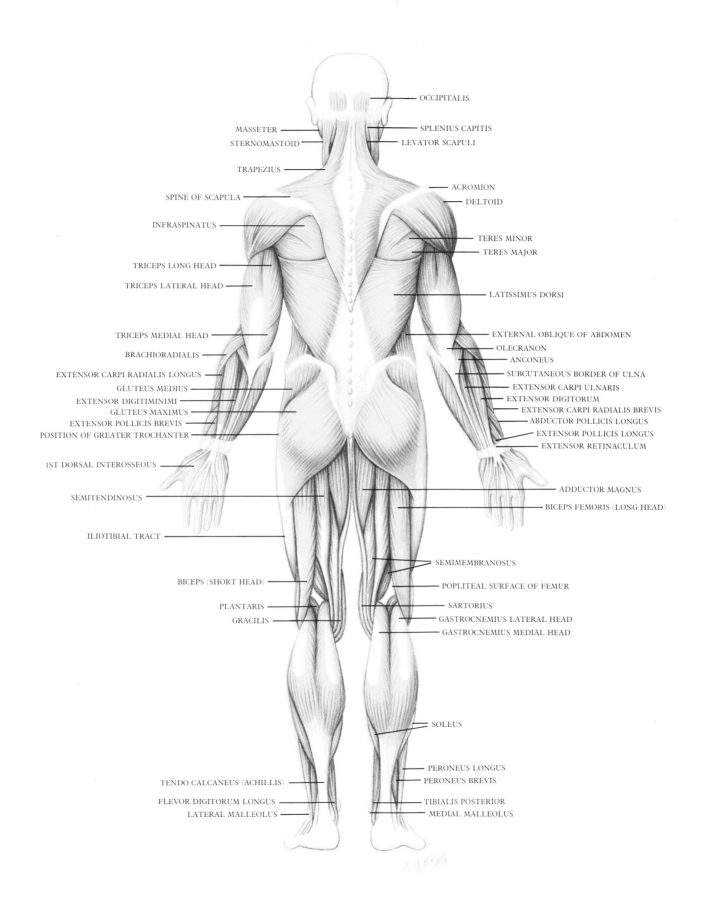

OCCIPITALIS

MASSETER

SPLENIUS CAPITIS

STERNOMASTOID

LEVATOR SCAPULI

TRAPEZIUS

SPINE OF SCAPULA

ACROMION

DELTOID

INFRASPINATUS

TERES MINOR

TERES MAJOR

TRICEPS LONG HEAD

TRICEPS LATERAL HEAD

LATISSIMUS DORSI

TRICEPS MEDIAL HEAD

EXTERNAL OBLIQUE OF ABDOMEN

BRACHIORADIALIS

OLECRANON

ANCONEUS

EXTENSOR CARPI RADIALIS LONGUS

SUBCUTANEOUS BORDER OF ULNA

GLUTEUS MEDIUS

EXTENSOR CARPI ULNARIS

EXTENSOR DIGITIMINIMI

EXTENSOR DIGITORUM

GLUTEUS MAXIMUS

EXTENSOR CARPI RADIALIS BREVIS

EXTENSOR POLLICIS BREVIS

ABDUCTOR POLLICIS LONGUS

POSITION OF GREATER TROCHANTER

EXTENSOR POLLICIS LONGUS

EXTENSOR RETINACULUM

1ST DORSAL INTEROSSEOUS

SEMITENDINOSUS

ADDUCTOR MAGNUS

BICEPS FEMORIS (LONG HEAD)

ILIOTIBIAL TRACT

SEMIMEMBRANOSUS

POPLITEAL SURFACE OF FEMUR

BICEPS (SHORT HEAD)

SARTORIUS

PLANTARIS

GASTROCNEMIUS LATERAL HEAD

GRACILIS

GASTROCNEMIUS MEDIAL HEAD

SOLEUS

PERONEUS LONGUS

PERONEUS BREVIS

TENDO CALCANEUS (ACHILLIS)

FLEVOR DIGITORUM LONGUS

TIBIALIS POSTERIOR

LATERAL MALLEOLUS

MEDIAL MALLEOLUS

7

PREFACE

For many medical and dental students, anatomy represents a period of learning facts based essentially on dried bones and cadaveric dissections, which bear little relationship with the living patient or even the dissections of operative surgery. The subject tends to become a chore which has to be tolerated in order to achieve the aim of working with living people. While the medical student does at least have the advantage of examining structures in three dimensions in the dissecting room or anatomy museum, these facilities are often not available to the other professional training groups for whom a knowledge of living anatomy is just as important as to the future doctor, e.g. physical and occupational therapists, nurses and other paramedical groups as well as physical educators, dance teachers etc.

The learning of anatomical structure is of little value unless it can be seen essentially as it exists and functions in the normal living person. To be of any value as anything but a morphological exercise, the anatomy must live, move, grow, age and exhibit all the variations evident in the community as well as the changes due to physical training, disease etc. The physician, surgeon, therapist, nurse, physical educator, artist must look at the skin covered individual and visualise what lies and functions beneath that skin. Only in this way can the clinician assess normal function and any variation from that normality be it from injury or disease.

Many structures can be seen readily from their surface contours and appearance; bony points, superficial muscles, tendons, veins etc. For deeper structures, their positions need to be known as from the surface and their normality assessed from a knowledge of their functions which can be tested clinically. Thus normal functioning of muscles (and their nervous control) can be tested from a knowledge of their positions and functions in the intact living body and, where pathology is suspected, how to test for that normality or otherwise is vital. It is also important to be able to assess the disability which might ensue from failure of structures.

In the physical fields the term kinaesiology has been coined to cover the study of muscle function and this particular aspect of living anatomy has been stressed within the overall functional control of the body.

It is fashionable, particularly among some physicians, to claim that they have forgotten most of the anatomy they ever knew and don't miss it. They dismiss the lifeless morphology in such statements and include their considerable knowledge of living anatomy as an integral part of their medical, clinical expertise. May we therefore offer this book in that light as an introduction to clinical medicine.

In examining the form and functioning of the body it has been necessary to limit the field to matters of more general importance and avoid the more specialist examinations. For this reason examination of the orifices of the body has been excluded. With the enormous developments in fibreoptics and other clinical weaponry for endoscopic examinations this has become an enormous field, well beyond the scope of a general book.

In producing a basically pictorial book of the surface of the body, it is always tempting to use dramatic lighting techniques and people with highly developed muscles. We have deliberately avoided these approaches. Our aim has been to produce good pictorial representation of the type of person whom the practitioner is likely to meet in everyday practice.

It has been a policy to leave many pictures unlabelled to persuade the reader to look and see. Copy pictures have been used to carry labels where considered advisable.

Although this book has been designed primarily with medical and paramedical personnel in mind it is hoped that, in view of its strong emphasis in kinaesiology, it will be of value to physical educators, teachers of dance etc. and also useful in life study for artists.

THE SKIN

Observation and examination of the body must begin with the skin, or, in the orifices, the mucous membranes. The skin is responsible for much of the health of the body. That health or lack of it is often evident in the appearance of the skin and it is prudent for the clinician to remember this fact.

The skin and subcutaneous tissues may do much to camouflage the deeper structures of the body but the clinician needs to be able not only to identify and locate these structures through the skin but also, in certain cases, to test their function and effectiveness. The skin must be closely related to the underlying structures but must move freely in accord with them without in any way restricting their movement. The body must have total skin cover. A major part of a plastic surgeon's activity is to replace skin after loss, whether by injury or necessary surgical excision, so as to give full protective covering for the body, by means of skin grafts or various forms of flaps. The new skin cover may then need to be manipulated to allow full freedom of mobility with, whenever possible, effective sensory response.

The skin contains the receptive components of much of the sensory awareness of the body, i.e. exteroceptive sensibility, and is linked by sensory nerves to the brain, either directly or through the spinal cord. In certain parts of the body this is especially important. The palmar surfaces of the hands for instance receive, under normal circumstances, such remarkably fine sensory stimuli that the resultant tactile awareness can give enormous amounts of information to the brain. The blind man can read braille through his fingers; the correct coin can be chosen from pocket or purse by touch. In fact, from this tactile awareness through the skin, the hands have been described as the eyes that see in the dark and around corners.

The character of the skin varies enormously over the body. This difference is particularly obvious at the lips where the relatively thinly keratinised vermilion region changes to much thicker hairy skin; here the shaven bearded area of a male (2).

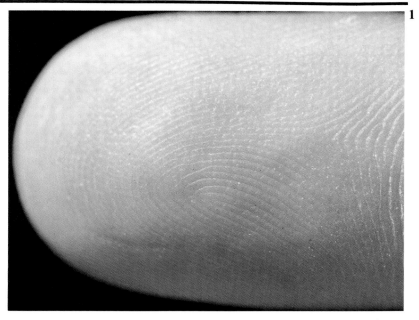

Beneath the dermal ridges which characterise the finger and palm prints are enormous numbers of touch end-organs, giving the potential of exquisite sensory awareness. Because of the need, a blind person makes much more effective use of this perception than the average sighted person. Note that in the special tactile areas of the body the skin is devoid of hairs. In the shaded area of the photograph the bright dots of sweat are obvious at the openings of the sweat glands.

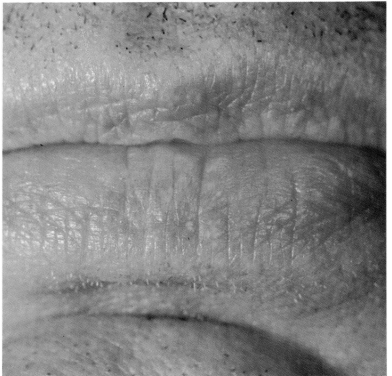

THE APPEARANCE OF THE SKIN

The appearance of the skin is so important to the majority of people, that vast amounts of money are spent in attempts to improve its quality and to prevent the ravages of time (and sometimes of disease or injury). The many skin colours, not only ethnic but even within an ethnic community, add to the vastness of the cosmetic supportive armamentarium.

As the skin must be related to the underlying structures but at the same time must be free to move and adjust with body movement, it needs to have a considerable intrinsic flexibility. The elasticity associated with this flexibility tends to be lost, as one of the ageing processes of the body, so that the skin becomes lined and sags in places and recovers poorly after deformation.

3

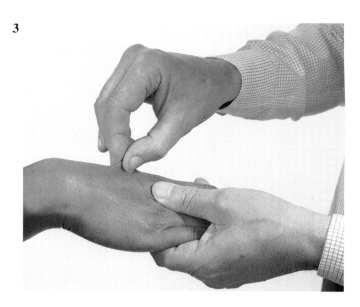

If the skin on the back of the hand is squeezed and lifted somewhat in a younger person, owing to the intrinsic elasticity it reforms to its natural resting state (**3** and **4**). If the same manoeuvre is carried out in an older person where the skin elasticity has been lost, the skin deformity remains until pulled out by movement; in this case flexion of the hand (**5**).

4

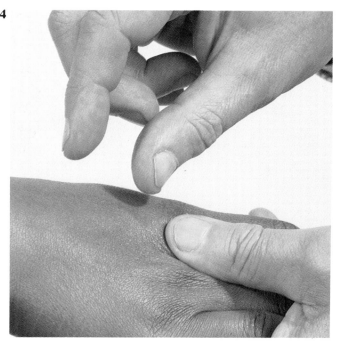

5

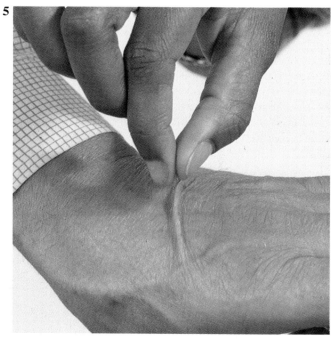

DEEP ATTACHMENTS OF THE SKIN

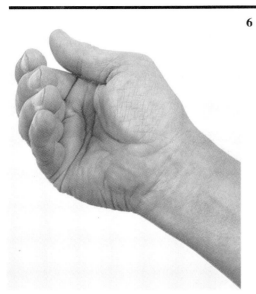

6

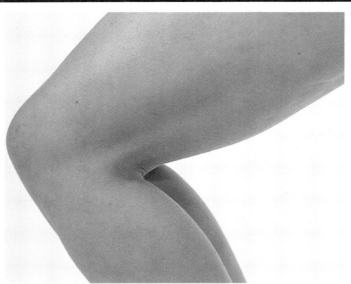

7 In the palm of the hand the skin is bound down to the underlying fibrous tissue (the palmar aponeurosis) in the central triangle between thenar and proximal flexor creases, as well as at the flexion creases (**6**). A similar arrangement is found in the various flexion creases in the limbs, as here at the knee (**7**), at the inguinal fold in the groin and similarly in the arms. Conversely where the extensor skin has to be pulled around a joint when flexed, the skin may be bound down in loose folds which are then taken up in flexion. This arrangement is particularly obvious over the finger joints (see page 138).

STRESS LINES IN SKIN

In certain places the skin must be bound down to the underlying deep fascia, as at the skin creases, to allow free movement without risk of interference by uncontrolled skin and subcutaneous fat.

The skin adjusts and follows the contours of the body regardless of movement. Although this is permitted by its intrinsic elasticity and its controlled binding, in certain places nevertheless skin is subjected to internal stresses, which vary from place to place. Langer showed that even in cadavers the skin is subject to stresses in certain directions and he plotted the stress lines. These are often known as Langer's lines. It has been shown that wounds along Langer's lines (i.e. with the stress in the same direction as the wound) heal with a minimum of scar, whereas when skin stresses tend to pull the wound edges apart the scar may become much thicker with the consequent risk of scar contraction. Langer's lines do not always correspond with the stress lines in life and so it is perhaps better to consider these as 'resting stress lines', i.e. stress in the living skin with the body at rest. In the flexor aspect of the elbow for instance the resting stress lines run transversely in the directions of the creases, but if the arm is at full stretch in extension, longitudinal stresses are imparted; hence the value in nursing repairing wounds with the skin in a resting position wherever possible.

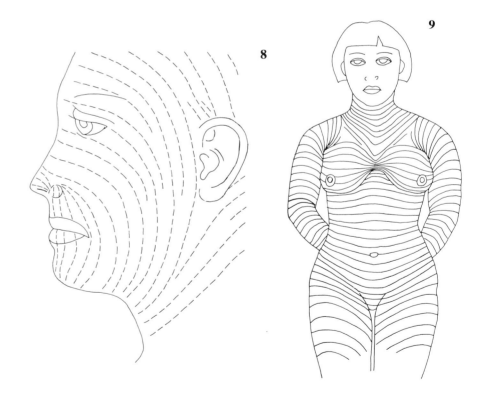

8

9

STRESS LINES IN SKIN

In certain areas, the face and neck and the ulnar **10** heel of the hand, striated muscle runs directly into the skin to generate movement, thus inducing dynamic stress lines in addition to the resting ones.

In the face the so-called muscles of facial expression are inserted directly into the skin. In the region of the eye they control lid closure while the orbital part pulls up the surrounding skin where it can help shade the eyes from the sun. Note how this has generated skin lines which have become accentuated by sun browning of the surrounding skin. See also **6** illustrating the effect of palmaris brevis in the hand.

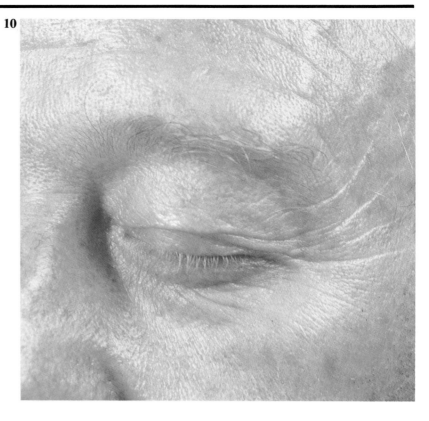

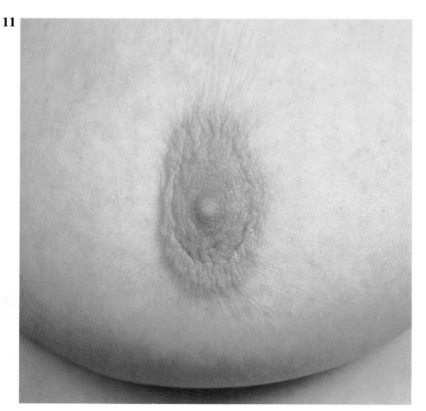

In other areas highly specialised involuntary muscle is incorporated into the skin to induce contraction in response to cold and other stimuli; e.g. the scrotum in the male and the nipples in both sexes.

HAIR

In certain areas hair is an obvious feature but over most of the body, apart from special sensory zones such as the palms of the hands, soles of the feet, lips etc., some degree of hair cover will be found. In many individuals and sites, particularly in women and children the hair may be fine and inconspicuous; in others, and particularly in males, it may be very obvious. In most parts of the body the hair, as in most mammals, is directional. Furthermore, as in these animals, the hair is controlled by tiny muscles to erect it in cold or fear, though in humans the most obvious effect is the production of 'goose pimples'.

In the scalp region hair becomes a prominent feature, showing considerable variations in structure and colour. As the hair is such an important feature of head and facial appearance considerable care is usually taken in its control.

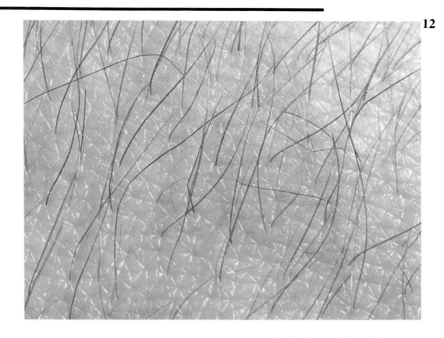

12

A magnified view of the skin on the back of a male forearm. Note the pits or follicles from which the hair grows and into which sebaceous glands open, as well as the other openings of sebaceous and sweat glands.

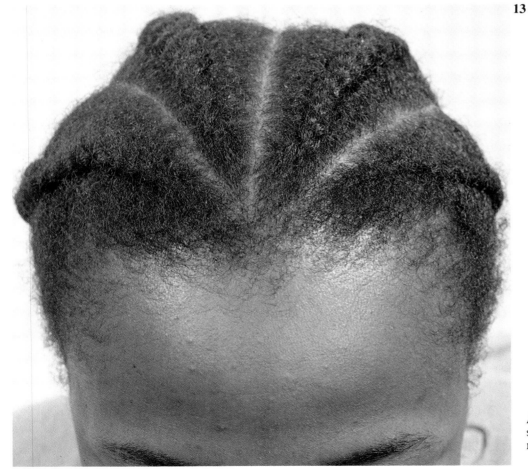

13

A form of hairdressing ideally suited to the short-growing curly negroid hair.

HAIR

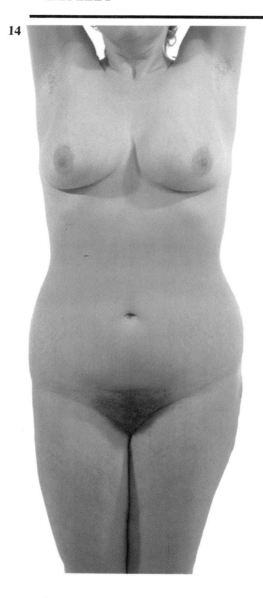

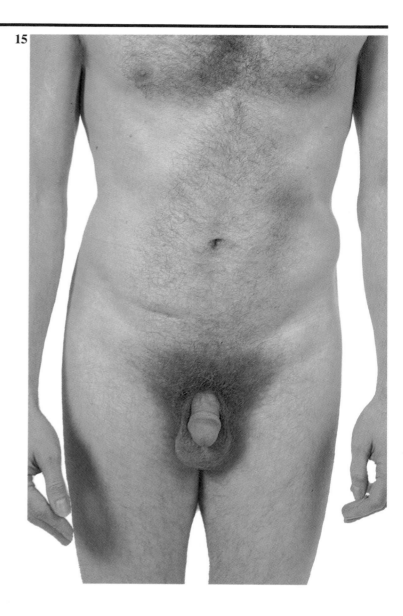

Characteristic patterns of male
and female body hair.

There is a tendency in certain males to go bald but this is an unusual and virtually always a pathological feature if it occurs in a female. Baldness is thus sex linked and familial.

With sexual maturity body hair becomes apparent in both sexes; in the axilla, the pubic region and in the male on the trunk and face. The pubic hair in the female tends to be limited to the mons pubis Veneris and to a lesser extent the labia majora, with a fairly sharp flat 'cut off' on to the abdomen, whereas that of the male is less sharp and tends to run up towards the umbilicus in the midline. In more generally hairy individuals the hair may continue centrally over the upper abdomen to increase in amount on the chest. The legs and to a lesser extent the arms may be quite hairy in the male. The face also becomes hairy in the male in the characteristic beard area. What is particularly interesting is that whereas a male may lose the hair on his head, that on his face and body continues to grow and the area may in fact increase with age. The ears may become quite hairy and the eyebrows more shaggy.

The sex hormones play an essential part in determining male and female characteristics, most obviously in the genitalia and the associated sexual structures. As we have seen, hair characteristics and patterns are sex linked. The male tends to have a heavier build with more bulky bone and musculature, though physical usage is also important. The male thus may give a more dynamic appearance with muscle contours showing through the skin. The female, however, is likely to have the muscular appearance smoothed out by subcutaneous fat to give the softer feminine curves. Where fat is increased in amount it is deposited somewhat differently between the sexes.

Fat is a feature of the female breasts and also the buttocks, lower abdomen, hips and thighs. Fat in the lower abdomen thus emphasises the relatively slim waist when compared with that of the male. The male tends to lay down fat more generally over the abdominal wall and in the mesenteries of the abdomen to give a protruding 'corporation', with loss of waist, though this is not the usual feature in a fit young man.

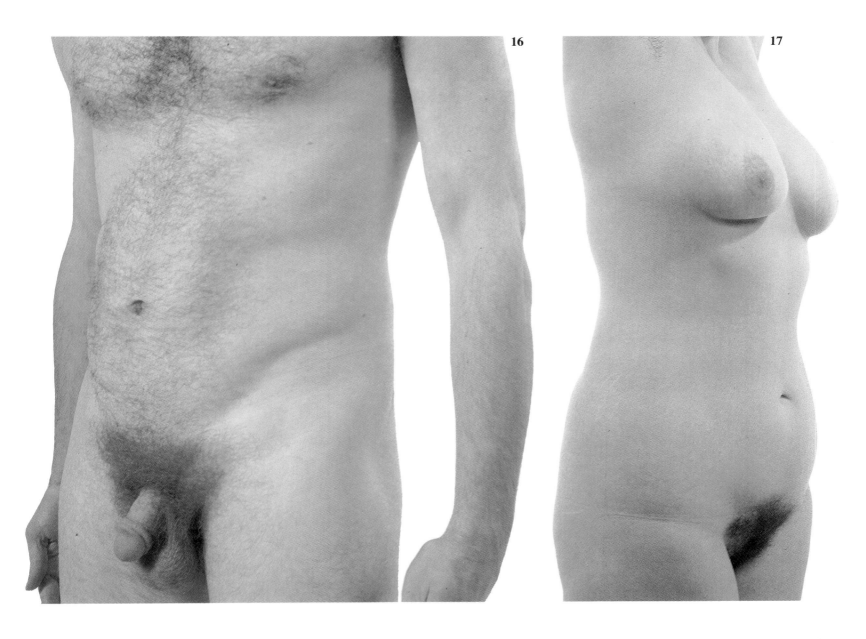

16   17

BONE AND MUSCLE

Much of the surface contour of the body is generated by the bony skeleton and the linking muscles. Of the axial skeleton the skull, part of the rib cage and the vertebral spines are readily palpable. The pelvis is mainly hidden but for certain prominent features. In the limbs certain bones run subcutaneously and are readily palpable whereas others are hidden by muscles except for their projecting features. Most of the surface skin overlies muscle, which may be masked by the covering skin and fascia unless put into activity and even then if there is little fat cover. In a muscular person some muscles may stand out, e.g. the deltoid at the shoulder and this is more likely in a male, for even in a slim athletic female there is still the likelihood of contour softening by the overlying tissues. Some individuals practise forms of muscle development, essentially by repeated isometric exercise of the individual muscles. This gives both remarkable bulk and isolated muscle control which makes observation of the muscles through the skin relatively easy. For the majority of the population, including even the athletically fit, examination is far less easy, as even continued hard training in most physical activities, leads to strong muscles rather than great bulk. Many outstanding athletes are remarkably slim (**18**).

Few people can isolate activity in an individual muscle and hence the examiner must be able to instruct the patient or subject to generate movements which will produce contraction in the muscle to be examined. It must be remembered that under normal circumstances muscles do not work in isolation but in groups. In fact even when the body is at rest all muscles in the body are contributing to its control though few may be showing action potentials of active contraction. Muscles are elastic structures exhibiting such elastic pull as is commensurate with their size.

The concept of group activity of muscles is important. The four muscles of the quadriceps group in the leg normally work as a team, giving not only powerful extension at the knee but also imparting an essential stabilising control over a potentially unstable joint. Pectoralis major gives the main power towards flexion-adduction at the shoulder joint but as much of its pull is downwards it would also be a most effective dislocator of the joint if it did not work synergistically with that weak flexor adductor but strong shoulder joint relocator, coracobrachialis.

Since even a highly trained athlete, gymnast or dancer is unlikely to be able to move most of the individual muscles in isolation, examination of muscles for their individual action and hence the normality of their nerve supply, must be linked with movement of the group as a whole and the activity (or lack of it) of the individual muscle assessed from this. Commonly it is necessary to compare the one side with the other if action of the muscle is not readily observable from the surface, though always remembering that the dominant arm may be stronger than the other as a result of occupation.

When examining muscles it is important to remember that some muscles run over only one joint and hence their activity and fine control is directed to that joint. Others run over more than one joint; the long flexors of the fingers and toes cross and theoretically control several, which would be totally inefficient. Muscles cannot exercise a high level of control over more than one joint. Therefore multijoint muscles will normally work with other muscles or sometimes ligamentous structures to control one or more joints in the chain thus limiting the number of joints over which they are acting at that particular time. The fingers cannot work effectively through the long flexors unless the wrist and mid-carpal joints are fixed by other muscles (**19**); conversely an unstable wrist inevitably means poor and weak digital function when the uncritical observer may put the blame on the digital muscles or joints.

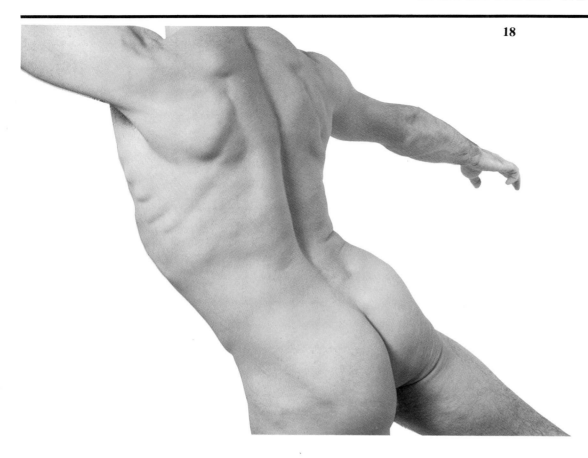

18

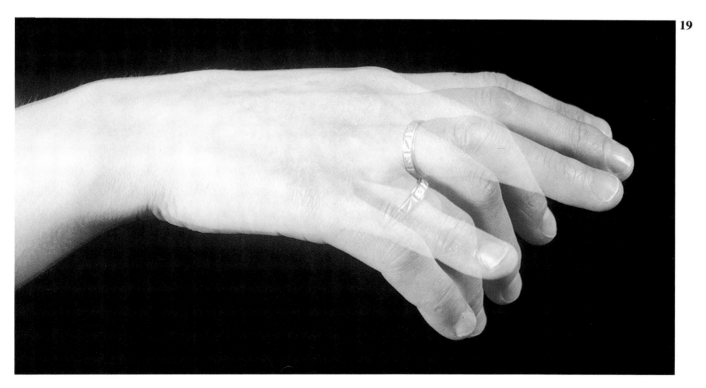

19

INSUFFICIENCY IN MUSCLES

Multijoint muscles may not be able to contract **20** or stretch enough to allow the full range of movement over all the joints over which they run. For instance, the hamstring muscles run over hip and knee joints, extending the hip and flexing the knee. But if the hip is extended they run out of power of contraction before the knee is fully flexed. They exhibit what is called active insufficiency. If, however, the hip is flexed somewhat the hamstrings could then flex the knee to an equivalent amount.

These same muscles can be made to exhibit the reverse effect, passive insufficiency, i.e., the muscles cannot stretch enough to cover the full range of both joints. Thus if the knees are kept straight, flexion at the hip is limited by the stretched length of the hamstrings (**21**). If, however, the knees are bent then hip flexion can continue (**22**).

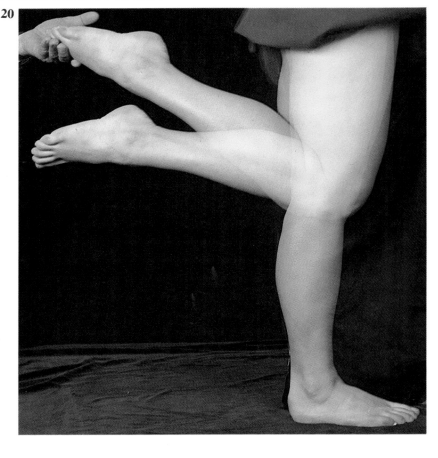

Cyclograph of knee flexion with the hip in extension. The subject cannot flex the knee actively any more but the examiner is able to take the knee to its full range of flexion.

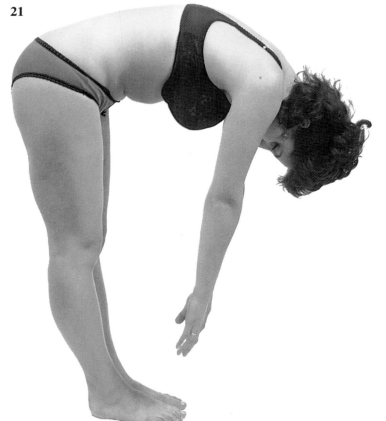

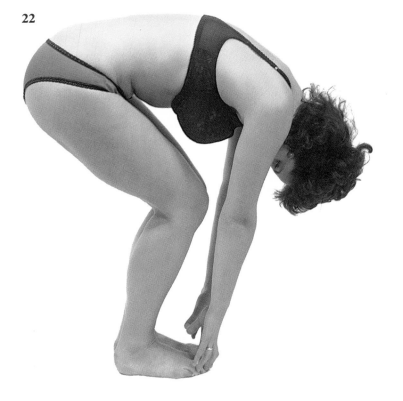

Active insufficiency can influence hand function. For maximal power the long digital flexors must work on a fixed wrist and preferably with some degree of extension. If, however, the wrist is flexed the power of flexion on the digits is weakened. This fact can be used practically in removing the knife from an assailant. The forearm is grabbed and the wrist forced into full flexion when it becomes virtually impossible to maintain a hold on the knife.

23

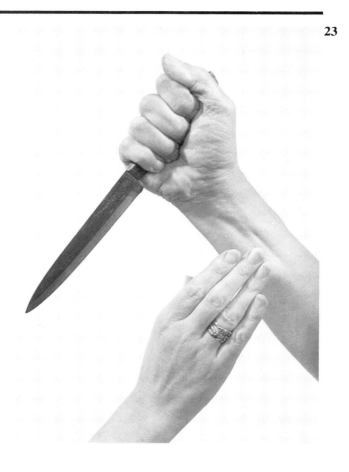

24

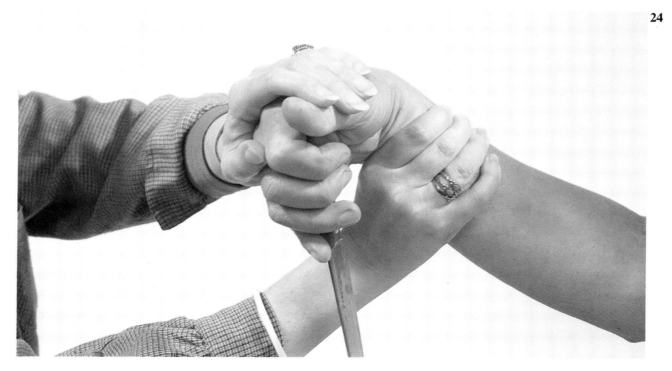

PROPORTIONS OF THE BODY

The proportions of the various parts of the body vary enormously with age. In the antenatal period the nervous system must form almost completely in anticipation of free living. Hence the nervous tissue of the brain, spinal cord and the peripheral nerves is virtually complete at birth though obviously growth in length of fibres will be necessary. Myelination of the nerves will then continue over the next 1½–2 years by which time the cranial cavity will be approaching adult size, the major growth changes to the skull thereafter being mainly bony. Growth of the head does continue to a considerable extent in the facial skeleton. Meanwhile the trunk and, to an even greater extent the limbs, will grow thus changing the body's proportions.

25

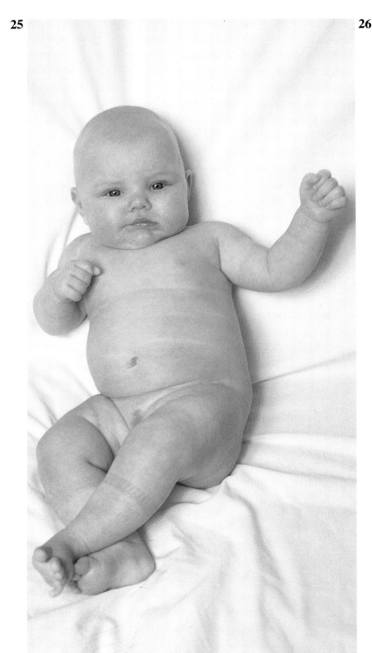

26

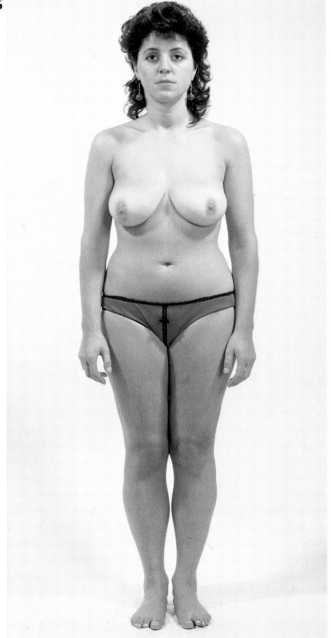

PROPORTIONS OF THE BODY

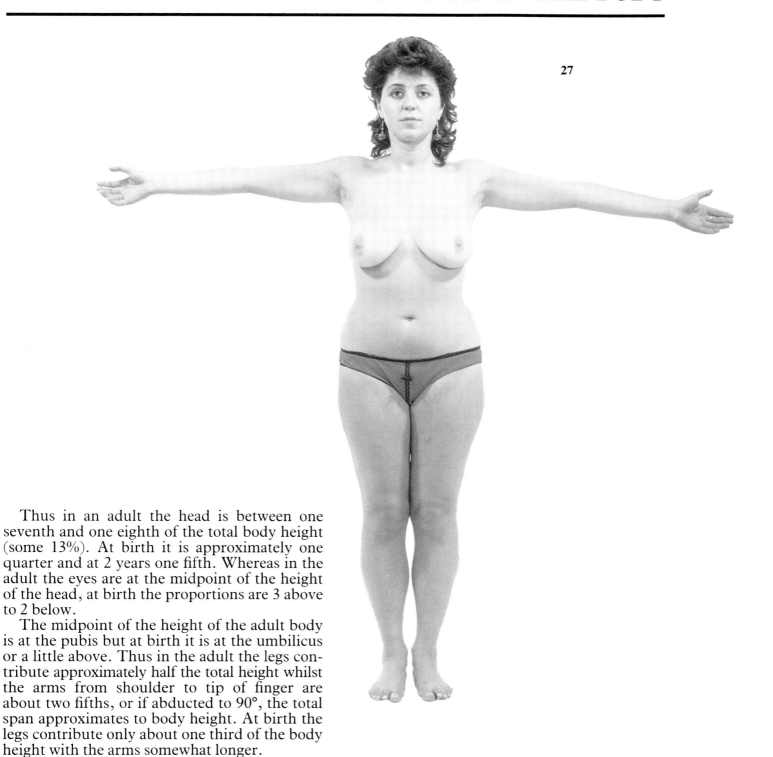

27

Thus in an adult the head is between one seventh and one eighth of the total body height (some 13%). At birth it is approximately one quarter and at 2 years one fifth. Whereas in the adult the eyes are at the midpoint of the height of the head, at birth the proportions are 3 above to 2 below.

The midpoint of the height of the adult body is at the pubis but at birth it is at the umbilicus or a little above. Thus in the adult the legs contribute approximately half the total height whilst the arms from shoulder to tip of finger are about two fifths, or if abducted to 90°, the total span approximates to body height. At birth the legs contribute only about one third of the body height with the arms somewhat longer.

An adult when kneeling would come up to the level of the axilla when standing, so the lower leg is the same height as from the axilla to the top of the head. The sitting height is a little over half the standing height.

FACIAL PROPORTIONS

Variations from the proper facial proportions are readily noticeable even if it is less easy for the casual observer to perceive what is wrong. For Leonardo da Vinci, analysis of facial as well as other bodily proportions was important and his approach towards ideal form is vital for anyone involved in facial surgery·or art.

The following details are largely based on Leonardo's observations.

In an adult the eyes should be at the mid-point of the vertical height of the head (**28**). Each eye should be the same width (A) as the distance between the eyes (B), which should also be the width of the lower part of the nose. The width of the mouth at rest should be the same as the distance between the irises of the eyes (**29**).

29

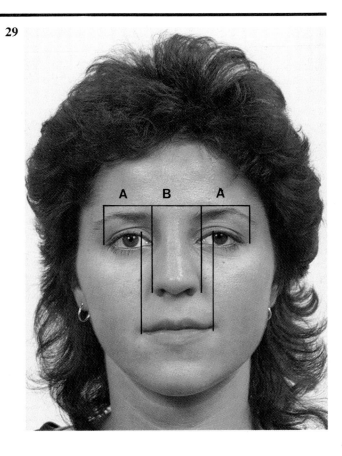

28

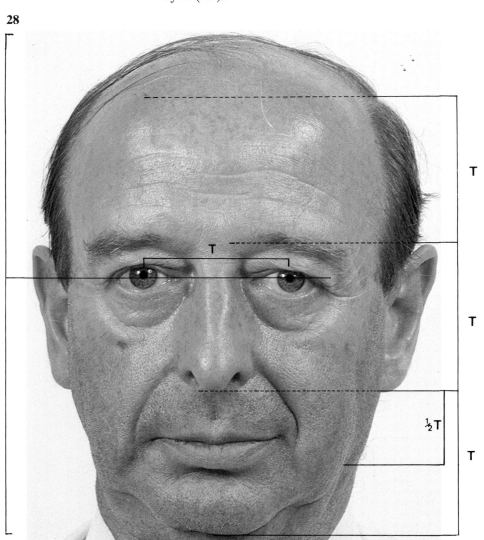

The upper tip of the ear should be level with the eyebrows and the glabella; the spine of the helix of the ear level with the root of the nose, the nasion; whilst the tip of the nose should be level with the lobe of the ear. The crease between lower lip and chin should be approximately midway between tip of nose and chin, and level with the angle of the jaw (**29**).

Many of the measurements of the face follow a 'rule of thumb'. The vertical height of the ear normally is the same as the length of the thumb, i.e. between the tip and the metacarpophalangeal joint (**30**). The same length measures the distance from the ear to the lateral aspect of the eye and from there to the midline (**31**). Similarly it fits the chin to the tip of the nose, from there to the glabella or eyebrows and from there approximately to the hair line. The lobe of the ear to the angle of the jaw is about half the thumb length as is also the width of the ear.

It is often said that the vertical height of the face, from chin to normal hair line, is equal to the length of the hand but this is so variable as to be of minor value.

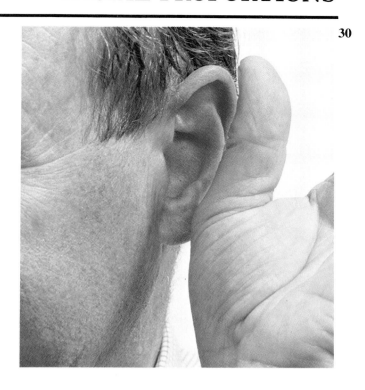

30

31

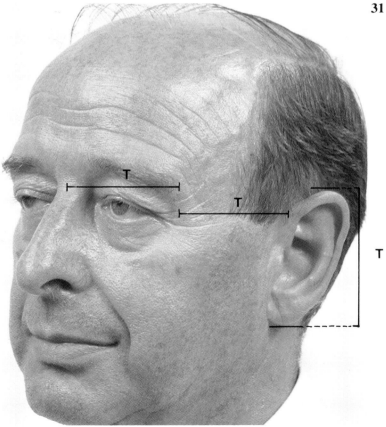

EXAMINATION OF BONY POINTS

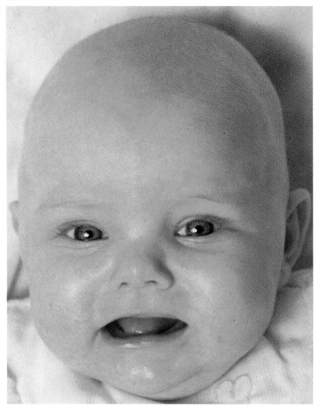

32

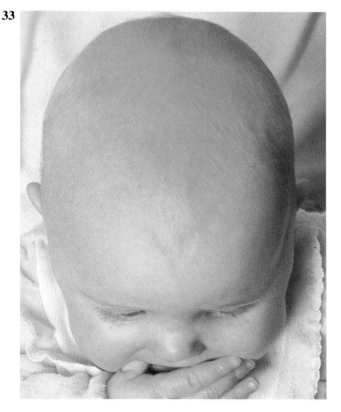

33

The major bony features of the face and head are relatively easy to examine in the normal state but may be much less so when covered by swollen tissues after injury.

The vault of the skull forms a continuous dome-like structure though rather flattened in the parietal region. At birth, however, the skull vault is made of bone little thicker than egg shell and even so is not completely ossified, leaving major membranous areas, the fontanelles. Immediately after birth the thin skull bones may override each other due to moulding during birth, producing sharp ridges, but this is only a temporary phenomenon of a day or so. Two fontanelles are quite easy to feel and may actually bulge a little when the baby cries. The anterior fontanelle is a diamond shaped area at the junction of the two parietal and frontal bones. The frontal bones are separated at this stage by the metopic suture, which begins to close in the second year with the fontanelle but may persist throughout life. The posterior fontanelle between the two parietal and the single occipital bone is triangular in shape; this is usually closed by the end of the first year. Two lateral fontanelles are present on each side. The anterior one is covered by temporalis muscle and therefore impalpable but the posterior one at the junction of temporal, parietal and occipital bones can usually be felt but less easily than those of the vault. In fact, the sutures at the sites of these fontanelles can often be felt throughout life if the overlying hair is not too thick.

The state of ossification of the bones of the skull, as well as the form of the facial skeleton can be seen in the four views of a skull of a newborn baby (A: anterior, B: lateral, C: posterior, D: from above). The positions of the fontanelles are readily seen by their membranous nature.
The anterior fontanelle is easily seen through the skin of this 5 month old baby. In the view from above it is also just possible to see the open interparietal suture though this and the fontanelles are very easy to feel in a child of this age.

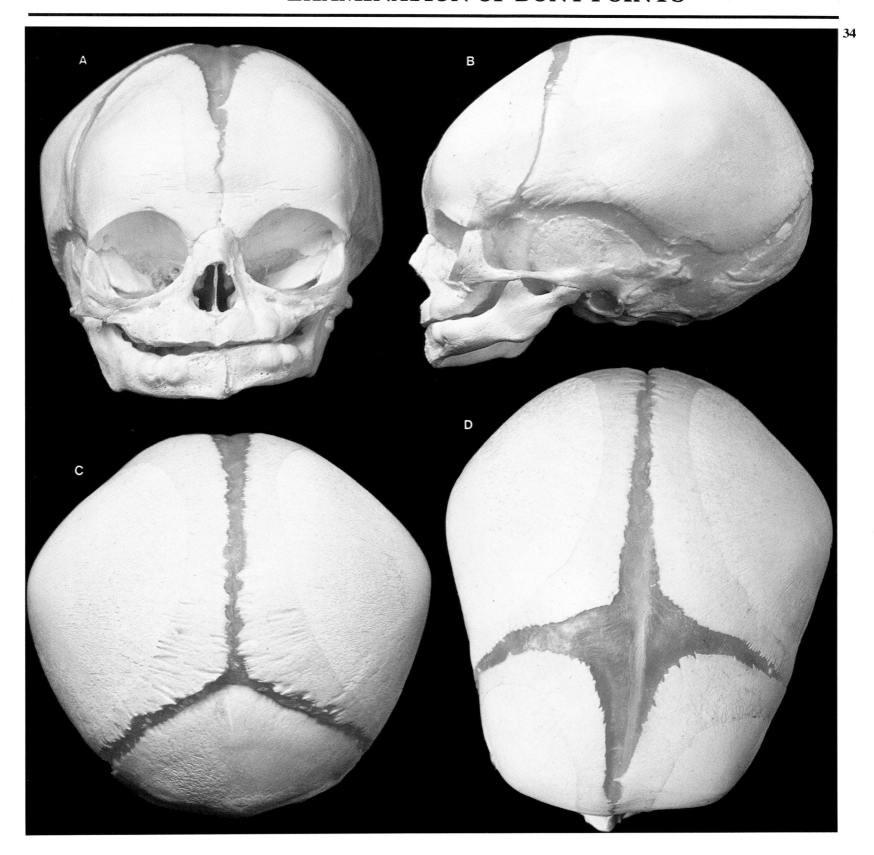

EXAMINATION OF BONY POINTS

1 Frontal process of maxilla
2 Frontomaxillary suture
3 Nasal bone
4 Frontonasal suture
5 Frontal prominence
6 Supraorbital foramen
7 Frontozygomatic suture
8 Zygomatic arch
9 Maxillozygomatic suture
10 Infraorbital foramen
11 Infraorbital margin
12 Nasal spine
13 Maxillary suture
14 }
15 } Upper incisor teeth
16 Canine tooth
17 1st premolar tooth
18 Mental foramen
19 Mental protuberance
20 Mental shelf

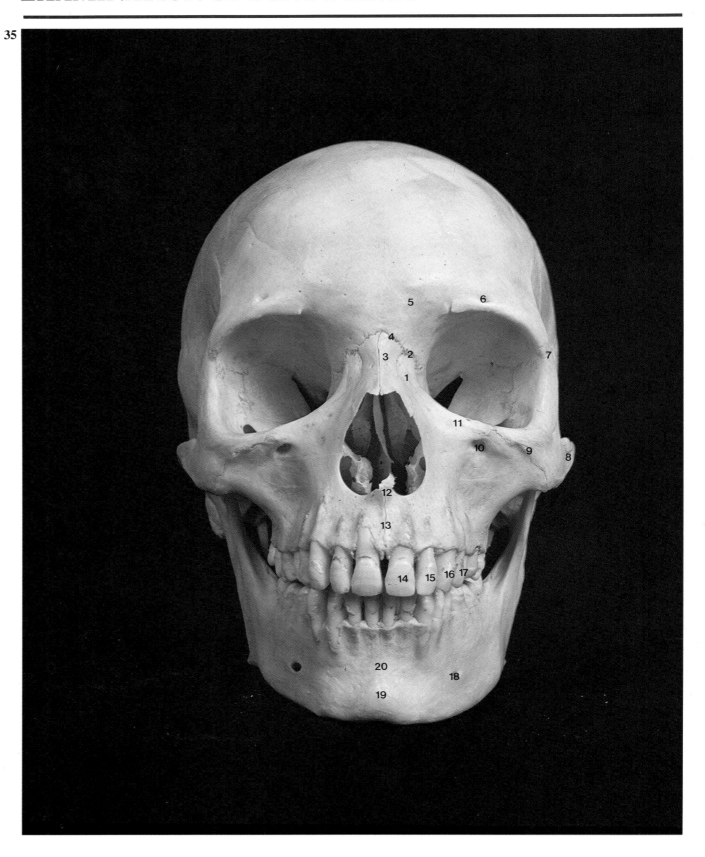

The margins of the orbit are readily palpable (**36**) and discontinuity of the infraorbital margin due to fracture can usually be felt unless the tissues are grossly swollen as they may be. (N.B. the two sides should always be felt for discrepancies.) The infraorbital foramen should be palpable and a little pressure here may produce the uncomfortable sensation of nerve compression.

Laterally the fronto-zygomatic suture may be felt just below the lateral tip of the eyebrow. Superiorly the supraorbital notch should be felt about an inch from the midline (or take three of the patient's fingers, place one in the midline and the third should overlie the notch). The notch may be closed over to form a foramen but again pressure produces discomfort from the supraorbital nerve.

37

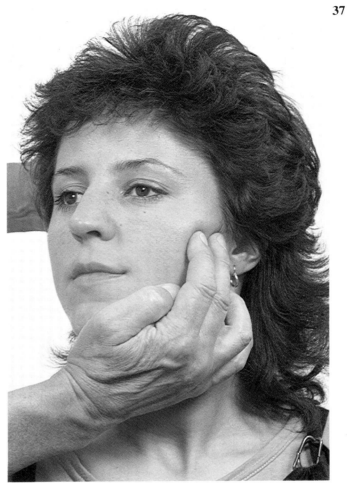

36

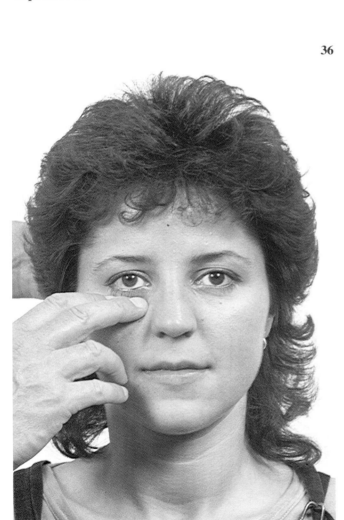

The zygomatic arch is readily palpable if approached from below (**37**). Posteriorly it bulges out in front of the ear level with the tragus. This is the zygomatic process of the temporal bone which joins the zygomatic bone in the arch. As the arch runs forwards it thickens considerably and its margin drops as it approaches the infraorbital region though the inferior margin is readily palpable virtually to the nose. From examination of the skull it would appear that the superior margin of the zygomatic arch and the lateral orbital wall should be readily palpable. However, the dense temporal fascia is attached to these edges rather like a drum skin so camouflaging them.

EXAMINATION OF BONY POINTS

The lower border of the mandible is readily palpable and as such forms the lower border of the face (**41**). In many females the lower edge runs smoothly round the curve of the angle to the posterior border of the ascending ramus; in males the angle projects down a little to produce a preangular notch though the difference is not entirely sex specific. A short distance up the ramus the parotid gland overlaps the mandible so that the details are lost between here and the head which projects in front of the tragus of the ear. Anteriorly the mental protuberance is obvious, producing a sloping shelf between chin and anterior margin of the alveolus. Examination of the mandible must include the teeth and the bite. The upper spade-like incisors should overlap the narrower lower, and laterally the upper outer cusps (buccal) should overlap the lower (**42**).

1 Occipitoparietal suture
2 Mastoid process
3 External auditory meatus
4 Temporal root of zygomatic arch
5 Head of mandible
6 Zygomatic process of temporal bone
7 Temporozygomatic suture
8 Frontozygomatic suture
9 Frontal prominence
10 Frontonasal prominence
11 Nasal bone
12 Frontal process of maxilla
13 Nasal spine
14 Alveolar margin of maxilla
15 2nd upper incisor
16 Canine
17 } Premolars
18 }
19 }
20 } Molars
21 }
22 Coronoid process of mandible
23 Angle of mandible
24 Mental foramen
25 Mental process of mandible

38

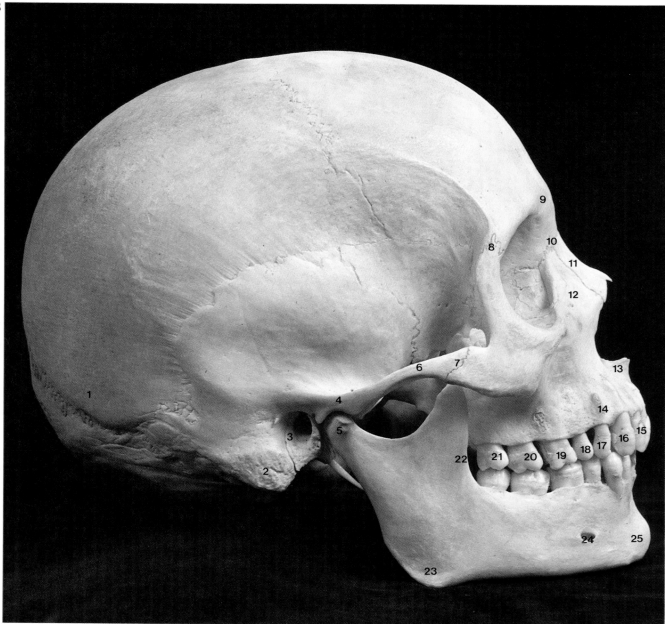

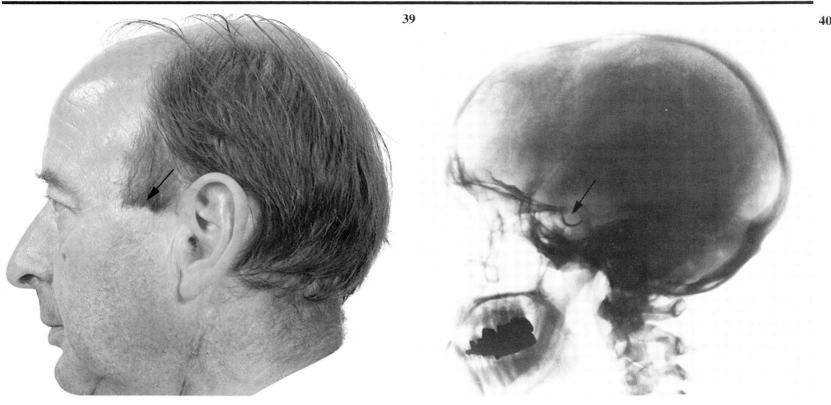

Surface projection (39) and radiograph (40) of the pituitary fossa.

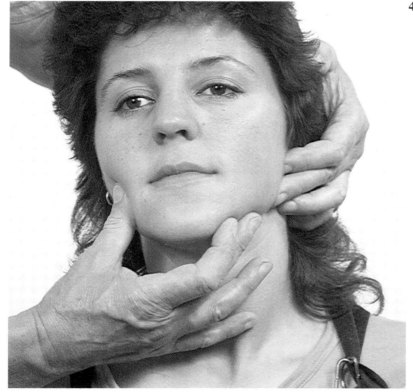

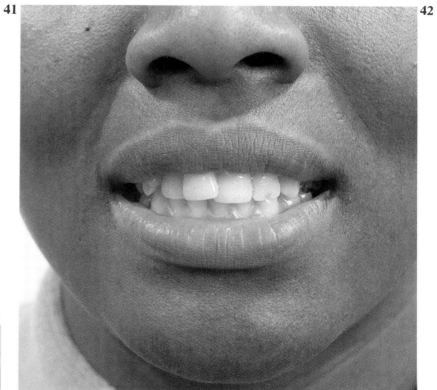

43

1 Nasal bone
2 Lateral cartilage underlying nasal bone
3 Lateral cartilage
4 Free edge of lateral cartilage forming nasal valve
5 Alar cartilage – lateral crus
6 Alar cartilage – medial crus

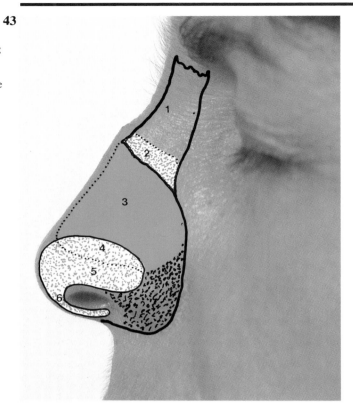

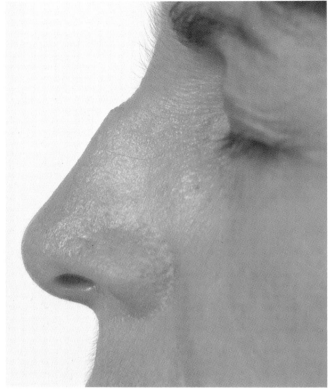

44

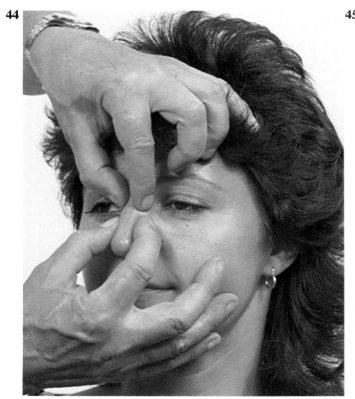

45

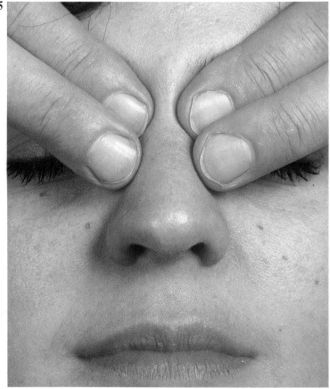

The structural support of the nose is both bone and cartilage. Above, the two nasal bones each articulate laterally with the frontal process of the maxilla and are supported beneath by the nasal process of the frontal bone and the bony septum (**38**). Below, two lateral cartilages are effectively fused along the bridge to the septal cartilage by the perichondrium to give a strong T-shaped section. Two alar cartilages control the two nostrils (**43**).

The nose should be examined from above for symmetry, from the side and from below as well as internally (**44** and **45**). Along the bridge it is possible to feel the junction between bone and cartilage as a slight ridge or groove but there may be quite marked discontinuity of line. Laterally the sharp margins of the nasal bone are readily identifiable due to the lateral cartilages being attached beneath the bone. Below, the lateral cartilages are overlapped by the alar cartilages which allows their lower margins to be pulled in to form the so-called nasal valve, the appearance of which may be accentuated in forced respiration by flaring of the nostrils (**46** and **47**). The nasal valve controls the direction of air flow into the nose.

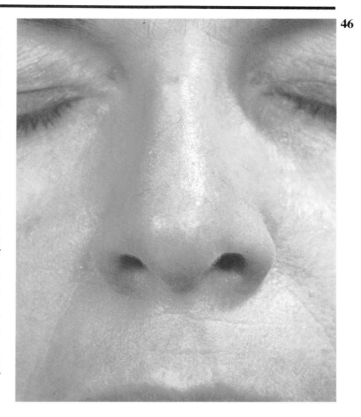

46

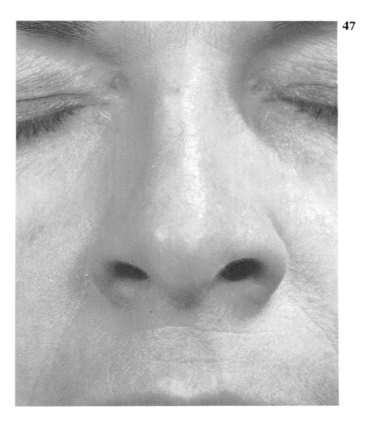

47

THE NOSE

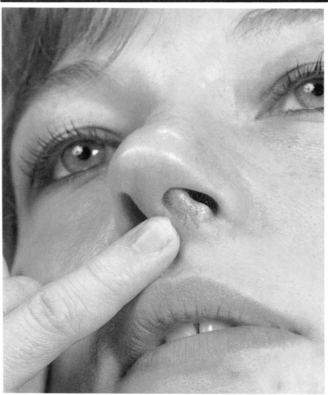

The alar cartilages are each curved around a nostril and each cartilage has a medial and a lateral crus. The two medial crura form the somewhat mobile support for the columella. They lie close together towards the nasal spine and are loosely attached together and deeply to the lower end of the septal cartilage. Because of their mobility they can be moved across to show the more rigid sharp edge of the septal cartilage (**48**). As the cartilages approach the tip of the nose they separate before curving round into the lateral crus. The groove between them can usually be felt and occasionally seen (**49**).

Although the alar cartilages support the margins of the nostrils towards the tip they do not follow the margins, leaving a membranous triangle (**49**).

1 Alar cartilage
2 Lateral crus
3 Medial crus
4 Membranous triangle
5 Septal cartilage
6 Nasal spine

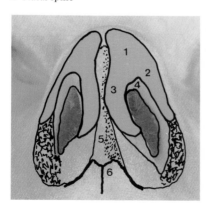

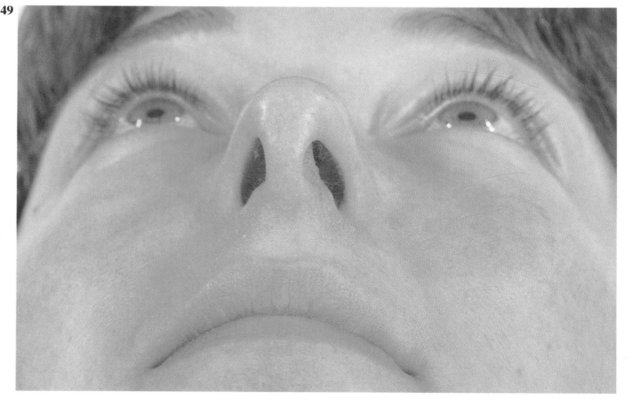

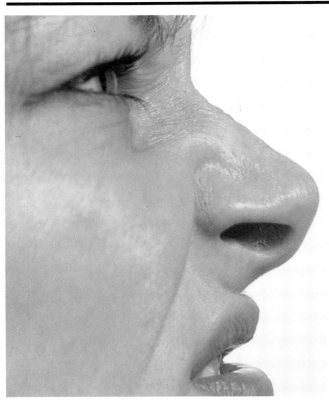

Both crura of the alar cartilages are controlled by the muscle nasalis. Levator labii superioris alaeque nasi pull up the lateral crus over the lower edge of the lateral cartilage (**50**) whereas depressor septi pulls the medial crus downwards (**51**). Overactivity of this latter muscle is sometimes responsible for the effect shown, occurring naturally.

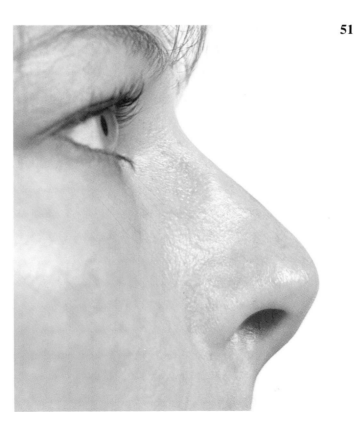

TEMPOROMANDIBULAR JOINT

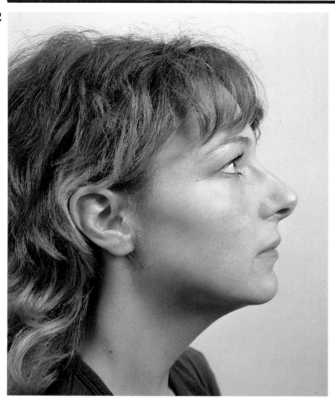

The temporomandibular joint is not a true hinge in humans as it is in many animals. The head of the mandible sits at rest in the articular fossa of the temporal bone but separated by the articular disc, which divides the joint cavity into two. The head of the mandible is like a transversely running cylinder and its lateral end can be felt when at rest, immediately in front of the tragus of the ear, below the root of the zygoma. As the jaw is opened, the head of the mandible is carried forwards onto the promontory and, in many people, as in this person can be seen forming a slight swelling below the zygomatic arch (53). As the masseter muscle is put on stretch the hollow normally apparent below the arch is also taken up.

As the jaw is closed and clenched the head is carried back into the fossa but owing to the powerful action of the masseter muscle the hollow below the zygoma is less pronounced and the bulge of the muscle can be seen over the angle of the mandible (54). It is interesting to note that the temporomandibular joint probably bears very little load on its joint surface even when in a powerful bite. The mandible is

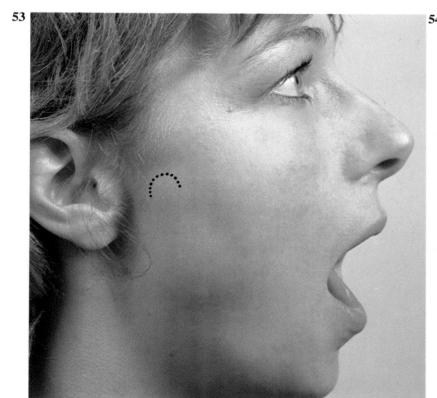

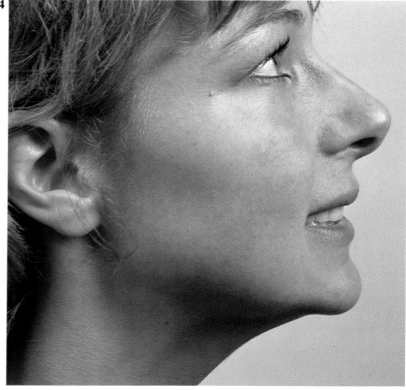

carried under the very precise control of its muscles and the whole system can be very rapidly readjusted to dental change.

It is usual to describe four muscles of mastication all supplied by the mandibular division of the trigeminal nerve (the only division of this essentially sensory nerve to carry motor fibres). These are the *temporalis, masseter, medial pterygoid* and *lateral pterygoid* but to these should be added the muscles below the mandible which open the jaw. Two of these, *mylohyoid* and the *anterior belly of digastric* are also supplied by the mandibular nerve through the mylohyoid branch of the inferior alveolar nerve. The first three muscles close the jaw and, importantly, return its head back to the fossa; the lateral pterygoid assists in opening the jaw by pulling the head of the mandible forwards as the inframandibular muscles pull the jaw downwards. As the two pterygoid muscles lie deep they are not readily available for direct palpation on activation as are the others. The temporalis muscle originates from the side of the head over the temporal bone, i.e. above the zygomatic arch and runs down deep to the arch into the tip and anterior border of the coronoid process. It is a wide fan shaped muscle whose posterior fibres run forwards and therefore retract the head of the mandible whilst the anterior fibres run vertically and pull the mandible up into a bite. In **55** the examiner's right index finger is feeling the contraction of the temporalis while the middle finger feels for the masseter. If the fingers were placed over posterior and anterior fibres of the temporalis as the wide open jaw was forcibly closed, the only activity felt would be in the posterior fibres (i.e. producing retraction and closure), the bulging showing activity of the anterior fibres occurring only on full closure. The examiner's left hand fingers overlie the submandibular muscles, particularly mylohyoid and the anterior belly of digastric and these can be felt acting when the subject is asked to open the jaw (particularly against resistance) or when asked to swallow. In the former case they pull the mandible down towards the hyoid bone and in the latter they pull up the hyoid bone to form a firm base for the floor of the mouth and the tongue.

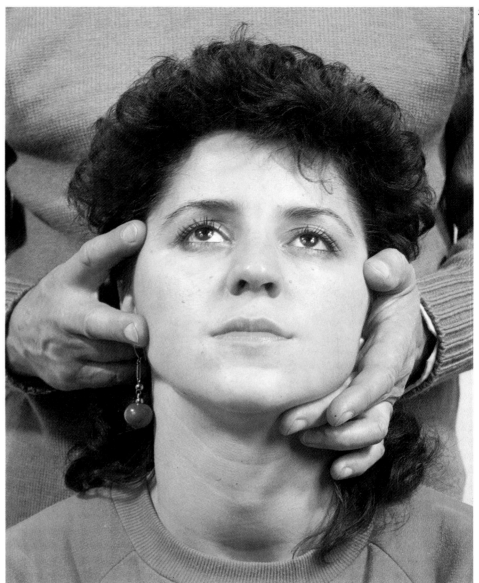

THE EYE

The eye is a globe supported and controlled by ligaments and muscles within the bony socket. Light enters the eye through the cornea and pupil and is focused on to the light receptive retina. The visual information is then transmitted to the brain by the optic nerve. Although the pupil looks dark, light shone into the eye can produce a red reflection from the human retina or greeny yellow from many animals' eyes. The cornea is a central transparent part of the globe while the surrounding white sclera is opaque. Behind the periphery of the cornea and in front of the lens is the circular iris, a variously coloured diaphragm, which expands and contracts due to activity of its intrinsic muscles to control the amount of light entering the eye through the pupil. The pupil is small in bright light, wider in poor light.

The lids protect the globe and fit closely except at the medial commissure where a small space forms the lachrymal lake. Here the lachrymal caruncle is obvious and also the remains of the third lid of many animals, the plica semilunaris. The lachrymal gland is below the upper lid on the lateral side.

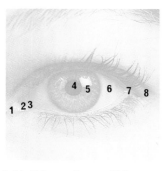

1 Medial commissure of lids
2 Lachrymal caruncle
3 Plica semilunaris
4 Pupil
5 Iris
6 Sclera (covered by conjunctiva)
7 Openings of glands on lid margins
8 Eyelashes

56

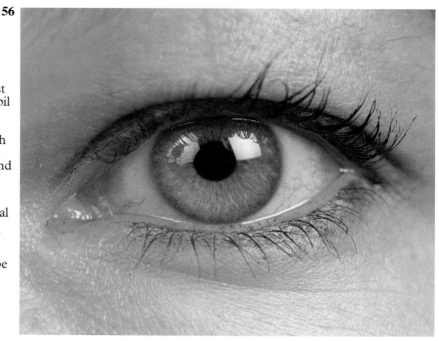

The normal upper lid should just touch the upper aspect of the pupil (when looking ahead) and the lower, the limbus (the junction between cornea and sclera). Each lid has several rows of hairs (lashes) except most medially, and glands opening onto its margin.

Each lid is supported by thin fibrocartilaginous plates, the tarsal plates. That to the lower lid is quite narrow and the lid can be everted easily to show the pink conjunctival sac (its colour can be used clinically to assess blood haemoglobin levels (57)).
The upper tarsal plate is quite large and has to be bent to evert the lid (58).

57

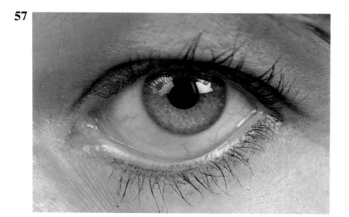

58

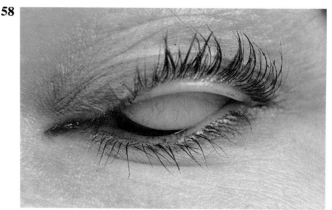

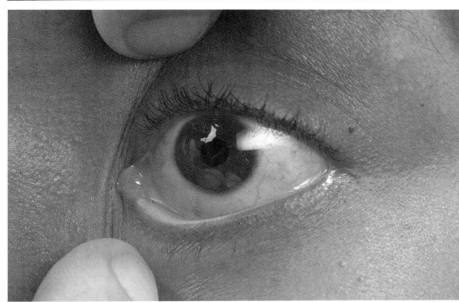

Note the puncta at the medial ends of each lid via which tears drain through the lachrymal apparatus into the inferior meatus of the nose.

The lids are lined by a thin serous membrane, the conjuctiva, which is continuous with the skin at the lid edge and is firmly adherent to the tarsi on their global surface. On the upper lid it extends as far as the orbital margin and on the lower lid almost as far, before being reflected on to the eyeball, the reflection being known as the fornix. Laterally the fornix is extended to the equator of the globe but medially it is limited by the lachrymal caruncle and the plica semilunaris. In **60** the lower lid has been retracted to show the reflection of the conjunctiva on to the globe. At first the conjunctiva lies loosely but at about 3 mm from the cornea it becomes more closely related, although still separable surgically up to the cornea. Here it fuses with the cornea at the conjunctival annulus some 1 mm over its edge from the corneal limbus. The rich vascularity of the lid and the sclera is evident with the vessels running between the conjunctiva and sclera. However, the blood vessels cease at the limbus, leaving the cornea avascular.

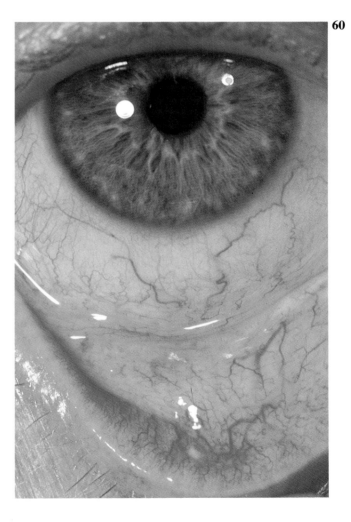

THE EYE

The posterior parts of the eye are lined with the pigmented retina and the vascular choroid. The retina is continued over the surface of the ciliary body and thence on to the posterior aspect of the iris. It is the retinal pigment which gives the basic blue colour to the iris (**61**). Additional colour of the iris is brought about by pigment laid down in the anterior layers; in small amounts (**56**) and in much greater amounts (**62**).

Much of the iris is made up of blood vessels. An outer anastomotic ring sends radial branches into the iris to form another anastomosis in the free margin, the circulus arteriosus iridis minor with a parallel venous circle. The architecture can be seen when not overlaid with pigment (**61**).

61

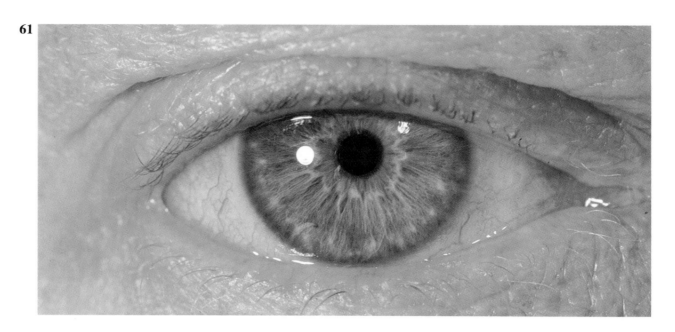

62

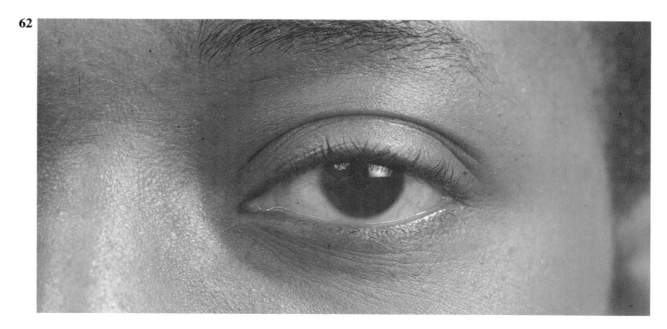

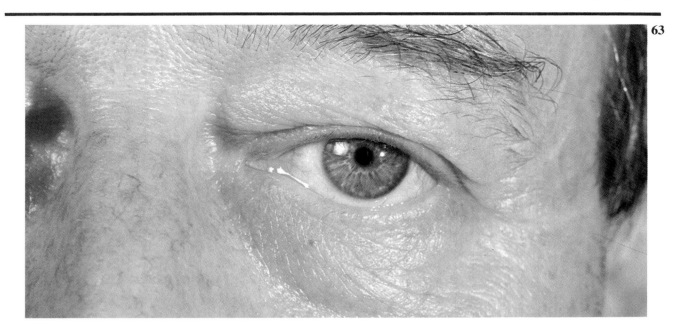

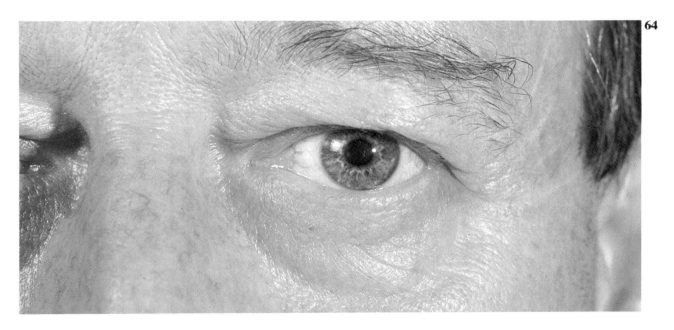

Intrinsic mucles of the eye are necessary for the control of the lens, for focus (accommodation) and in the iris, for light intensity. The lens lying behind the iris is controlled by ciliary muscles acting against the intrinsic elasticity of the lens itself with the object of focusing incident light on to the retina. The effectiveness of the system can be examined by assessing long and short vision. The iris musculature can be observed in action more readily. Circular muscle, controlled through the parasympathetic nerves, constricts the pupil in response to bright light (**63**); in lower light intensities the pupil dilates under sympathetic control (**64**).

THE EXTRAOCULAR MUSCLES

The six extraocular muscles are responsible for the balanced positioning of the eyes in the socket and also for their movement. As muscular balance is vital, any loss of power in a muscle will lead to over-effectiveness of the antagonist which is likely to produce diplopia (double vision) and strabismus (squint). The six muscles are innervated by three nerves. The third cranial nerve, the oculomotor, supplies four of the muscles, the superior, inferior and medial recti and the inferior oblique together with the voluntary component of the elevator of the lid, levator palpebrae superioris. The fourth cranial nerve, the trochlear supplies the superior oblique whilst the sixth, the abducent, supplies the lateral rectus.

The *lateral rectus* runs in the axis of the eye globe and hence pulls it laterally (i.e. abducts the eye) whilst the *medial rectus* has the opposite effect. The other four muscles all pull from a position medial to the axis. Thus the *superior rectus* elevates the globe but pulls it medially as well, with the *inferior rectus* pulling downwards and medially. The *superior oblique* pulls in effect from the front close to the nose by running around a pulley at this site, thus producing movement downwards and outwards; the *inferior oblique* turns the eye upwards and outwards.

Loss of the pull of a muscle will lead to the eye being carried in the direction of the antagonist with resultant double vision. Thus loss of the power of the lateral rectus either directly or through loss of its nerve supply (abducent) will lead to internal strabismus due to the uncontrolled action of the medial rectus. Loss of the superior oblique (trochlear nerve) will mean the loss of downwards and outwards pull. However, as the other muscles can give some semblance of balance the loss may only become obvious to the observer when the patient is asked to look downwards and outwards, and cannot do so. Loss of the oculomotor nerve leaves only the lateral rectus (abduction) and the superior oblique (abduction-depression) so that the eye is left looking outwards and a little downwards. In addition, as the nerve also supplies the levator palpebrae superioris, there will be ptosis (drooping) of the upper lid and, owing to loss of the parasympathetic fibres, the pupil will be dilated (due to unopposed sympathetic action) with loss of light reflex and loss of accommodation and convergence.

Many minor cases of muscular imbalance pass unnoticed unless special ophthalmological tests are carried out. More gross levels can readily be observed by asking the subject to hold the head still and follow the finger towards the periphery of vision (**65–70**). Notice how in the vertical movement the upper eyelids adjust likewise.

In order to maintain binocular vision the eyes work in parallel only in long distance viewing. As the object moves closer, the eyes must converge so that when the object is close the eyes appear to be squinting (**70**). Thus by definition a strabismus or squint must be one which is uncontrollable or, if minor only controllable by an effort. In the latter case the squint is likely to become obvious when the subject is tired or visually relaxed.

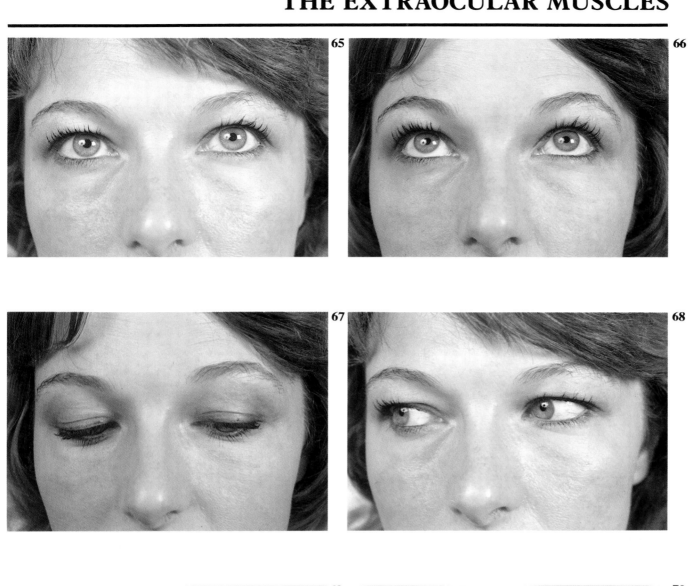

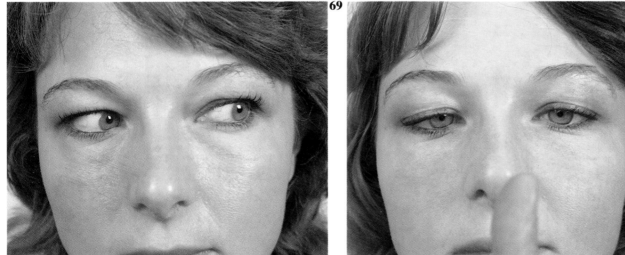

THE EXTERNAL EAR

The external ear, the auricle or pinna, is built upon a single piece of elastic fibro-cartilage which shows the essential contouring of the ear. Many deformities of the ear such as 'bat ears' are secondary to deformity of the cartilage and therefore any surgical treatment is bound to fail unless the cartilage is included. The cartilage of the pinna is continuous with the cartilaginous portion of the external acoustic meatus which in turn is joined to the margins of the bony meatus by fibrous tissue.

The skin of the ear is thin and bound to the underlying cartilage, particularly on the lateral aspect. The skin has numerous sebaceous glands particularly on the conchal surface. The acoustic meatus is guarded by stiff hairs growing particularly on the tragus, antitragus and incisure. The hairs commonly become more numerous in older males when they can give a very bushy appearance to the hollow of the ear. Hairs may also become more evident along the margin of the helix and can grow quite long.

The details of the auricle or pinna are shown in **71**. The concha and antihelix form a collecting shell or trumpet for the reception of sound waves approaching the acoustic meatus. This formation gives a stiff base to the pinna which is carried through from the antihelix particularly into the inferior crus. The concha is in part traversed by the crus of the helix. The region above it is called the cymba conchae and this overlies the suprameatal triangle of the temporal bone to which this part of the ear is attached. The bone can be felt through the cymba and deep to the trigone lies the mastoid antrum. From the cymba the hollow can be felt to continue anterosuperiorly into the scaphoid fossa. The helix is quite firm superiorly and particularly anteriorly where its spine is firmly attached by fibrous tissue to the underlying bone, from whence its crus sweeps downwards and backwards into the concha. Inferiorly, opposite the tragus, the helix becomes less firm and here the cartilage becomes separated from that of the antihelix by a fissure, the fissura antitragohelicina. The helix thus has an inferior cartilaginous tail which ends at the upper edge of the lobule. The lobule contains no cartilage and is essentially a variably shaped dependent mass of fibrofatty material.

1 Helix
2 Auricular tubercle
3 Scaphoid fossa
4 Triangular fossa
5 Crura of antihelix
6 Crus of helix
7 Concha
8 Tragus
9 Antihelix
10 Intertragic incisure
11 Antitragus
12 Tail of helix
13 Lobule
14 External acoustic meatus

71

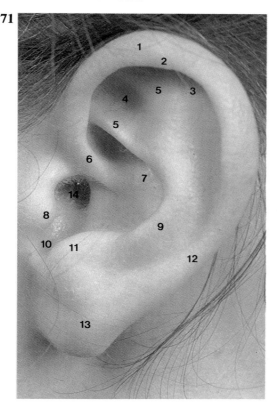
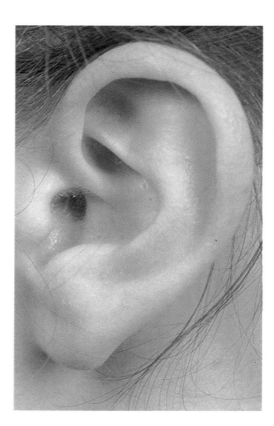
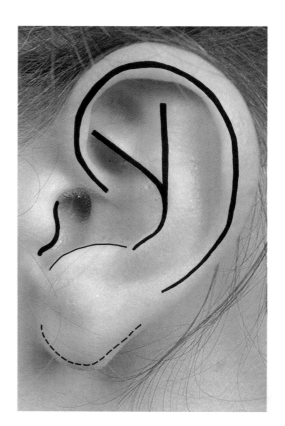

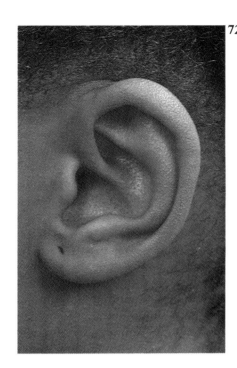 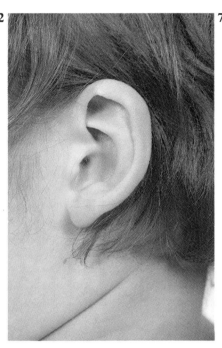 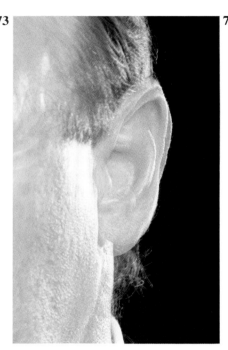

In the upper part of the outer rim of the helix a prominent tubercle is present from about the sixth month of intrauterine life, the auricular or Darwin's tubercle, a feature also of the ears of monkeys. This may persist into adult life (**71** and **73**) but in many cases although it may be possible to feel a prominence in the cartilage of the helix no external sign may be seen. **72** shows only a slight fullness at the site.

The ear is equipped with both external and internal sets of muscles, the former positioning the pinna in relation to the head and the latter varying the shape of the pinna. Both sets of muscles are supplied by branches of the facial nerve. In man the external muscles can often produce some movement as shown in the cyclograph (**74**), but the range is usually small. Surprisingly perhaps, it has been shown that these muscles, for all their minimal movement, respond by electromyographically recordable activity to sound stimulation. The intrinsic muscles can only be seen to act in a small number of people and in these the most obvious is a slight ability to pull the superior part of the helix towards its spine.

The sensory nerve supply of the ear is somewhat complicated for although C2 and C3 nerve roots supply much of the surface, cranial nerves are also involved. Furthermore there is a considerable overlap and variability in areas supplied. The greater auricular innervates most of the cranial (posterior) surface and much of the lateral aspect of the helix, antihelix and lobule whilst the lesser occipital supplies the upper part of the cranial surface. The auriculotemporal nerve, a branch of the mandibular division of the trigeminal, supplies the tragus and the crus and part of the helix. The vagus together with fibres from the glossopharyngeal as well as some from the facial nerve supply part of the concavity of the concha and the posterior part of the external auditory meatus and drum. Some fibres from these nerves also supply a small area around the junction of the cranial surface and the mastoid process.

MUSCLES OF FACIAL EXPRESSION

This is a name commonly given to those muscles in the face controlled through the facial (7th cranial) nerve. The name, although strictly correct, is unfortunate for although the muscles do influence facial expressions, their most important functions are control of the eyelids and of the cheeks and mouth.

Orbicularis oculi is a muscle system controlling closure of the eyelids and the periorbital tissues. It has two major components. The palpebral part consists of fine rapidly acting muscle responsible for closure of the eyelids (**75**). In blinking the closure is so rapid that the person is usually unaware of the action. The same component of muscle is responsible for maintaining the lids and hence the lachrymal puncta in contact with the globe. As lid movement is important for normal flow of tears, both across the globe and thence through the lachrymal apparatus, a subunit of the muscle, the lachrymal part, runs behind and into the lachrymal sac assisting in this flow.

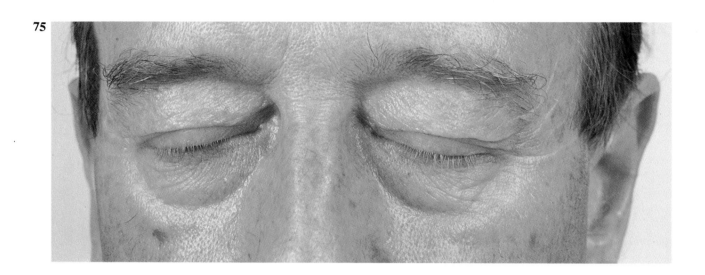

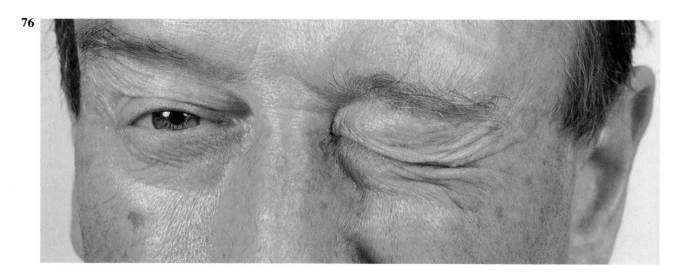

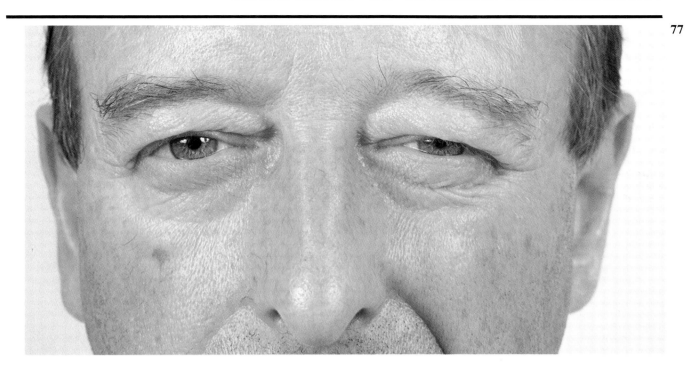

77

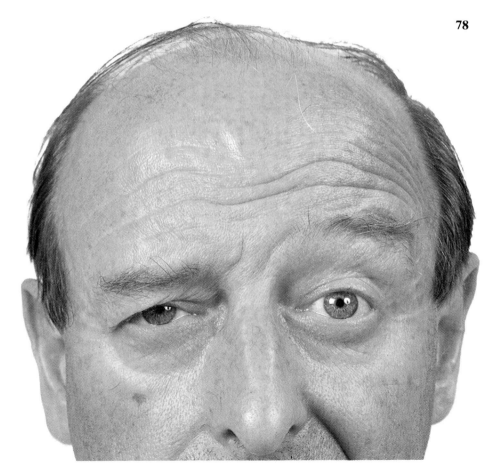

78

The orbital part is redder, cruder, slower acting muscle responsible for bunching up the periorbital tissues (**76**). The muscle also works to shade the eye against bright light (**77**).

Levator palpebrae superioris is the elevator of the lid and the direct antagonist of the palpebral part of the orbicularis oculi, while the *frontalis* pulls up the forehead on the scalp. **78** shows the orbital part in action on one side as an eye shade and the frontalis elevating the brow on the other. Whereas *occipitalis* controlling the galea aponeurotica of the scalp at the back is attached to bone, its counterpart *frontalis* is not and intermingles with the orbital part of the orbicularis oculi to be inserted into skin. For this reason fluid collecting under the galea of the scalp is free to track down into the eyelids.

MUSCLES OF FACIAL EXPRESSION

The action of the muscle around the eyes is linked with the development of skin creases around the lids. With age and loss of skin elasticity the lids tend to become baggy. This is, however, not entirely due to the skin elasticity. The lid muscle overlies soft fatty tissue and this increases in amount, pierces the muscle and increases in the subcutaneous tissues (**79**). Hence plastic surgery to take away the bags involves removal of not only surplus skin but also the fat both superficial and deep to the muscle.

79

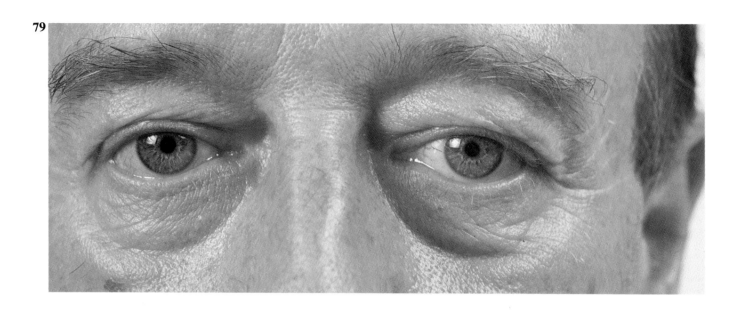

Buccinator is the sheet of muscle controlling the cheek, the muscle on each side being continuous with the superior constrictor of the pharynx through the pterygomandibular raphe. Its fibres run to the mouth, producing the smile of **80**. It holds the cheek against the teeth and thus, with the tongue, controls food in the mouth, preventing it collecting outside the teeth. In controlling the cheek buccinator plays an important part in dental hygiene.

80

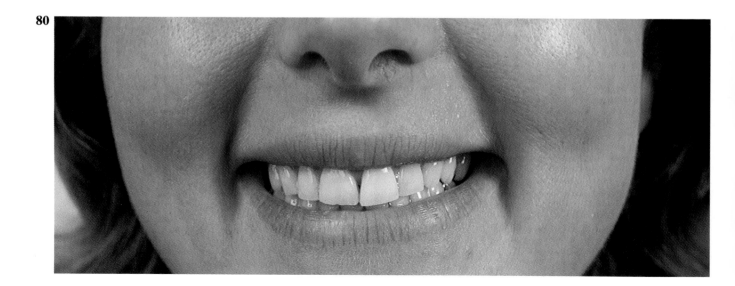

MUSCLES OF FACIAL EXPRESSION

As the buccinator muscles approach the mouth they divide, some of the fibres interdigitating to provide many of the fibres of *orbicularis oris*. Other muscles join in above and below to form the complex system responsible, with buccinator, for controlling lip movement as well as providing firm closure of the mouth. Orbicularis oris should therefore be considered primarily as a sphincter of the mouth while at the same time giving insertion for those muscles acting upon it.

81

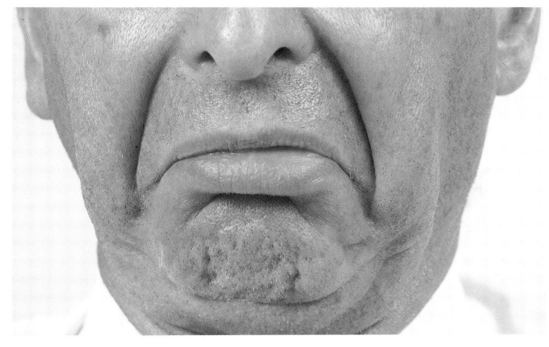

Buccinator acting with depressor anguli oris and mentalis on the mouth.

82

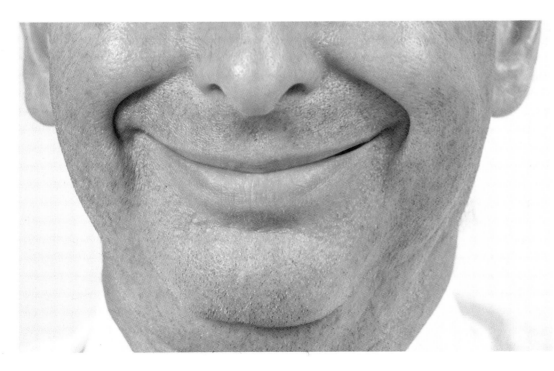

Buccinator with levator anguli oris.

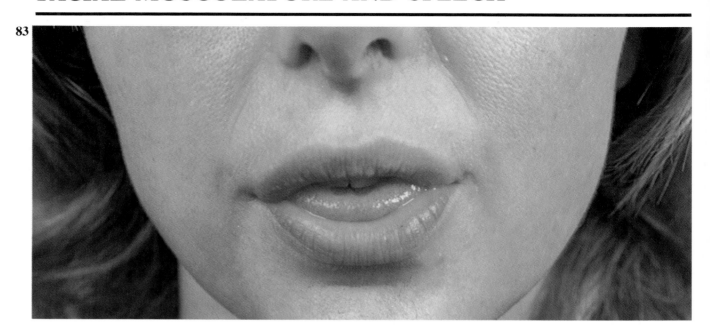

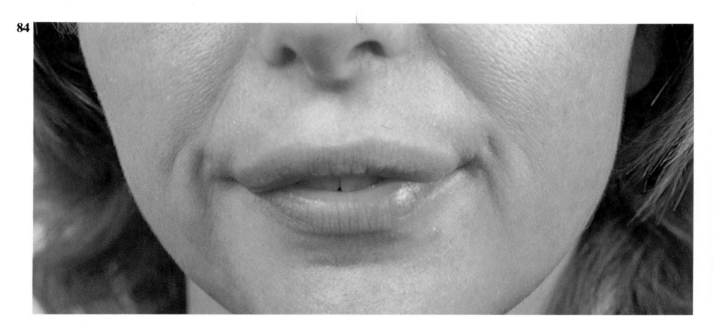

The production of sound, both volume and pitch, is primarily a laryngeal function (phonation). The modification of the sound into the basic components of speech (articulation) is supralaryngeal.

Sphincteric control of both the pharynx with the soft palate and the tongue with the palate are necessary to allow the explosive 'g' 'k' and 't' sounds. A juxtaposition of tongue with palate,

keeping an open palatopharyngeal sphincter is required for the sounds 's' 'n' 'ee' and 'r' which thus need fine lingual control. Apposition of tongue and teeth is required for 'th' (**83**).

Other sounds require the activity of the lips, either to produce a complete initial seal as for 'p' and 'b' or the lower lip pressed against the upper teeth for 'f' and 'v' (**84**).

Open lips with linguopalatal approximation are required for 'ee' and 'y' (**85**) whilst rounded constricted lips are needed for 'o' and 'oo' (**86**).

Thus in addition to an effective larynx, speech requires fine control of the pharynx, soft palate, tongue, cheeks and lips with an equally effective breath control from the respiratory muscles and, in particular, the diaphragm.

85

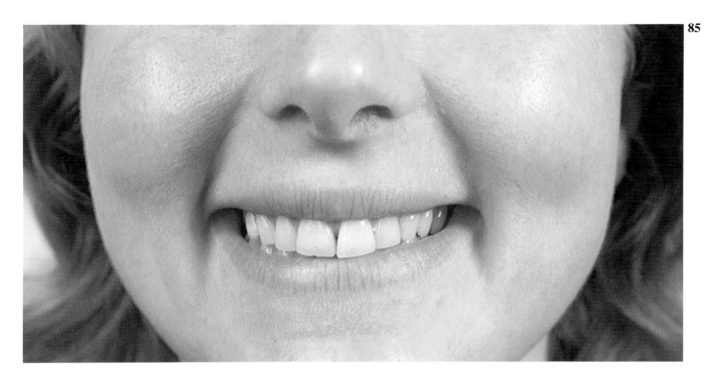

86

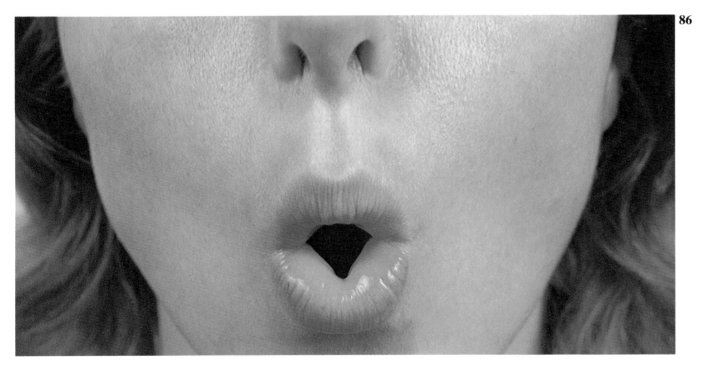

THE CRANIAL NERVES

The cranial nerves of the head are not always limited in their effect upon the region. Furthermore, they do not always exhibit the mixed motor and sensory functions characteristic of the spinal nerves. Some are purely special sensory in function while others carry important parasympathetic fibres.

The *olfactory nerves* linked to the olfactory bulb are distributed to the upper part of the nasal mucosa and carry olfactory (smell) stimuli. Thus testing for intactness of this nerve depends upon satisfactory detection of various scents. It should be noted that although taste is usually associated with the tongue many of the components of taste are derived from nasal olfactory stimulation via the posterior choanae and the pharynx.

The *optic nerves* transmit visual impulses from the retina to the brain and failure results in loss of vision. The normal neural pattern of the body is that the one side is represented on the other side of the brain (excepting the cerebellum where representation is on the same side). With optic representation this pattern appears confused by the partial cross over of fibres of the optic nerves at the chiasma. However, if the macula, which has bilateral representation is excluded, it will be evident from **87** that it is not so complicated. In effect, light from the right side is received on the nasal side of the right and temporal side of the left retina. With the cross-over of stimuli from the nasal retina at the chiasma, those from the right eye now join those from the left to go to the left side of the brain.

Oculomotor, Trochlear and *Abducent nerves* are all motor in function, controlling the extraocular muscles whose functions and examination have been described with the eye. In addition the oculomotor nerve also carries parasympathetic fibres to the intrinsic ocular muscles, of which the pupil constrictors are the easiest for rapid examination. N.B. Sensory (kinaesthetic proprioceptive) fibres from the extraocular muscles travel with the motor nerves only for a short distance before transferring to branches of the

87

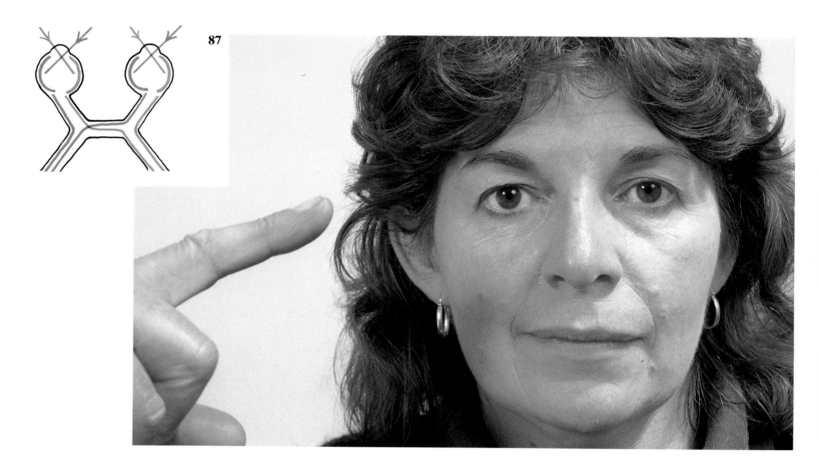

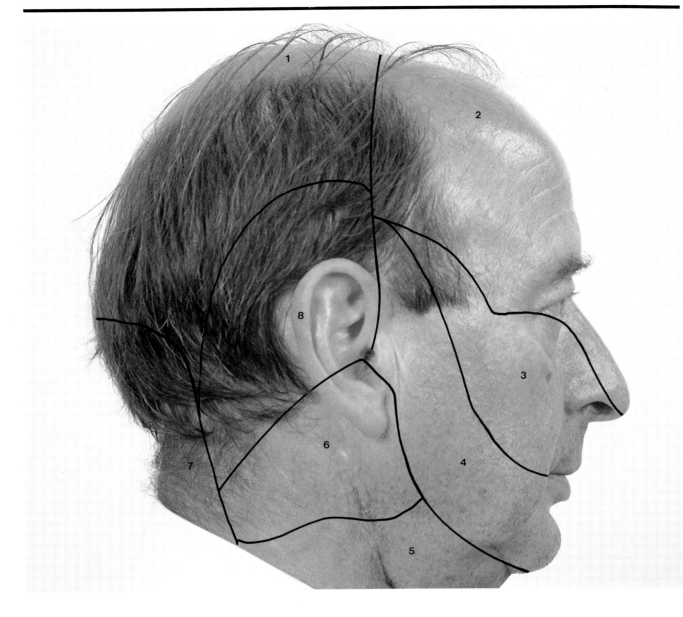

1 Greater occipital
2 Ophthalmic division of trigeminal
3 Maxillary division of trigeminal
4 Mandibular division of trigeminal
5 Transverse cervical
6 Greater auricular
7 C3
8 Lesser occipital

ophthalmic division of the trigeminal nerve.

The *trigeminal nerve* as its name indicates divides into three sensory divisions, the ophthalmic, maxillary and mandibular, the latter also having a motor root running with it. The sensory divisions supply areas of the face indicated by their names (**88**).

The *ophthalmic division* travels through the orbit, supplying the eyeball, conjunctiva, upper lid, the skin of the forehead (supraorbital and supratrochlear nerves) up to the vertex of the scalp, the external nose and the mucosa of the anterior part of the nose, frontal and ethmoidal sinuses.

The *maxillary division* runs into the pterygopalatine fossa from whence it supplies the meninges, nasal mucosa, palate, the upper teeth, maxillary sinus and skin of the anterior part of the cheek and upper lip.

The *mandibular division* supplies skin of the temporal region, part of the ear, lateral cheek and chin mucosa of the cheek, the anterior two thirds of the tongue and the lower teeth.

THE CRANIAL NERVES

From time to time it is necessary to carry out local injections of sensory nerves for regional anaesthesia and therefore the siting of the nerves from the surface is important.

The main ophthalmic division may need to be anaesthetised but as this is in the specialist ophthalmological field the details are not included here. It is worth noting, however, that as the optic nerve runs close by, it may also be included in the anaesthetic field.

The *supraorbital nerve* runs on to the forehead at the supraorbital notch or foramen with the supratrochlear a little medial to it, directly above the medial commissure of the lids. The supraorbital notch is usually not difficult to feel on the supraorbital margin about one finger's breadth lateral to the medial commissure of the eye or two fingers' breadth from the midline. Alternatively, taking three fingers of the size of the subject's if one is placed in the midline between the eyebrows, the third will overlie the notch. If pressure is exerted at this point the effect can be quite unpleasant if too firm. In fact pressure on this nerve has been described as one way of producing a reaction in a person whose collapse is thought to be hysterical.

Local anaesthetic block of these nerves may be effective for the anterior part of the scalp and forehead but often a local infiltration is necessary because of the nerve overlap (**89**).

The main trunks of the *maxillary and mandibular nerves* may need to be blocked on occasions. Both lie deep, the maxillary nerve in the pterygopalatine fossa, whose entrance lies anterior to the lateral pterygoid plate, whilst the mandibular division leaves the skull through the foramen ovale near the root of the free edge of the plate. The plate lies deep to the mandibular notch. Thus for the *maxillary nerve* the needle is inserted above the notch of the mandible and below the zygomatic arch about 1 cm in front of the head of the mandible (**90**). When the lateral pterygoid plate is reached the needle is then directed anteriorly and superiorly until the fissure is entered. For the *mandibular nerve* the needle is directed upwards and backwards until it just passes the free edge of the plate. It must be remembered that this is a very vascular area with the rich pterygoid plexus of veins and therefore veins may be damaged with local bleeding. It is important to check, as always, that the injection it not into a vein.

89

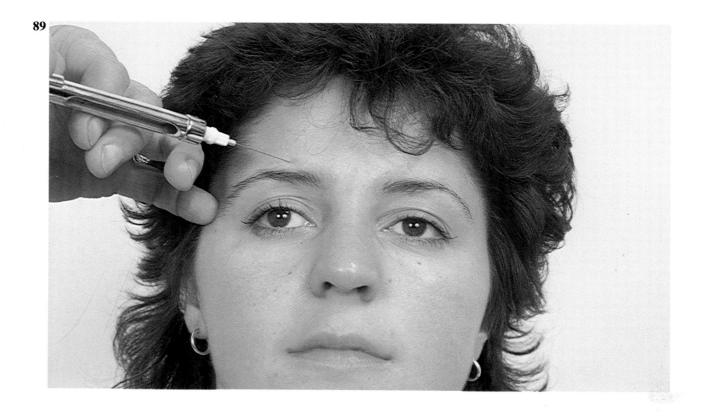

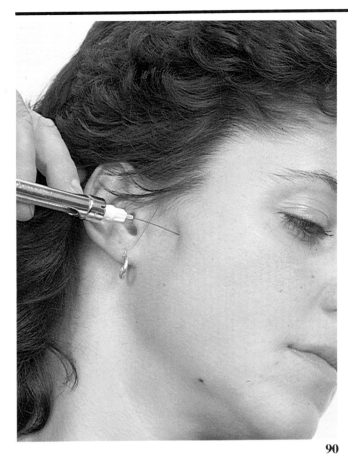

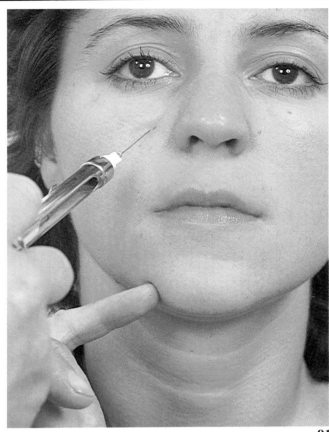

90 **91**

The *infraorbital nerve* may also need to be blocked. The infraorbital foramen may be palpated by placing one finger against the alar of the nose with an adjoining finger overlying the foramen, and pressure again producing an unpleasant sensation, if too severe. It is also described as being midway between the alar and the outer canthus of the eye (**91**). The foramen also lies in a straight line between the supraorbital notch and the mental foramen (which lies above the pointing finger in the picture).

Of the branches of the mandibular division the *auriculotemporal nerve* runs behind the head of the mandible, passes through the parotid gland (which it supplies) to run upwards over the zygomatic arch just behind the superficial temporal artery. As this artery can be palpated over the zygoma and temporal fascia (see arteries page 59) the nerve's position should be easy to find.

The *lingual and inferior dental nerves* run together inside the mandible. The lingual nerve is accessible and vulnerable as it lies under the buccal mucous membrane, level with the roots of the third molar tooth.

The inferior dental nerve is easy of access for nerve block, a manoeuvre regularly practised to anaesthetise the mandibular teeth. The nerve enters the mandible behind the third molar tooth. With the jaw opened wide the pterygomandibular raphe is put on stretch so fixing the mucous membrane for easy passage of the needle (**92**). The needle is taken backwards and somewhat laterally, level with the occlusal surface of the mandibular teeth, running close to the bone to the midpoint of the ramus. Sometimes the thick tendon of temporalis muscle at its lowest point interferes with the needle's progress and a more medial insertion may be needed. As the lingual nerve runs so closely, it may also be included in the area of anaesthesia, so influencing the anterior part of the tongue, as well as the mandibular teeth and skin of the chin as expected. The nerve to myohyloid is also likely to be included, affecting swallowing.

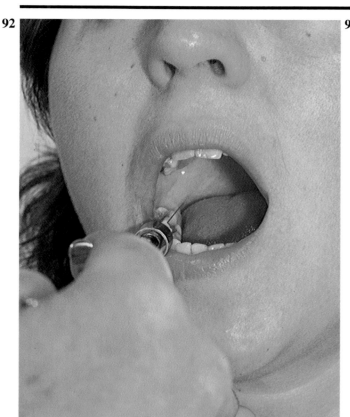

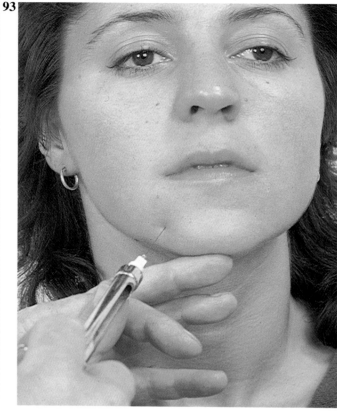

The inferior dental nerve sends a *mental branch* from the bone through the mental foramen to supply the skin of the chin and the lower lip. The foramen can often be felt about level with the second premolar tooth and, in the adult with teeth, midway between the gingival margin and the lower border of the mandible (**93**). It is about one finger's breadth anterior to the border of the masseter and the facial arterial pulse.

The *motor component of the mandibular nerve* supplies the four large muscles of mastication, temporalis, masseter, medial and lateral pterygoids, together with mylohyoid and the anterior belly of digastric, as well as the tensores tympani and veli palatini. The examination of these muscles has been dealt with on page 35.

The *facial nerve* carries both parasympathetic and taste fibres but these leave the main trunk within the skull so that when the nerve leaves the stylomastoid foramen it is largely motor. Since such sensory fibres as it carries at that stage are of uncertain function it is usual to describe it from there on as being essentially motor. The stylomastoid foramen lies in front of the mastoid process, superficial and a little posterior to the styloid process. The styloid process gives resistance if the finger is pressed between the mastoid process and the mandible just below the external acoustic meatus. The posterior belly of digastric runs downwards and forwards here also. Surgically the facial nerve can be found by running anterior to sternomastoid muscle at its attachment to the mastoid process just below the cartilaginous external acoustic meatus, until the nerve comes into view (**94**). It is now common practice to find the nerve in this way prior to removal of the parotid gland. The nerve gives small posterior branches to supply occipitalis and the auricular muscles and, lateral to the styloid process, branches to the posterior belly of digastric and stylohyoid muscles, and then enters the parotid gland. Here it divides in a very variable manner to emerge from the gland as five named branches. It commonly divides first of all into upper (temporofacial) and lower (cervicofacial) divisions which then further divide into the five branches or sets of branches. The upper division gives *temporal* and *zygomatic* branches (which are commonly multiple); the lower gives the *mandibular* and *cervical*, with the *buccal* coming from this or from both (**95**). The mandibular is the most stable in its course, running along the lower border of the mandible before entering the face with the facial artery to supply the muscles of the lower lip. The cervical branch supplies platysma, the buccal, buccinator and orbicularis oris, the zygomatic, lower parts of orbicularis oculi, nasal muscles and elevators of the upper lip, whilst the temporal supplies muscles of the forehead and the major part of orbicularis oculi. These muscles have been described under muscles of facial expression (pages 44–47).

Loss of the nerve supply presents major problems for the patient. As the muscles controlling the mouth are normally balanced on the two sides, loss of one side leads to the mouth being pulled across to the normal side, interfering with buccal function of feeding and particularly of speech in the production of labial sounds. Loss of the upper branches leads to inability to wrinkle the brow, but far more important, loss of lid closure, the lids falling away from the globe so that the puncta are no longer in contact with the globe for the collection of tears, which consequently pour on to the face.

The *vestibulocochlear nerve (auditory or acoustic)* is the nerve responsible for hearing, from the cochlea, and for balance impulses from the semicircular canals of the inner ear.

The *glossopharyngeal nerve* contains both motor and sensory as well as parasympathetic fibres. Sensory fibres come from the posterior third of the tongue (including taste), the tonsillar area and the oro and laryngopharynx. Loss of the nerve thus gives some sensory loss in these areas. The nerve supplies only one muscle, the stylopharyngeus, an elevator of the pharynx and larynx and hence of some importance in swallowing. Secretomotor fibres, given off early, eventually reach the parotid gland in the auriculotemporal nerve. Isolated loss of the nerve is unusual but perhaps the most obvious feature of loss is reduction in the gag reflex from the tongue, palate and pharynx.

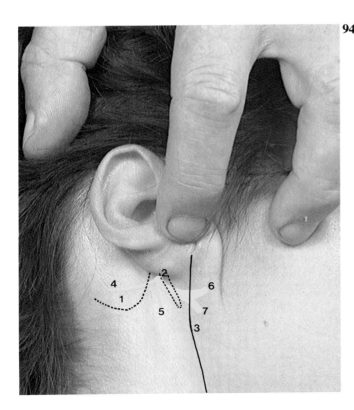

94

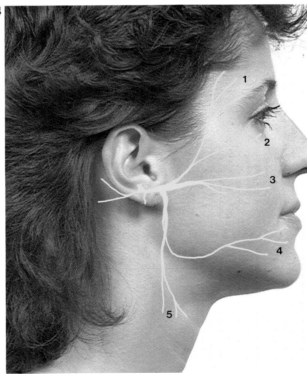

95

1 Mastoid process
2 Styloid process
3 Mandible
4 Facial nerve posterior branches
5 Stylohyoid branch
6 Upper division
7 Lower division

1 Temporal
2 Zygomatic
3 Buccal
4 Mandibular
5 Cervical

THE CRANIAL NERVES

The *vagus nerve* is large and complex and much of its influence is outside the head and neck through its parasympathetic fibres supplying the thoracic and abdominal viscera. It leaves the skull with the glossopharyngeal and accessory nerves through the jugular foramen which lies 1 cm deeper and a few mm anterior to the facial nerve (**94**). It can also be described as being 2 cm deep to the notch below the tragus of the ear (intertragic incisure) (**97**). Thereafter the vagus nerve runs down the neck along with the internal and common carotid arteries and the internal jugular vein, within the carotid sheath (**98**). Although the courses of the two nerves are dissimilar in the root of the neck relative to the other structures, the surface positions are essentially the same and both cross behind the sternoclavicular joints, into the thorax. Here the right one runs anterior to the first part of the subclavian artery and thence behind the brachiocephalic vein, moving medially towards the trachea; the left maintains a more vertical course.

Close to the jugular foramen the vagus is joined by the cranial part of the accessory nerve and the conjoined nerve supplies palatal and pharyngeal muscles through the pharyngeal branch. It also gives sensory supply to the epiglottis and upper larynx and motor supply to the cricothyroid muscle via the superior laryngeal branch, and the remainder of the laryngeal muscles and sensory supply to the lower larynx from the recurrent laryngeal branch.

Loss of the pharyngeal branch would effectively paralyse both soft palate and pharynx inducing dysphagia and, through the failure of the palate, a typical cleft palate form of speech. Movement of the soft palate is readily elicited by observation of the palate as the patient is asked to say a sound such as 'ah' (**96**).

Paralysis of the laryngeal nerves and particularly the recurrent one leads to dysphonia.

The *accessory nerve* is made up of the two totally unrelated parts which travel together for a very short distance. The cranial part links

96

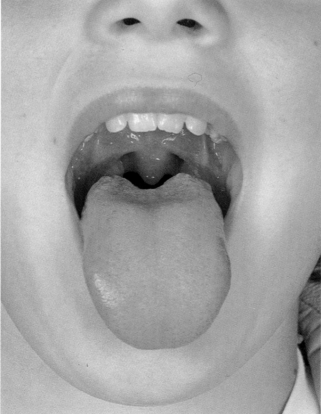

97

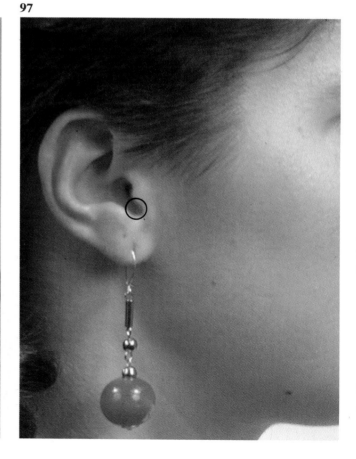

with the vagus (see above). The spinal part leaves the upper five segments of the spinal cord dorsal to the normal motor roots and, joining together enter the cranial cavity through the foramen magnum and then leave with the cranial part. When the cranial part joins the vagus, the nerve carries on to enter the deep surface of sternomastoid, which it supplies, before leaving about half way down its posterior border to run across the roof of the posterior triangle of the neck to enter and supply trapezius about 5 cm (2 in) above the clavicle. The surface marking therefore of the nerve can be drawn as a line from below the tragus to that point on the trapezius (**98**). Action of sternomastoid is shown on page 66 and of trapezius in **99** – lifting the shoulder against resistance. In classical block dissection of the neck to clear lymph nodes in carcinoma, the sternomastoid is removed and with it the nerve. Thus trapezius usually loses its motor nerve supply with dropping of the shoulder.

The *hypoglossal nerve* supplies the muscles of the tongue (except for palatoglossus). If one nerve is lost, that half of the tongue atrophies and if the patient is asked to put out the tongue as in **100**, it deviates to the side of the lesion.

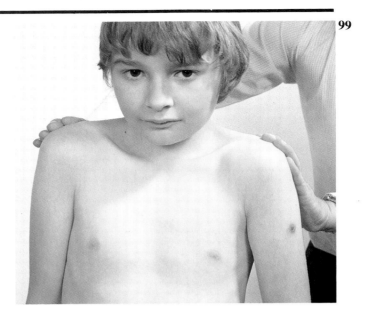

99

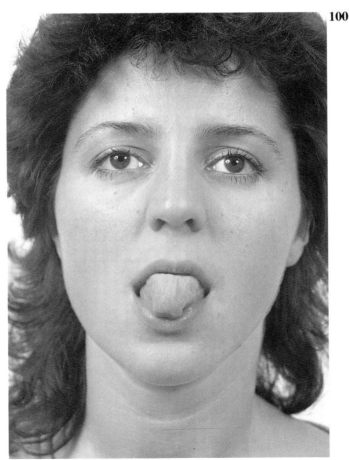

100

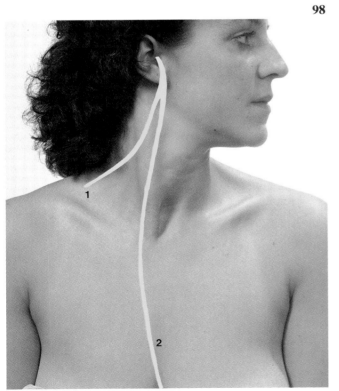

98

1 Accessory nerve
2 Vagus

BLOOD VESSELS OF THE FACE AND HEAD

The face and head have an extremely rich blood supply (**101**). On the face the arterial supply and anastomoses from one side to the other are so good that if the facial artery or one of its branches is cut, both ends of the cut vessel will bleed in a pulsatile arterial manner, instead of just at the cardiac end as in most cases.

The facial artery is the main superficial artery to the face. It leaves the external carotid artery just behind the angle of the mandible immediately after the lingual (which runs deep to the mandible to supply the tongue where its pulsations can often be seen or felt on the underside near the tip). It runs upwards for a short distance before looping to turn downwards behind the submandibular gland, the posterior surface of which it commonly grooves. It then runs up over the surface of the gland to pass into the face over the mandible at the anterior border of the masseter muscle. If the subject clenches the jaw, the muscle can be felt more easily, and its anterior border identified where the artery can be felt pulsating over the bone (**102**). The facial vein also crosses the mandible at this site together with the mandibular branch of the facial nerve and lymphatics. If there is facial inflammation a lymph node may become swollen and palpable at this site also.

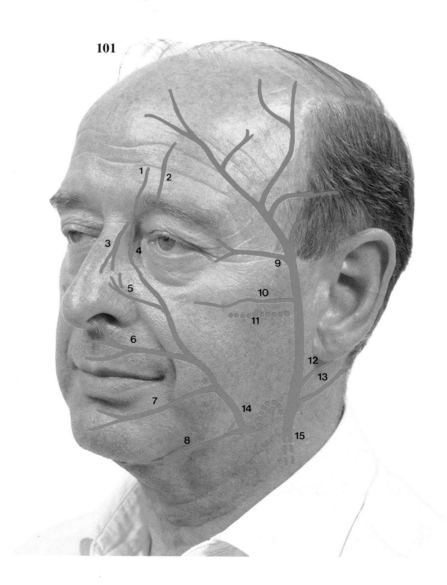

101

1 Supratrochlear
2 Supraorbital
3 Dorsal nasal
4 Angular
5 Nasal
6 Superior labial
7 Inferior labial
8 Mental
9 Superficial temporal
10 Transverse facial
11 Maxillary running deep
12 Posterior auricular
13 Occipital
14 Facial
15 External carotid

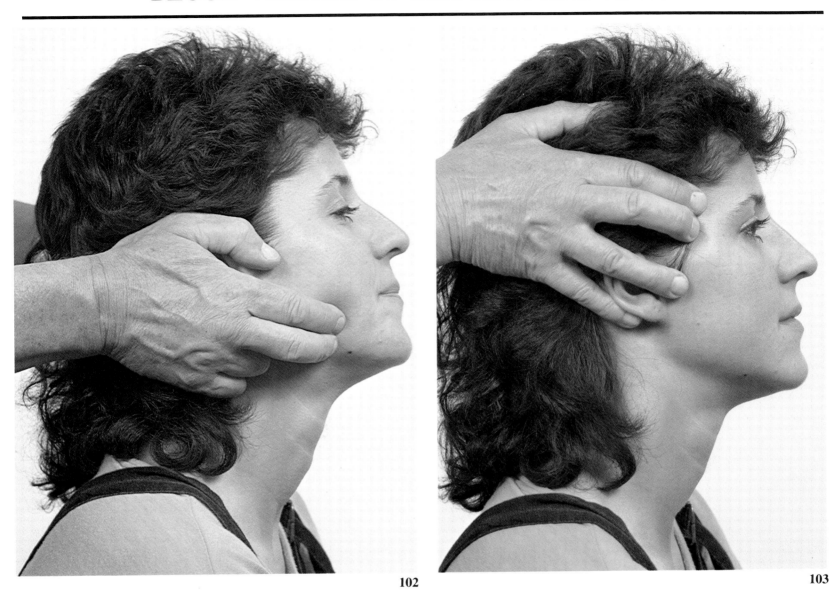

102 **103**

From the mandible the artery follows a very irregular course across the face towards the inner canthus of the eye, giving branches as it goes to the upper and lower lips and the nose, and linking with the deeper transverse facial artery. The branches to the lips are particularly large and anastomosing with those of the other side. The pulsations of the labial arteries can often be felt by holding the lip between finger and thumb.

The *superficial temporal artery* is the other major artery whose pulsations can easily be felt in the face. It is the terminal branch and continuation of the external carotid artery after its last branch, the maxillary, has left it in the substance of the parotid gland, to run forwards deep to the neck of the mandible. The superficial temporal artery leaves the substance of the gland, runs in front of the ear over the zygomatic arch and thence over the tense temporal fascia. Here it should be easy to feel (**103**). The artery then divides into frontal and parietal branches, the former supplying the forehead region and the latter the parietal scalp, and each anastomoses with branches of the opposite side.

BLOOD VESSELS OF THE FACE AND HEAD

The *supraorbital and supratrochlear* arteries are branches of the ophthalmic which leave the orbit, pierce frontalis muscle and run up on to the forehead. It is often possible to feel the pulsations of the supraorbital artery about 2.5 cm (1 in) from the midline (see supraorbital nerve, page 52).

The *occipital artery* supplies the posterior part of the scalp. It appears from beneath the sterno-mastoid muscle to run on to the scalp between the origin of that muscle and trapezius. It can readily be felt pulsating as it crosses the superior nuchal line some four fingers' breadth behind the ear.

104

1 Facial artery
2   submental branch
3   inferior labial branch
4   superior labial branch
5   internal nasal branch
6   external nasal branch
7   angular branch
8 Supratrochlear artery
9 Supraorbital artery
10 Superficial temporal artery
11   parietal branch
12   frontal branch
13   transverse facial branch
14 Posterior auricular artery
15 External carotid artery

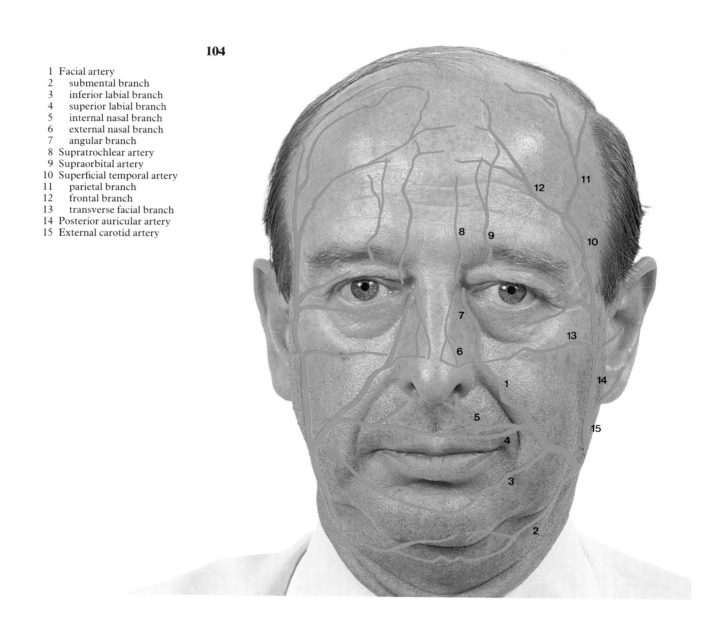

AXIAL (VASCULAR) FLAPS IN THE FACE

In view of the rich vascularity of the face it is often possible to carry out repair of tissue loss by local axial flaps, i.e. flaps based on the axis of blood vessels (105). The superficial temporal artery allows the whole forehead to be transposed on the frontal branch for repair of cheek or chin whilst particularly in a bald person the anterior scalp can likewise be transposed on the parietal branch, filling the defect in the scalp with a split skin graft. Very narrowly based flaps on the supratrochlear or supraorbital vessels allow quite long forehead flaps to be turned down to repair a nose or the adjoining area. So rich is the supply from the facial artery that quite narrowly based flaps can be taken even without great regard for vessels, in a way that would be impossible in other parts of the body.

105

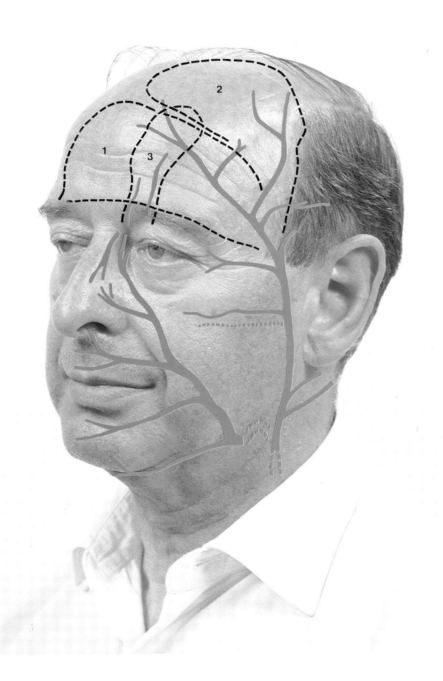

1 Whole forehead flap including frontal branch of superficial temporal artery
2 Anterior scalp flap on parietal branch of superficial temporal artery
3 Forehead flap on supratrochlear and supraorbital vessels.

THE SALIVARY GLANDS

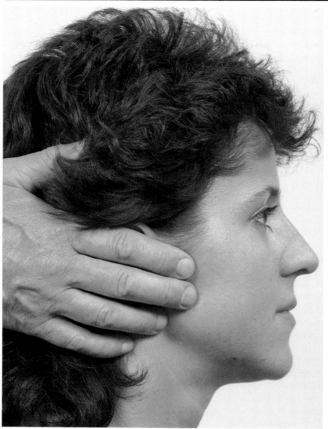

106

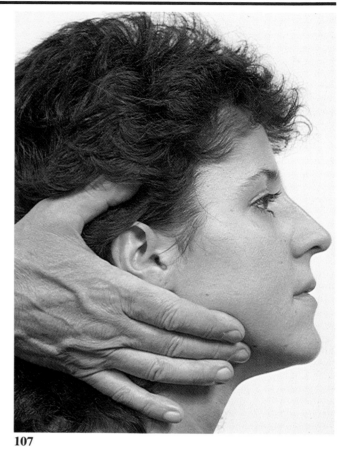

107

The three major salivary glands on each side are the parotid which is mainly serous, the submandibular (mixed mucous and serous) and the sublingual (which is largely mucous but with some serous secreting cells). In addition numerous small glands are scattered around the mouth in the palate, cheeks, lips and the posterior part of the dorsum, the periphery and the underside of the tongue.

The *parotid* is the largest of the three glands. Its major part lies tucked in the space between the anterior aspect of the mastoid process and the sternomastoid muscle, posteriorly, and the ramus of the mandible, anteriorly. Superiorly it runs up to the external auditory meatus and down almost to the angle of the mandible. Deeply it is limited by the styloid process and the stylomandibular ligament but it can come into close contact with the pharyngeal wall. The most obvious portion in a dissection is that which goes forward over the surface of the

masseter on to the cheek, and this is the easiest portion to examine (**106**). Normally because of its dense capsule which is continuous with the fascia over masseter it is not easy to identify in the normal state, though the lower border may be felt as a thickening over the surface of the masseter. Hence any readily palpable gland is probably indicative of some form of pathology. Occasionally small lymph glands may become swollen over the surface of the gland and also at the anterior border of the masseter.

The duct runs forward (often linked with small accessory parotid glands) level with the upper part of the lobe of the ear, to the anterior border of the masseter. There it turns inwards, pierces buccinator, which gives it some compressional control, and then forward a little between muscle and mucous membrane to open level with the junction of root and crown of the second upper molar tooth. The opening can be seen and felt quite easily in most cases.

THE SALIVARY GLANDS

The submandibular gland lies superficially beneath the mandible in a hollow in front of the angle and in the space between it and the mylohyoid muscle. Although enclosed in a split in the deep investing fascia of the neck this is not so dense as that over the parotid, and the outlines of the gland may be felt by careful examination (**107**). Again, superficial to it, submandibular lymph nodes may be felt if these become swollen.

From this superficial position, the submandibular gland wraps around the posterior edge of the mylohyoid muscle to run deep and forwards for a little way between this muscle and hyoglossus. From here the duct runs forwards to open at the sublingual papilla with the openings of the sublingual gland (**108**).

The *sublingual gland* lies superficially in the floor of the mouth deep to the mucosa of the sublingual fold to the side of the frenulum. It fills the space above the mylohyoid between the genioglossus medially, the mandible anteriorly and laterally and the deep part of the submandibular gland posteriorly (**109**).

108

109

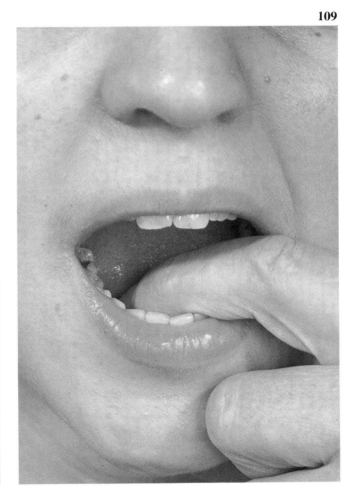

1 Underside of tongue
2 Plica fimbriata
3 Frenulum linguae
4 Lingual vein overlying
  lingual gland
5 Sublingual papillae
6 Sublingual fold over
  sublingual gland

THE NECK

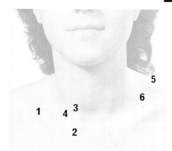

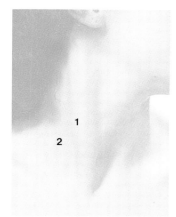

1 Clavicle
2 Medial end clavicle
3 Sternal head of
  sternomastoid muscle
4 Clavicular head of
  sternomastoid muscle
5 Trapezius muscle
6 Posterior triangle of
  the neck

1 Sternal head of
  sternomastoid
2 Clavicular head of
  sternomastoid

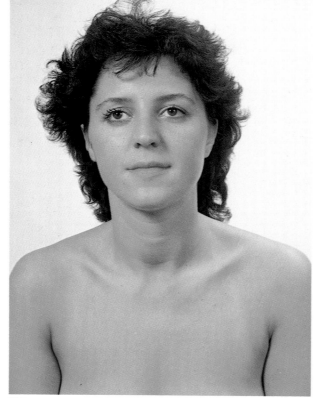

110

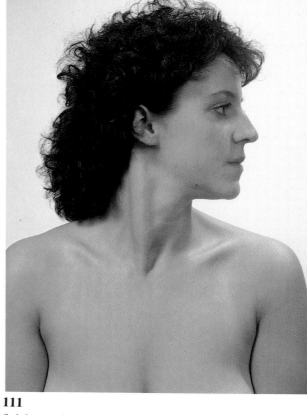

111

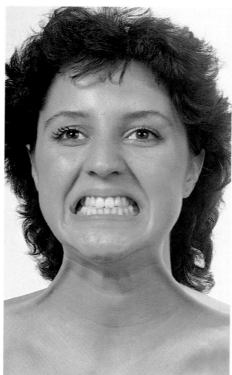

112

At rest the superficial muscles of the neck are relatively inconspicuous. The clavicle is usually obvious with its prominent medial end, though the lateral end is masked by deltoid. The sternal attachment of sternomastoid muscle stands out as a rounded tendon but the clavicular attachment is only just visible and often totally inconspicuous. The upper border of trapezius muscle shows on the shoulder, producing a hollow between it and sternomastoid, the posterior triangle of the neck.

Even more superficial is the platysma muscle. This human equivalent of the panniculus carnosus muscles of many mammals (useful for twitching the skin etc.) is relatively afunctional in humans. It stands out in rather variable patterns in different people when under stress. Like the facial muscles the platysma is supplied by the facial nerve.

Rotation of the head brings sternomastoid into activity. The sternal part stands out as a rounded column (1), while the clavicular head is now more obvious (2). The latter, though, is flat muscle as distinct from the rounded column and tendon of the sternal part.

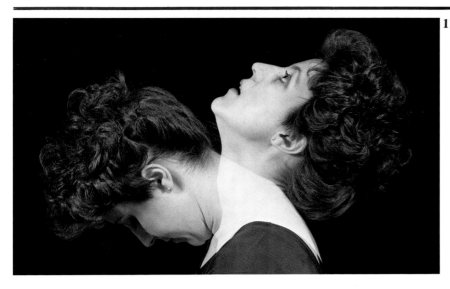

113 The mobility of the neck generates the relatively free movement of the head. The muscles and joints of the neck have a remarkably fine nervous control which, under normal circumstances, gives fine control and adjustment of the head on the trunk. Unfortunately the neck also allows for bad posture and, usually associated with this, osteoarthrosis of the neck vertebrae is common and may be extensive, with consequent functional and often neurological damage.

Flexion and extension are remarkably free, allowing flexion to bring the chin onto the chest and a considerable range of extension limited by the neural arches and muscle control.

114

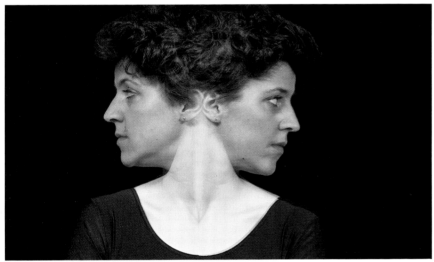

Rotation occurs throughout the neck with some 60–80 degrees in each direction. About half this rotation occurs between the axis and atlas vertebrae with the other half in the remainder of the neck.

115

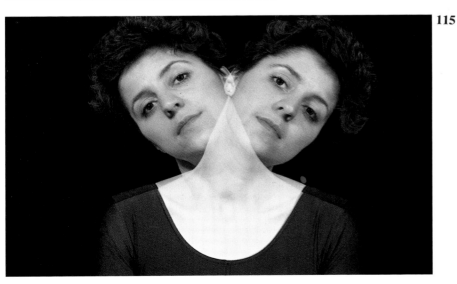

Lateral flexion is less free due to the lateral masses of the vertebrae but if a little rotation is allowed the range is very much increased. Note that a small amount of rotation has occurred in this case to allow the range achieved.

STERNOMASTOID MUSCLE

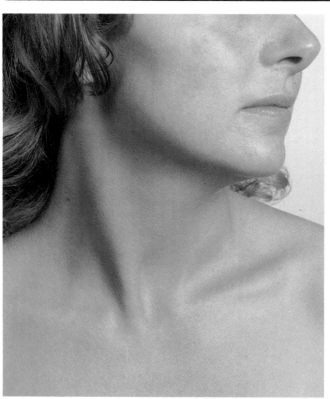

Sternomastoid is a somewhat complicated muscle running from the mastoid process and superior nuchal line of the head to the manubrium sterni and the clavicle. Although the cranial attachment is in a continuous line with that of trapezius posteriorly, as it runs downwards it divides. A superficial anterior and medial portion forms a rounded muscle and tendon running to the manubrium, which stands out distinctly when the muscle contracts. The deeper and more lateral component forms a flat muscle which runs to the medial third of the clavicle and is usually much less obvious even on contraction.

Contraction of a single muscle turns the head to the opposite side and facing upwards (**116**). To produce a more powerful contraction a hand can be used to resist the turning of the head but in this subject such a manoeuvre was unnecessary. Contraction of both muscles pulls the back of the head downwards, so that the subject looks upwards and cranes the neck somewhat. Note how well both lower attachments to the clavicle and the sternum stand out in this case, with this manoeuvre (**117**).

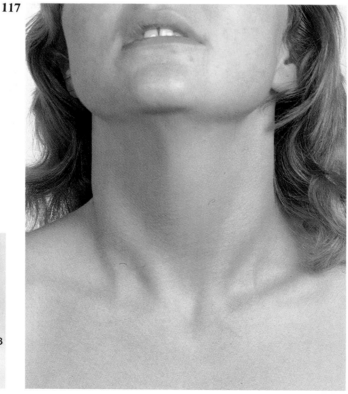

1 Sternal head of sternomastoid
2 Clavicular head of sternomastoid
3 Suprasternal notch
4 Supraclavicular fossa

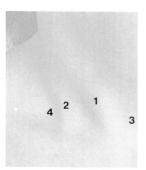

Even when the head is carried across to the opposite side at rest (**118**) the tension in the sternal head is evident and emphasises the suprasternal hollow in which, in this case, there is a prominent suprasternal jugular venous arch linking the variably sized anterior jugular veins. These veins run superficial to the infrahyoid strap muscles and drain by running behind sternomastoid either into the external carotid at its lower end or, slightly more medially into the subclavian. Posteriorly the anterior margin of trapezius, also on stretch, as is the overlying skin, delineates the posterior triangle of the neck (though the anterior border, the posterior border of sternomastoid, is less evident). However, the external jugular vein can be identified and so also can the skin raised by the stretched upper trunk of the brachial plexus.

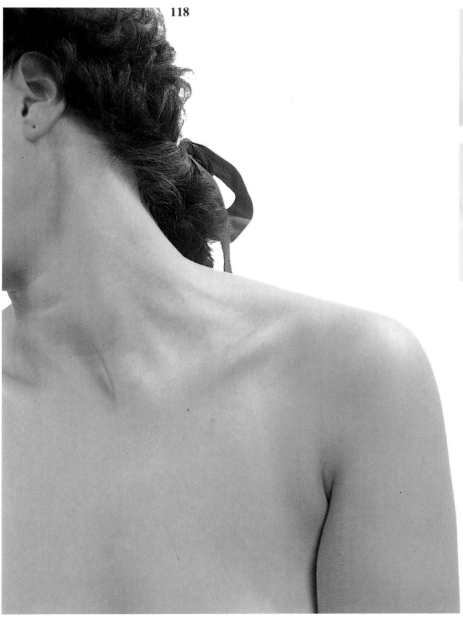

118

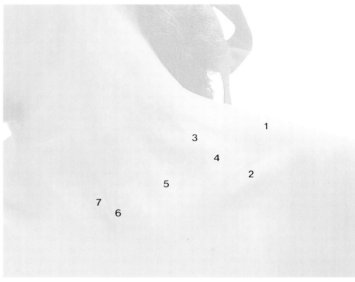

1 Trapezius
2 Clavicle
3 Brachial plexus (upper trunk)
4 External jugular vein
5 Clavicular head of sternomastoid
6 Sternal head of sternomastoid
7 Suprasternal jugular venous arch

THE POSTERIOR TRIANGLE

The posterior triangle of the neck is not exactly posterior, except relative to the sternomastoid muscle and the anterior triangle lying in front of it. It is bounded by the anterior margin of trapezius, the posterior border of sternomastoid and the clavicle below (**119**). The two muscles normally meet at their attachment to the skull along the superior nuchal line and here the occipital artery may be felt pulsating, having emerged from beneath sternomastoid to run up into the scalp.

The lower part of the triangle is most obvious, being the supraclavicular fossa.

Although splenius capitis and levator scapulae form the floor of the upper and posterior part of the triangle they mostly lie beneath trapezius. Scalenus medius forms the major part, running from the posterior tubercles of all the cervical transverse processes (usually) into the first rib. More anteriorly the scalenus anterior completes the floor with the phrenic nerve running down over its surface. The roots and trunks of the brachial plexus run down from between these muscles behind the clavicle and may raise a ridge, especially when the head is leaned to the opposite side.

The external jugular vein runs down across the triangle to pass deep to the clavicle lateral to sternomastoid's attachment.

The omohyoid muscle and tendon runs across obliquely from beneath sternomastoid about level with the cricoid cartilage towards its insertion by the suprascapular notch; it may produce a ridge if the shoulders are raised (**120**).

119

1 External jugular vein
2 Posterior border of sternomastoid
3 Omohyoid muscle
4 Scalenus anterior (crossed by phrenic nerve)
5 Scalenus medius
6 Anterior border of trapezius
7 Brachial plexus
8 Clavicle

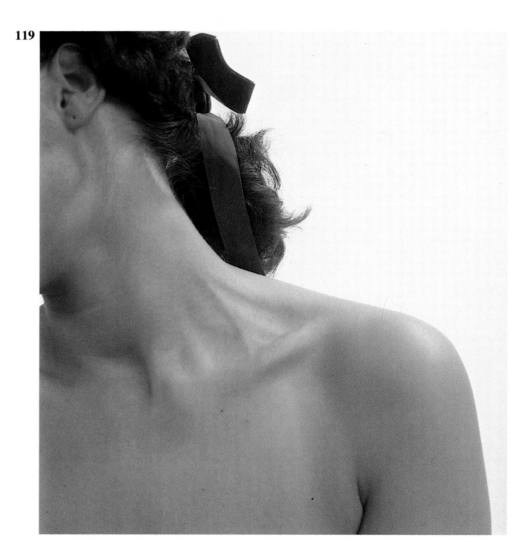

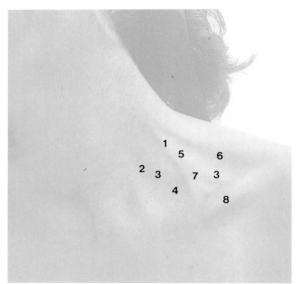

120

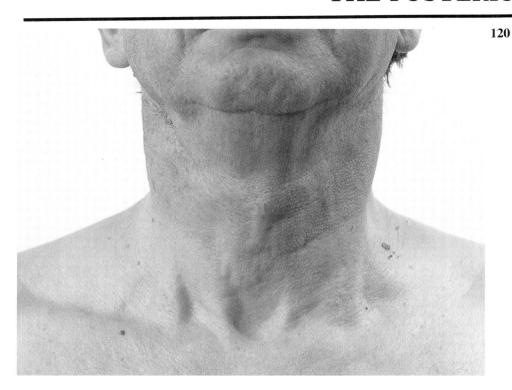

The transverse processes of the cervical vertebrae may be palpated. The second can be felt through sternomastoid about 1 cm (½ in) below the mastoid process and thence in line down to C6 above the middle of the clavicle (**121**). Pressure over the processes usually gives the sensation of nerve pressure from the emerging cervical nerves.

If the finger is pressed down behind the middle of the clavicle, the subclavian artery should be felt pulsating against the first rib. Sometimes the artery can be felt pulsating against the transverse process of C6 in those cases when it makes a high loop. The same pressure behind the clavicle should also compress the trunks of the brachial plexus.

The accessory nerve runs across the triangle from a point midway down the posterior border of the sternomastoid to enter trapezius about 5 cm (2 in) above the clavicle, whilst the several supraclavicular nerves (C4) emerge from behind sternomastoid at about the same point to run down over the clavicle where they can sometimes be felt by rolling the finger along the bone.

Supraclavicular lymph nodes, although not normally palpable, lie in the supraclavicular fossa and if swollen may become apparent.

121

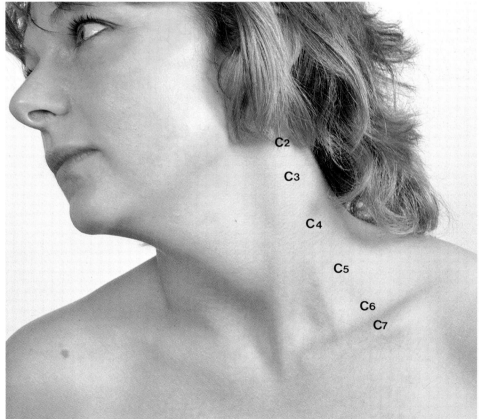

THE CERVICAL NERVES

The cervical nerves give, as do most spinal nerves, both anterior and posterior primary rami. The posterior primary rami supply the muscles and skin of the back though the supply of C1 is entirely muscular. C2 gives a much larger sensory supply than most and this forms the greater occipital nerve. It pierces trapezius to supply the back of the head. It can generally be palpated crossing the superior nuchal region at the back of the head close to the attachment of trapezius, about midway between the mastoid process and the midline. At this point it is readily available for local nerve block. It may be involved in neural pressure at the site, giving pain to the back of the head.

The anterior primary rami of the upper four cervical nerves form a plexus, so supplying cervical muscles and skin of the neck and of the shoulders (C4). The phrenic nerve also arises mainly from C4 with small contributions from C3 and larger ones (sometimes running separately) from C5 to give all the motor and most of the sensory supply to the diaphragm.

C2 arises above the transverse process of the axis and C3 and C4 above their respective vertebrae. The major branches appear from

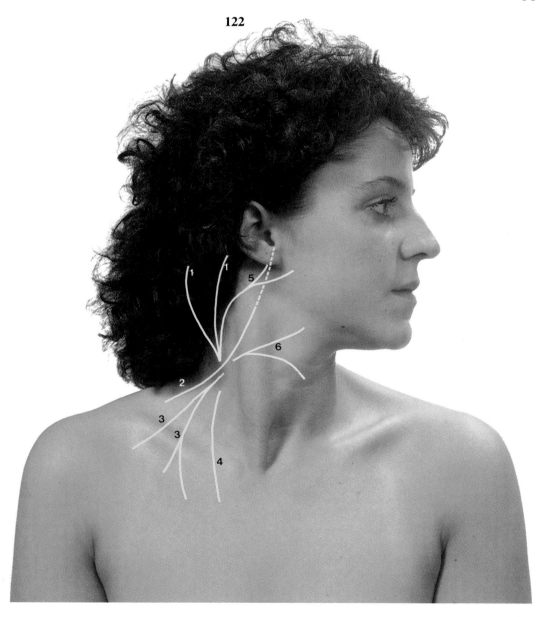

122

1 Greater and lesser occipital
2 Accessory
3 Supra clavicular
4 Phrenic
5 Greater auricular
6 Transverse cervical

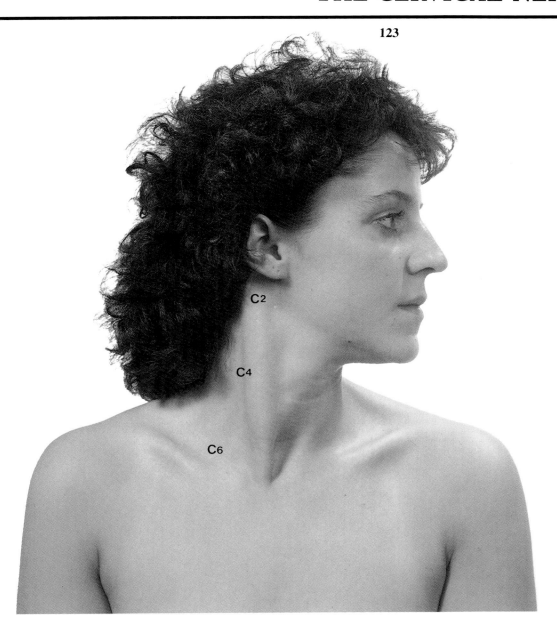

123

behind sternomastoid muscle (**122**). The supra-clavicular nerves leave at about the middle of the muscle as does the accessory nerve. The greater auricular turns upwards and anteriorly over the muscle, a little higher, towards the angle of the mandible, to supply skin over the angle, the parotid gland, the lower two thirds or so of the back of the ear plus the lobular region anteriorly.

Cervical nerve block depends on the localisation of the transverse processes of the upper cervical vertebrae (**123**). The processes are relatively superficial. That of C2 is about 1 cm below the mastoid process. That of C4 is about the middle and just behind the posterior border of sternomastoid. The external jugular vein usually runs off the surface of sternomastoid close to C4. C3 is approximately midway between. C6 can be felt above the middle of the clavicle (the so-called carotid tubercle).

As would be expected anaesthetisation of the cervical roots is likely to block the cervical sympathetic chain also producing lid lag on that side.

THE CERVICAL NERVES

The phrenic nerve starts its course behind sternomastoid but runs down over the surface of scalenus anterior behind the lower part of sternomastoid. If the clavicular head of sternomastoid is pulled forwards and the area infiltrated towards the anterior tubercle of C6 the nerve should be effectively anaesthetised (**124**). Conversely it is sometimes necessary to stimulate the phrenic nerve electrically to induce diaphragmatic respiratory movements. The electrodes can be applied at the same site as for the local injection.

The roots and trunks of the brachial plexus lie in the posterior triangle of the neck, the divisions behind the clavicle and the cords in the axilla. The upper and middle trunks are readily accessible in the triangle but the lower trunk lies close to the first rib behind the clavicle. If a line is drawn from the middle of the posterior border of sternomastoid to the middle of the clavicle this should overlie the trunks and roots beginning with C5 (plus usually some of C4) down to T1 beneath the clavicle. If the head is held to the opposite side a ridge raised by the trunks can be felt.

Local nerve block of the brachial plexus can be done in several sites. A supraclavicular approach is excellent but there is always the danger of pneumothorax due to perforation of the suprapleural membrane (Sibson's fascia) if the syringe is disconnected from a needle which has pierced the fascia. At the midpoint of the clavicle the external jugular vein passes beneath it and the subclavian artery can be felt (**125**).

The plexus should run immediately behind the pulse but it is usual to make the injection 1–2 cm above the clavicle and pointing downwards and backwards (**126**). It is important to be sure that the needle is not in a vessel or the lung before injecting the anaesthetic. To avoid risk of penetrating the lung a somewhat higher interscalene injection may be done. It is important that the injection is within the fascial sheath to allow the anaesthetic to track down to lower levels.

An axillary approach to the plexus is also possible but here the disadvantage is the spread-out nature of the cords around the artery (see page 105).

124

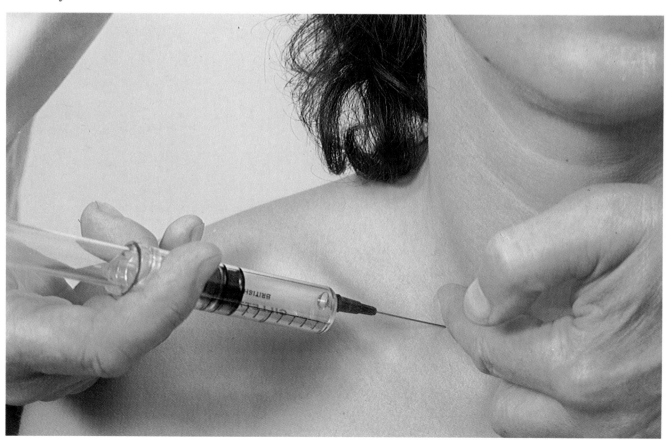

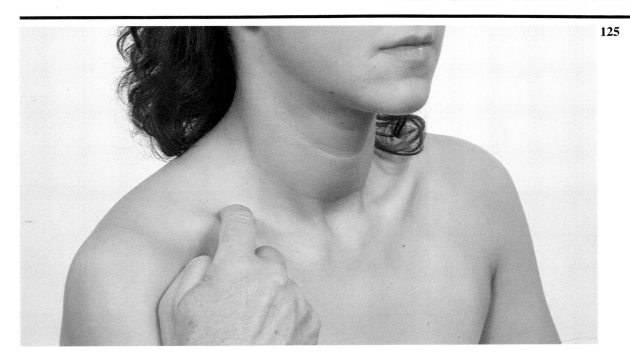

125

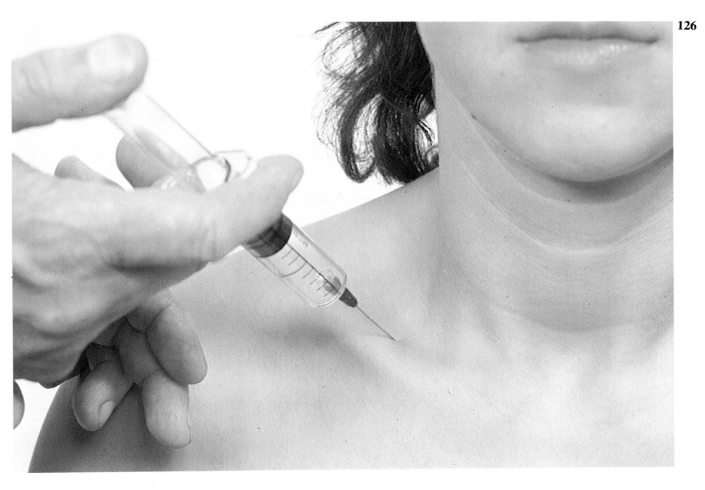

126

THE LARYNX

The prominence of the larynx is often visible in the neck as 'Adam's apple' and as that colloquial name suggests, it is a feature most obvious in adult males (129). The readily visible component is the thyroid cartilage with its upper border and the vertically running angle between the two laminae. The vocal cords or ligaments are attached to the back of the thyroid cartilage and run backwards to the arytenoid cartilages mounted on the posterior lamina of the cricoid. At puberty the male larynx grows in size so that the cords which are some 12.5–17 mm in length in women are 17–23 mm in men. The thyroid cartilage thus projects further forwards and its angle becomes sharper, from 120° in a child or woman to 90° in a man.

127

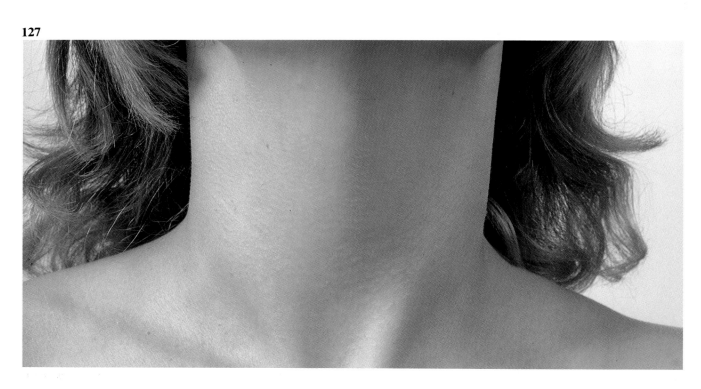

128

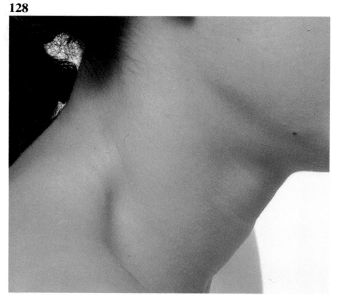

129

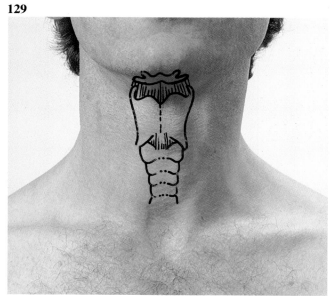

If the head is fully extended (**130**), the upper part of the thyroid cartilage is midway between chin and sternum but in a natural position it is tucked more closely under the chin. In an adult the arch of the cricoid cartilage is level with the 6th cervical vertebra and the hyoid level with C3–4. In a newborn baby the larynx is much higher, with the epiglottis level with the soft palate, but it sinks as the face and neck grow.

Palpation of the larynx should be carried out very gently. Gentle palpation not only increases tactile sensibility but pressure on the larynx, particularly in the region of the cricoid, produces a very unpleasant sensation for the patient.

The hyoid bone is a base for muscle attach-ments and therefore is not easy to palpate anteriorly but if the finger is moved more to the side then it is much easier. One way is to take the two greater cornua gently between finger and thumb. It is important to realise that the hyoid bone is tucked up under the mandible. If the finger is carried down it then comes to rest on the projecting shelf of the upper aspect of the thyroid cartilage. Whilst examining the hyoid between finger and thumb the superior cornua of the thyroid may be felt approaching it from below. If the finger now runs down the vertical angle of the thyroid it will drop into a small shallow depression before meeting another small prominence, the anterior arch of the cricoid.

130

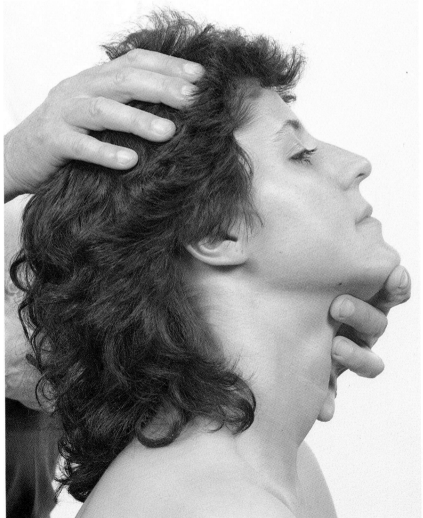

The examiner's index finger rests on the chin, the middle finger to the side of the hyoid bone, the ring finger on the upper part of the thyroid cartilage and the little finger on the cricoid.

131

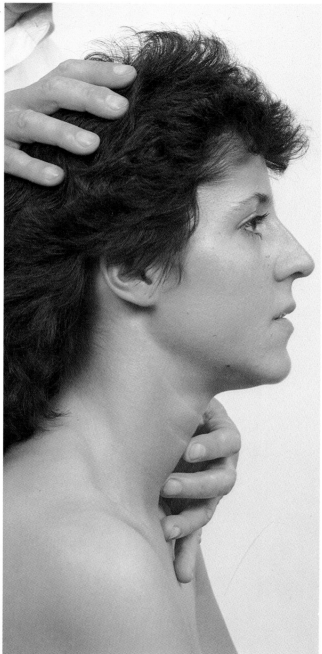

The strap muscles of the neck run down on either side of the midline from the hyoid to sternum and hence cover the lobes of the thyroid gland. However, with gentle palpation it is often possible to feel the slight thickening of the isthmus of the gland crossing the 2nd and 3rd tracheal rings just below the cricoid swelling (**132**).

During swallowing the larynx is raised by muscles controlled by the vagus and cranial accessory nerves through the pharyngeal branch, as well as the glossopharyngeal nerve controlling stylopharyngeus, and then returned by the strap muscles (C2 and C3). The larynx also tends to be raised in singing a high note but a trained singer should be able to relax the muscles and so prevent the larynx being raised.

132

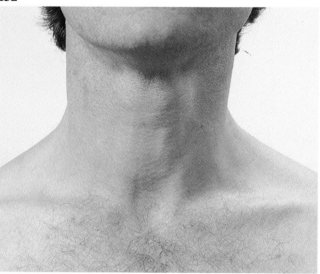

Because of the greater prominence of the larynx in a male it is sometimes possible to see the outlines of the thyroid gland to some extent even when normal.

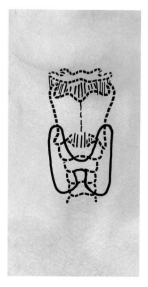

The index finger rests in the hollow between the thyroid and cricoid cartilages, the middle finger on the isthmus of the thyroid gland, the ring finger on the suprasternal notch and the little finger over the manubriosternal joint (sternal angle of Louis).

SUBMANDIBULAR REGION

This is a region where subcutaneous fat is laid down in many people and particularly with the sagging skin of increasing age. In a young person, however, when the skin is put on stretch it is often possible to identify a number of structures and these can be used as indicators for the whereabouts of others (**133**).

133

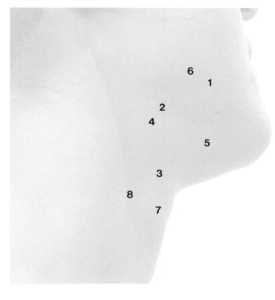

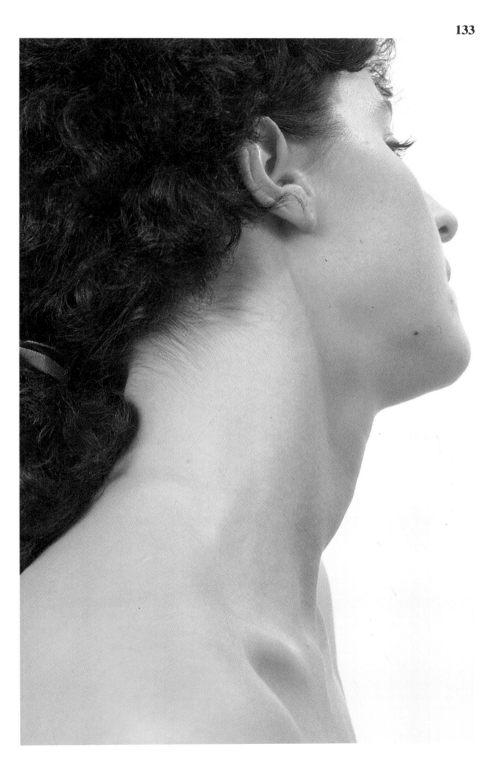

1 Mandible
2 Submandibular gland
3 Hyoid bone
4 Posterior belly of digastric
5 Anterior belly of digastric
6 Anterior border of masseter
7 Thyroid cartilage
8 Superior cornu of thyroid cartilage

GREAT VESSELS OF THE NECK

The neck is an important transit zone for vessels linking the brain and the heart as well as for local head and neck supply. The vertebral vessels including the rich venous vertebral plexus supply much of the brain as well as the cervical spinal cord. The vertebral artery from the first part of the subclavian usually enters the foramen transversarium of the 6th cervical vertebra, the transverse process of which can be felt a little above the middle of the clavicle.

The common carotid arteries run upwards. That on the right side is formed behind the sternoclavicular joint by division of the brachiocephalic into it and the subclavian artery. On the left side the common carotid leaves the arch of the aorta behind the left side of the manubrium sterni and runs upwards, likewise behind the sternoclavicular joint. The arteries then follow a more or less straight course towards the ear where the internal carotid branch enters the skull about 1 cm or so deep to and a little behind the head of the mandible (or deep to the intertragic notch of the ear).

The common carotid artery normally divides behind the superior cornu of the thyroid cartilage into internal and external branches (**134**). The internal carotid artery runs at first anteromedial to the internal carotid and later more laterally to end in the parotid gland behind and deep to the neck of the mandible. Here it divides into its terminal branches; the superficial temporal continues in line over the zygomatic arch (see page 58) while the maxillary artery runs forwards deep to the neck of the mandible.

The first branch of the external carotid, the superior thyroid artery, leaves to run to the upper pole of the thyroid gland immediately after but often just before the division, whilst the ascending pharyngeal leaves the medial aspect shortly thereafter. The lingual artery leaves the anterior aspect at about the level of the greater cornu of the hyoid bone followed almost immediately after by the facial artery, usually tucked under the angle of the mandible. Just above the greater cornu of the hyoid bone the occipital artery runs backwards under cover of the sternomastoid muscle to appear on the scalp just medial to its attachment. As the occipital artery leaves, the hypoglossal nerve appears from between the arteries and the internal jugular vein to loop round the origin of the occipital artery and then run forwards over the external carotid, under cover of the posterior belly of digastric muscle. The posterior auricular artery runs backwards from the external carotid shortly after the occipital, or may leave as a common stem, the main artery now entering the parotid gland to reach its final division.

134

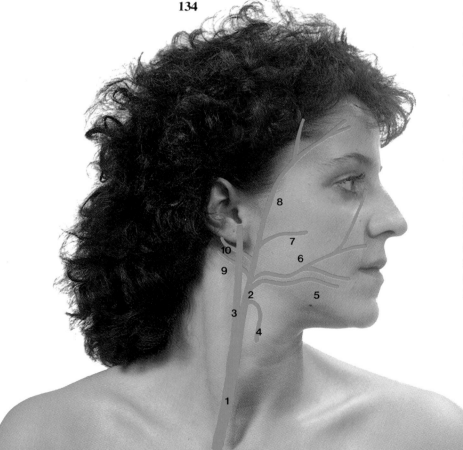

1 Common carotid
2 External carotid
3 Internal carotid
4 Superior thyroid
5 Lingual
6 Facial
7 Maxillary
8 Superficial temporal
9 Occipital
10 Posterior auricular

135

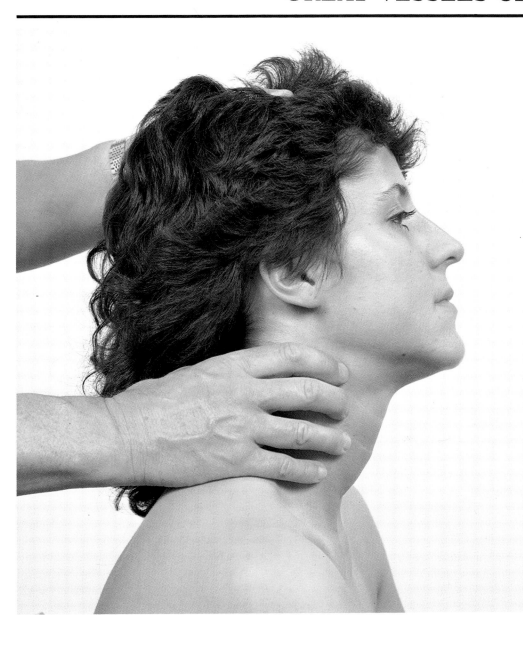

The carotid sinus and body are both found at the division of the common carotid artery and hence are close to and just behind the superior cornu of the thyroid cartilage.

The carotid arteries can be felt in the neck by pressing in front of the sternomastoid muscle towards the transverse processes of the cervical vertebrae (**135**).

One intracranial artery of importance from its surface marking is the middle meningeal which may rupture following head injury. This artery enters the skull through the foramen spinosum which is level with the middle of the upper border of the zygomatic arch. It then follows a course laterally within the skull for a variable distance before dividing into frontal and parietal branches. Looked at from the lateral side this will be only a few millimetres higher than the zygomatic arch of entry into the skull. The frontal or anterior channel then continues more or less vertically while the parietal (posterior) branch runs backwards and slightly upwards from the middle of the zygomatic arch.

GREAT VESSELS OF THE NECK

The great veins of the neck run both superficially and deeply. The major venous channel from the brain other than the vertebral venous plexus and vein is the internal jugular vein (**136**). It leaves the skull as a continuation of the sigmoid sinus through the jugular foramen, just lateral to and a few millimetres behind the internal carotid artery. So once again the inter-tragic notch makes an effective surface marking. It runs down with the internal and then the common carotid arteries, running deep to sternomastoid in the lower half of the neck and there becoming more directly lateral to the common carotid artery. In the root of the neck it crosses in front of the subclavian artery and joins the subclavian vein behind the sternoclavicular joint, to become the brachiocephalic vein. That on the right side continues downwards while that of the left crosses behind the upper part of the manubrium sterni to join the right one, to form the superior vena cava.

The internal jugular vein receives the facial and a branch from the retromandibular vein and usually superior and middle thyroid veins as well as lingual and pharyngeal veins. The middle thyroid vein is particularly important surgically for, although not always present (about 50% of cases), it is a short vein which runs over the common carotid artery to the internal jugular vein from which it can easily be torn in thyroidectomy while mobilising tissues in the neck, if the surgeon is not aware of the danger.

136

1 Internal jugular vein
2 Subclavian vein
3 Left brachiocephalic vein
4 Right brachiocephalic vein
5 Superior Vena Cava

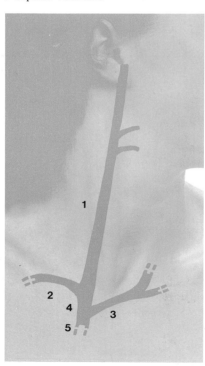

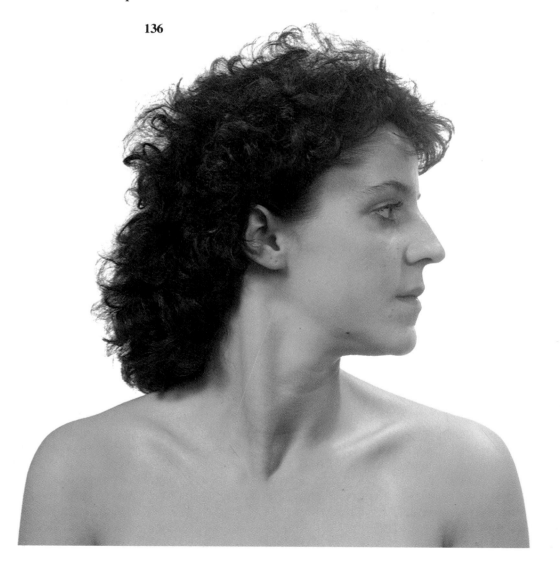

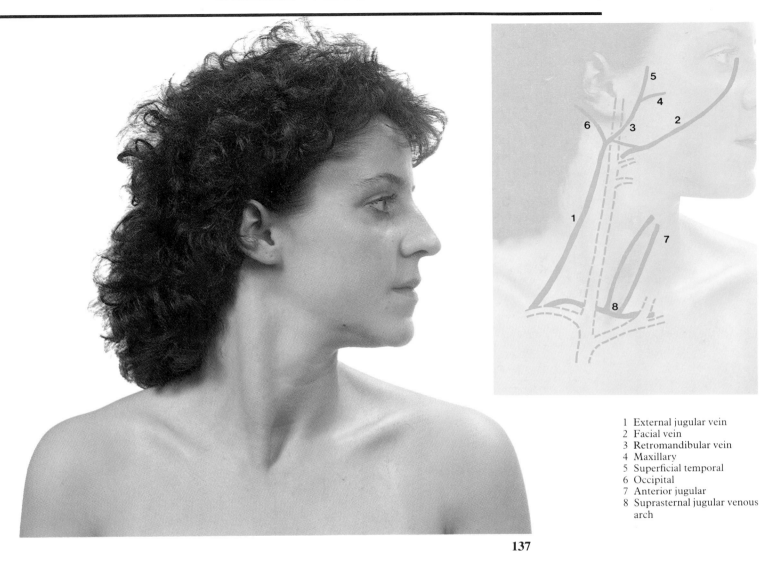

1 External jugular vein
2 Facial vein
3 Retromandibular vein
4 Maxillary
5 Superficial temporal
6 Occipital
7 Anterior jugular
8 Suprasternal jugular venous
  arch

137

The external jugular vein begins in the parotid gland, most commonly by union of the superficial temporal and maxillary veins, together with posterior auricular and a link branch with the facial (see internal jugular vein). It thus runs from behind the angle of the mandible over the surface of sternomastoid muscle to sink behind the middle of the clavicle to join the subclavian vein, or in about 30% of cases the internal jugular vein.

Anterior jugular veins run down from the submental region, following a variable course and of variable size to the lower neck where they are usually linked by a jugular venous arch. They drain below the arch into either the terminal part of the external jugular or slightly more medially into the subclavian vein (**137**).

It is worth noting that the jugular arch with the inferior thyroid veins (draining to the left brachiocephalic) and the deeper position of the trachea, makes this an unsuitable position for an emergency tracheostomy, although excellent for an elective procedure. The emergency approach should be above where the larynx and trachea are superficial and with no important structures in the midline. The choice rests with going between the thyroid and cricoid cartilages (laryngostomy) or through the upper rings of the trachea (high tracheostomy) either dividing or pulling down the isthmus of the thyroid gland.

CENTRAL VENOUS CATHETERISATION

With the frequent need for central venous catheterisation in modern medicine a knowledge of the major veins in the neck has become more important, together with the sites of ready approach. Although the veins at the antecubital fossa are useful there may be difficulty in threading the catheter through the veins to the heart. Thus approach through the internal jugular or subclavian vein may be needed with preference for the right side for easier passage to the heart. Furthermore accurate positioning of the needle is vital to prevent unnecessary damage to these important veins.

The internal jugular vein runs deep to the sternomastoid muscle in the lower part of the neck (**138**) and so it can be approached about midway down the anterior border of the muscle just lateral to the carotid pulse (1). Although the vein is behind sternomastoid, this muscle divides into sternal and clavicular attachments leaving a gap through which the needle can be passed in a downwards and medial direction (2). This position is better in a conscious patient.

Alternatively the subclavian vein may be approached, as it runs over the first rib behind the medial third of the clavicle, either from above the clavicle (3) or below (4). The available position is at the junction of the medial and intermediate thirds of the clavicle. From above, this will be at the lateral border of sternomastoid and the needle passed downwards and medially while from below it is passed upwards and medially. In either case it is important to remember how close the vein is behind the clavicle.

138

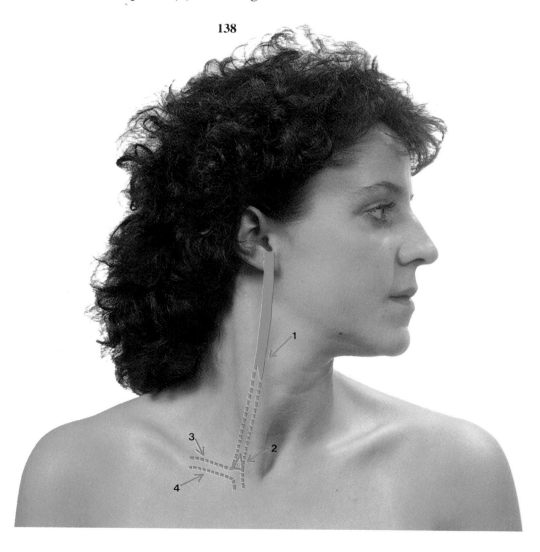

LYMPHATICS OF THE HEAD AND NECK

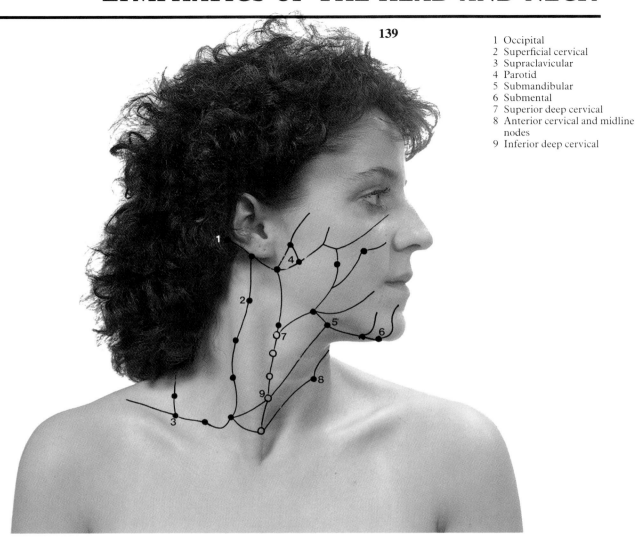

139

1 Occipital
2 Superficial cervical
3 Supraclavicular
4 Parotid
5 Submandibular
6 Submental
7 Superior deep cervical
8 Anterior cervical and midline nodes
9 Inferior deep cervical

The lymph glands are not normally palpable but it is important to know where to examine in case of swelling, either from infection or malignancy (**139**).

Superficial glands are found around the face and head, on the cheek at the anterior border of masseter, and on the parotid and over the mastoid and occipital regions of the head. At a slightly lower level submental glands drain the tip of the tongue, the lower lip and mouth while the submandibular glands receive from the submental and also from the tongue, mouth, cheek, upper lip and nasal cavity. More posterior lymphatics drain into nodes along the external jugular vein which in turn drain into the deep cervical nodes as do lymphatics from the pharyngeal and tracheal regions.

The deep cervical nodes lie along the internal jugular vein and form the main collecting system for the head and neck. They are usually described as superior and inferior deep cervical groups, including in the former, the jugulodigastric or tonsillar node and in the latter the jugulo-omohyoid node. The majority of nodes tend to lie deep to the sternomastoid muscle and lymphatics run in its fascial sheath. However, the anterior of the superior nodes including the jugulodigastric can be felt anterior to the upper part of the sternomastoid, whilst the posterior of the lower group may be felt along the posterior border of the muscle, i.e. in the posterior triangle, where supraclavicular nodes may also be felt in the hollow above the clavicle.

SHOULDER GIRDLE AND JOINT

The legs are mounted on a firm pelvis but the arms are designed to work with maximal controlled mobility on the trunk. Thus movement between leg and trunk is limited to the ball and socket hip joint. In the case of the arm, however, there is considerable mobility between shoulder girdle and trunk as well as at the shoulder joint itself.

From the point of view of true joints, the shoulder girdle is very weakly mounted onto the trunk at the sternoclavicular joint (**140**).

This is an essentially non-loadbearing joint divided into two parts by a central fibrocartilaginous disc. Furthermore whereas most synovial joints designed for load have hyaline cartilage over their bearing surfaces, the sternoclavicular joint (like the similar temporomandibular joint) has fibrocartilage. The axis of movement is not within the joint itself but some 2–3 cm (1 in) along the bone so that the medial end of the clavicle moves in the opposite direction from the point of the shoulder (**141**). Thus

140

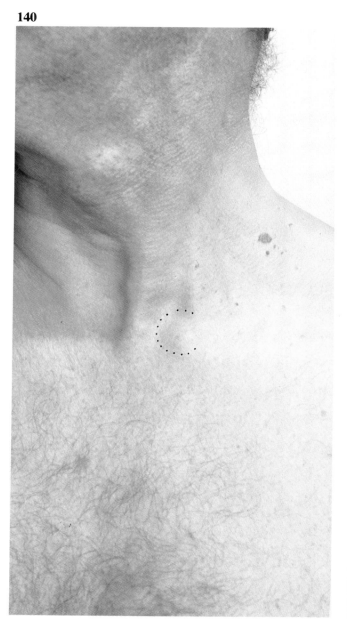

141

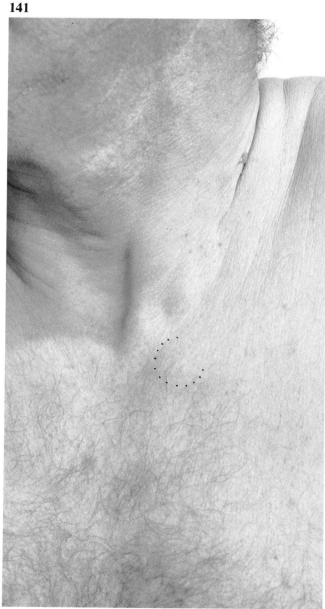

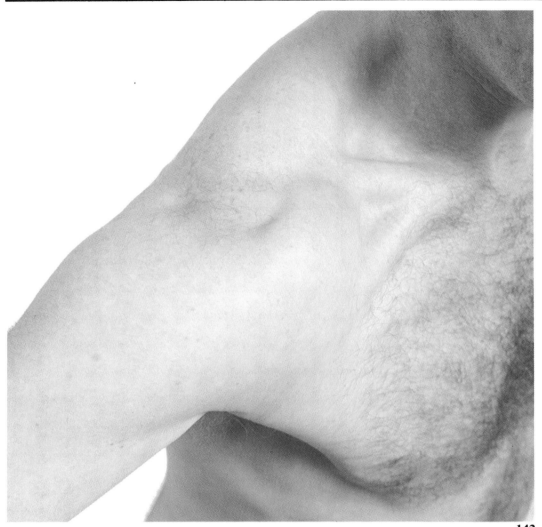

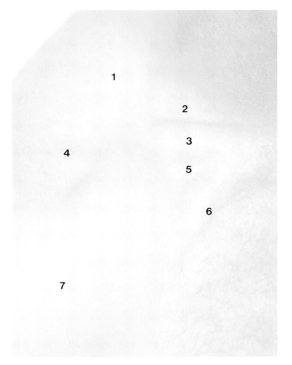

1 Trapezius
2 Supraclavicular fossa
3 Clavicle
4 Acromion
5 Infraclavicular fossa
6 Clavicular head of pectoralis
   major
7 Deltoid

142

as the shoulder is raised, the medial end of the clavicle is lowered. The clavicle thus moves on an axis around the attachment of the costo-clavicular ligament, under the dynamic postural control of the subclavius muscle. The bones of the shoulder girdle are almost exclusively controlled by the muscles linking them with the trunk and this is almost as true for the shoulder joint where a large humeral head fits into a small shallow glenoid fossa offering little more than a fulcrum for muscle control of the humeral lever.

The medial end of the clavicle curves around the upper chest wall, overlying the first rib and then a reverse curve produces the hollow of the shoulder as the lateral end fits, by a small plane joint, into the acromion. The acromion, a curved continuation of the spine of the scapula, gives the bony contour to the shoulder (**142**).

The acromioclavicular joint allows minimal movement between clavicle and scapula, mainly rotation, during abduction and adduction of the arm and otherwise these two bones move virtually in unison on the trunk around the costo-clavicular axis. The bony continuum of clavicle, acromion and spine of the scapula are readily palpable and visible in a slim person, though in a fat person the spine or the scapula may become hidden. However even in such a person the inferior angle of the scapula, usually very obvious, is normally palpable, particularly if the shoulder is moved.

SHOULDER GIRDLE AND JOINT

Below the lateral aspect of the clavicle, the coracoid process of the scapula can usually be felt though it is overlaid by the anterior fibres of the deltoid muscle. Just medial to the deltoid swelling a small gap between that muscle and the clavicular fibres of pectoralis major produces an infraclavicular fossa, emphasised dramatically when both muscles are put into action (**142**). From this intermuscular gap a narrow groove may be seen on the anterior aspect of the shoulder between these two muscles, the delto-pectoral groove containing the cephalic vein which, slightly lower in the region, lies in the groove between deltoid and biceps brachii muscles. Having reached the infraclavicular fossa the vein then pierces the clavipectoral fascia to join the axillary vein.

If the deltoid muscle is palpated a little below the acromion, the two humeral tuberosities may be felt, particularly if the arm is rotated a little to help identify the contour changes. With the arm in the usually described anatomical position (i.e. with the palm of the hand facing forwards) the greater tuberosity lies laterally and the lesser anteriorly, but in the more relaxed and commonly functional position as shown in **143** the greater tuberosity is anterior and the lesser medial.

143

1 Trapezius
2 Supraclavicular fossa
3 Acromion
4 Acromioclavicular joint
5 Clavicle
6 Coracoid process
7 Infraclavicular fossa
8 Deltoid
9 Deltopectoral groove
10 Pectoralis major
11 Cephalic vein

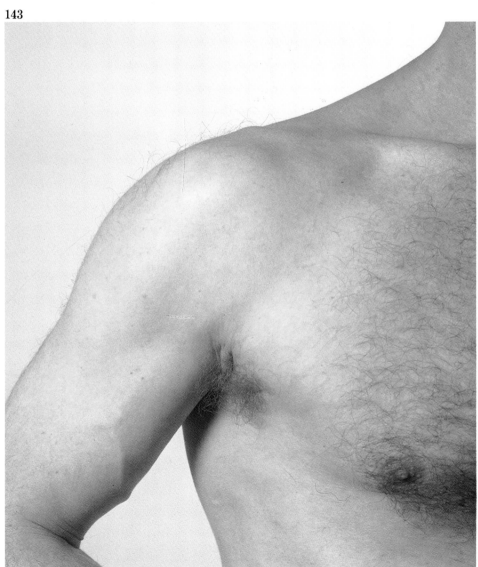

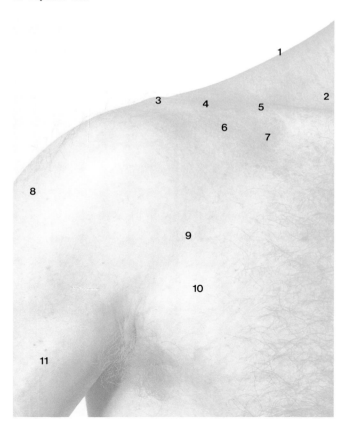

144

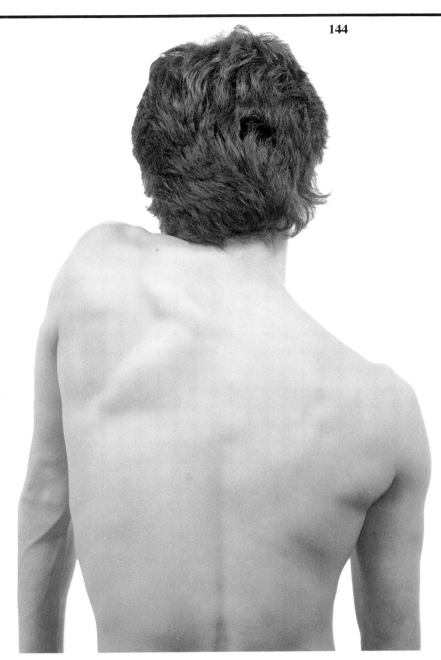

Examination of movements at the shoulder should be designed to differentiate between those of the shoulder girdle and those of the joint. However, as some muscles act over both and some movements are a combination of movements at both, this is sometimes a little difficult to achieve in practice.

At the shoulder girdle, elevation and depression indicate movements of the scapula without rotation. Similarly protraction carries the scapula around the chest wall so that the shoulder faces forwards, whilst retraction pulls the scapula towards the spine (i.e. bracing the shoulders). Upwards and downward rotation of the scapula indicates the direction of movement of the glenoid and these movements are normally a component of abduction and adduction of the arm (though produced separately in **144**).

145

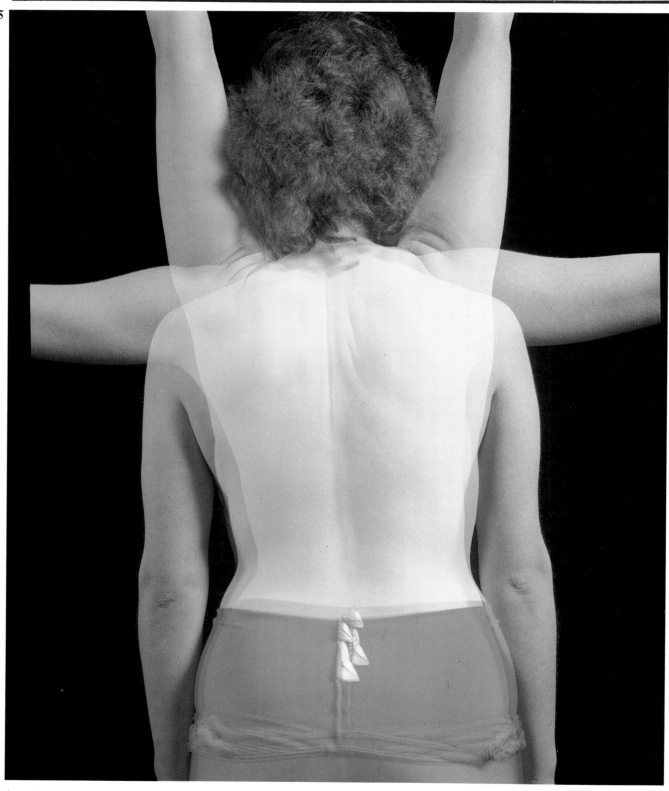

A cyclograph showing range of abduction at the shoulder girdle and joint.

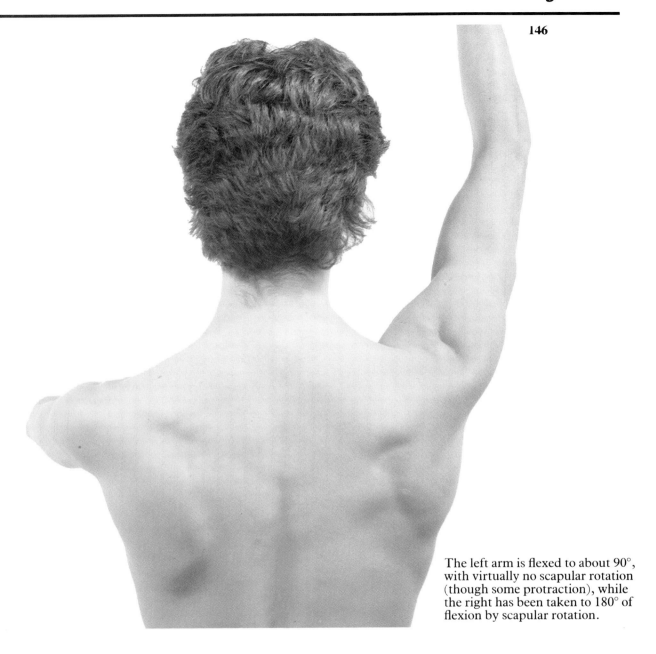

146

The left arm is flexed to about 90°, with virtually no scapular rotation (though some protraction), while the right has been taken to 180° of flexion by scapular rotation.

Movements at the shoulder joint are registered relative to the position of the scapula. Hence abduction and adduction are in the plane of the scapula which, with the scapula in its normal position, will be a little in front of the plane of the trunk. Abduction of the arm is a combined movement at both joint systems; a little over 90° being possible at the shoulder joint and a little less by upward rotation of the scapula. The relative contributions at any position vary somewhat with the individual but the shoulder joint contributes the greater amount as the arm moves from the side (**145**).

Flexion and extension are strictly at right angles to the plane of the scapula. Flexion is mainly at the shoulder joint for some 90° but the range available is increased by upward rotation of the scapula (**146**).

Medial and lateral rotation at the shoulder joint are also important and powerful movements.

MUSCLES CONTROLLING THE SHOULDER GIRDLE

Two important muscles run into the clavicle from the head and neck region, the sterno-mastoid into its medial end (see page 66) and the trapezius running into its lateral third. The *trapezius* is a large triangular muscle covering the neck and shoulder region, the two muscles together making a trapezium (**147**). The muscle has a long attachment to the superior nuchal line on the occiput (medial to sternomastoid), the ligamentum nuchae in the neck and the spines and supraspinous ligaments of the seventh cervical and all the thoracic vertebrae. The cranial fibres run to the lateral third of the clavicle with the progressively lower fibres being attached to the acromion and along the spine of the scapula to its medial end. The cranial fibres can either extend the head on the neck and turn it to the opposite side, or, if the head is fixed, raise the point of the shoulder; the intermediate fibres will brace the shoulders (adduct the

scapula) whilst the lowest will pull down the medial aspect of the scapula. Each part can work separately in conjunction with the other muscles of similar function, or the whole muscle will rotate the scapula so that the glenoid faces upwards. This rotation of the scapula accounts for much of the movement of the arm, particularly to the side, and can give reasonable movement to the arm even after fixation of the shoulder joint.

Even when standing at rest the trapezius is required to act to support the shoulders. Loss of the spinal accessory nerve supply to the muscle, as after a classical block lymph gland dissection of the neck, leads to dropping of the shoulder, with the scapula rotating somewhat downwards. The muscle is thus vital for good postural control of the shoulder girdle as well as in the more dynamic role of controlling the shoulder girdle as a base for arm movement.

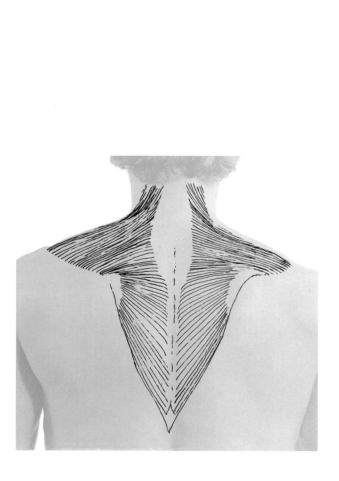

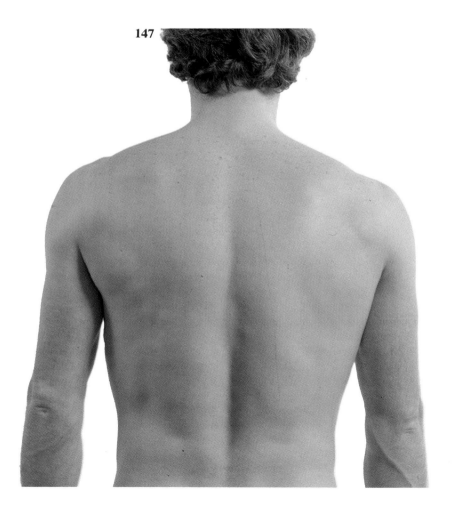

147

148

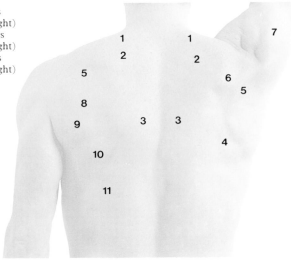

1 Upper fibres of trapezius
 (contracting firmly on right)
2 Middle fibres of trapezius
 (contracting firmly on right)
3 Lower fibres of trapezius
 (contracting firmly on right)
4 Rhomboideus major
5 Spine of scapula
6 Supraspinatus bulging
 under trapezius
7 Deltoid
8 Infraspinatus
9 Teres minor
10 Teres major
11 Latissimus dorsi

While maintaining good postural control of the trunk the right arm has been abducted through some 180°. The left scapula remains in a normal resting position but with firm muscle control, the glenoid pointing laterally. The right scapula has been rotated through some 70–75° under the activity of trapezius with the remaining arm movement occurring at the shoulder joint. Activity is obvious in deltoid, the major abductor at the shoulder joint, and no doubt in supraspinatus, though this muscle is masked by trapezius.

149

True abduction at the shoulder should be in the plane of the resting scapula as in **148**, thus carrying the arm in front of the plane of the trunk. If the arm is to be abducted in the plane of the trunk the scapula must be retracted as well as rotated. Note not only the retracting middle fibres of trapezius but also of the rhomboideus muscles running to the medial border of the scapula acting to pull the scapula into the plane of the trunk as the remainder of trapezius acts to rotate it upwards. The trunk has been allowed to move somewhat to the left to balance the weight of the abducted arm (**149**).

MUSCLES CONTROLLING THE SHOULDER GIRDLE

When the shoulder girdle is held in a relaxed state it must be supported from above against gravity and this is primarily a function of trapezius. Other muscles tend to be essentially inactive, even serratus anterior which controls the scapula against the chest wall. Note the slight prominence of the inferior angle of the bone together with the lower part of its medial border (150). This is lost when the scapula is stabilised for activity (151). If serratus anterior is lost as a functioning muscle, the scapular prominence becomes much more marked, leading to the so-called 'winging' of the scapula, a feature of division of the lateral thoracic nerve supply to the muscle.

In a female the muscular features are likely to be somewhat masked by subcutaneous fat but nevertheless the details can still be identified in the abducted right shoulder. The left arm is held in a relaxed but slightly flexed position, with some protraction of the scapula, giving a prominence to the medial border of the scapula.

150

151

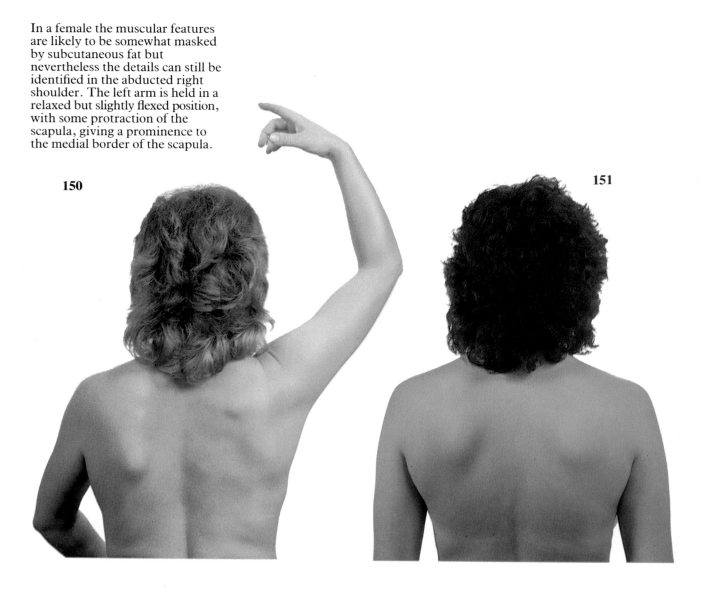

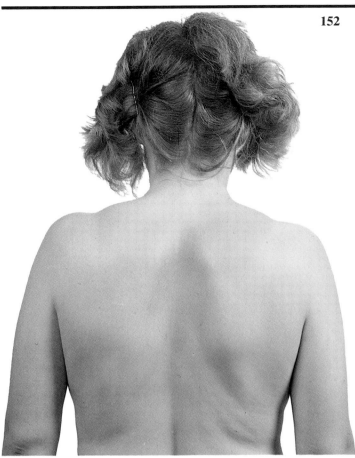

152 Elevation of the shoulders is brought about by the upper fibres of trapezius combined with levator scapulae. The bulge brought about by contraction of the upper fibres of trapezius is obvious. However levator scapulae runs down beneath it from the transverse processes of the upper cervical vertebrae to the superior angle of the scapula thus contributing to the bulk. In paralysis of trapezius, the levator scapulae then raises a prominent ridge when in action. As both elevators have a medially directed pull, the superior angles of the scapulae have become approximated. Note that the lower fibres of trapezius are inactive, giving a hollow between the lower parts of the scapulae. Levator scapulae is innervated from cervical 3 & 4 with a branch from the nerve to the rhomboids (C5).

153

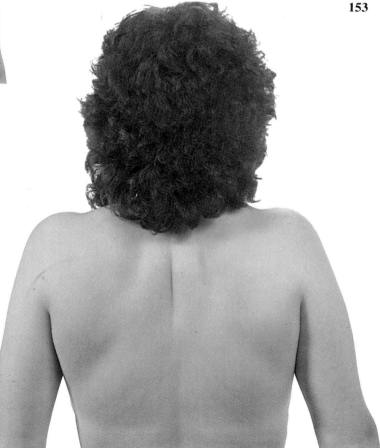

Depression of the scapula is brought about by the lower fibres of trapezius together with latissimus dorsi, some of whose fibres are attached to the scapula although most run to the humerus.

Retraction of the scapula, or bracing the shoulders is brought about by the intermediate fibres of trapezius together with the rhomboids lying beneath. As the rhomboids run downwards from the spine to the medial border of the scapula and mainly to the inferior angle there is a tendency for the scapula to be elevated with retraction. Note how the inferior angle of the scapula has been pulled into the chest wall by the action of rhomboideus major. Loss of the nerve supply to the muscles (C5) allows the scapula to fall away from the chest due to the pull of the arm muscles arising from the scapula giving particular prominence to the angle of the scapula, an exaggeration of the state in **150**.

MUSCLES CONTROLLING THE SHOULDER GIRDLE

Protraction of the scapula is brought about by serratus anterior muscle. This muscle arises by eight digitations, one from each of the upper eight ribs. The muscle runs backwards around the chest wall, under the scapula, to be attached to the under side of its medial border. As a postural muscle it contributes, with the rhomboids, to holding the scapula against the chest wall but most importantly it acts with the other muscles controlling the shoulder girdle to form a fixed base on which the arm can move accurately. This is effectively illustrated in **154–155**. In **154** the arm is held forwards and resting on a fixed object in relaxation. The medial border of the scapula is prominent particularly towards the angle. In **155** the arm is pressed down forcibly and, although serratus anterior plays no active part in the movement, the digitations (1) can be seen in active contraction, acting with other muscles to stabilise the shoulder girdle.

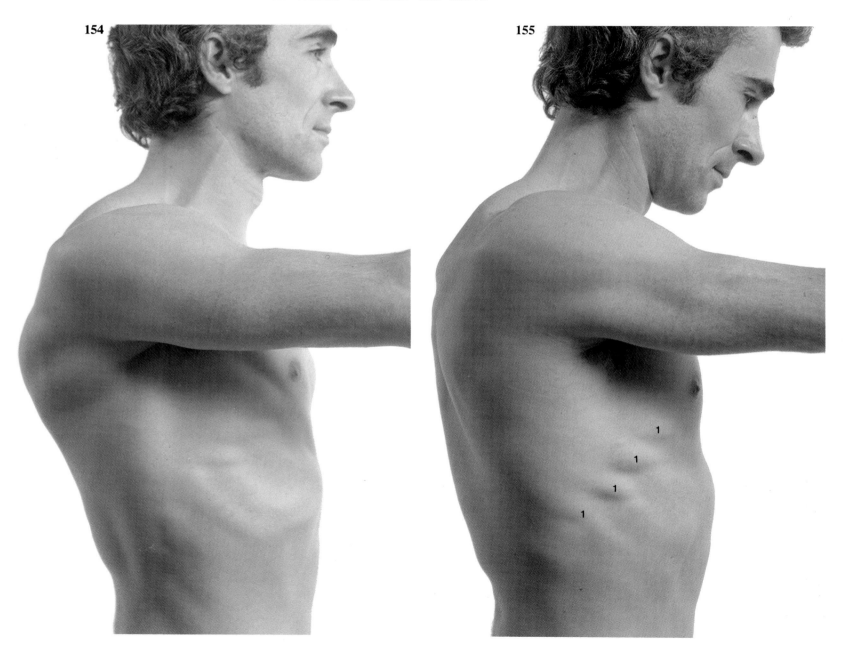

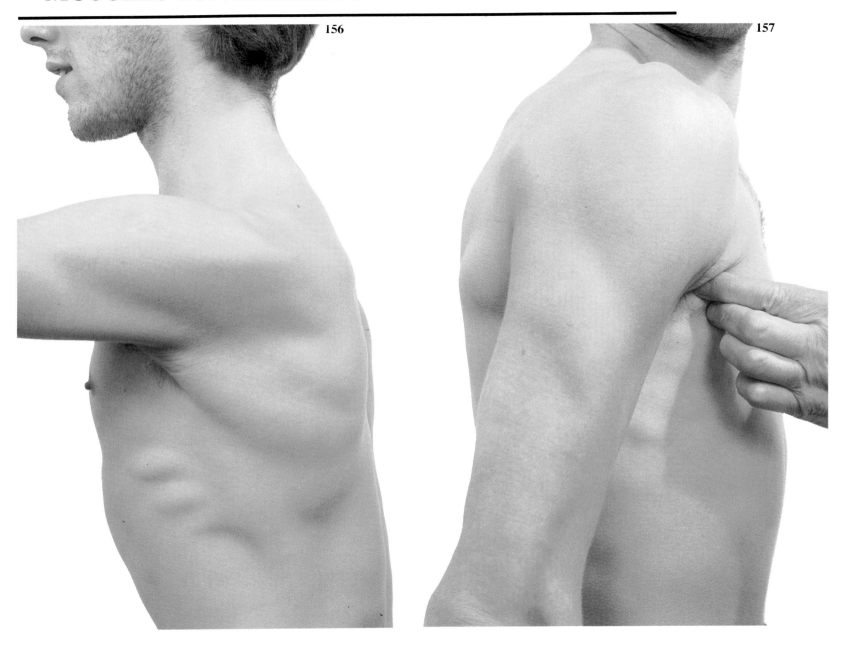

Isotonic contraction of serratus anterior leads to protraction of the scapula, as when pushing. Since 4–5 of the digitations all go to the inferior angle of the scapula, the muscle also has an upwards rotating action (**156**).

Pectoralis minor also acts as a protractor of the shoulder girdle but running upwards and laterally from the 3, 4 and 5 ribs to the corocoid process of the scapula, it also depresses the shoulder. It commonly acts together with the overlying sternocostal part of pectoralis major with which it runs in the anterior wall of the axilla. However as pectoralis major acts on the humerus, this muscle can be inactivated by allowing the arm to hang freely at the side as the shoulder is protracted. Pectoralis minor can then be felt contracting in the posterior part of the anterior wall of the axilla (**157**). It is supplied by the medial pectoral nerve (C8 and T1) from the medial cord of the brachial plexus.

MUSCLES ACTING OVER THE SHOULDER GIRDLE AND JOINT

Two large and very powerful muscles act over both joint systems. *Pectoralis major* is also a wide fan-shaped muscle but perhaps is better considered as having two separate parts, a clavicular and a sternocostal. The clavicular part comes from the medial third or so of the clavicle and runs down to the crest of the greater tubercle of the humerus (lateral lip of the bicipital groove). The sternocostal portion comes from the second to sixth costal cartilages and the related sternum. These fibres also run to the crest but with the lower fibres passing up deep to the clavicular ones, i.e. the sternocostal fibres reverse their original position with the lowest fibres going up behind the upper ones to be inserted high up close to the joint capsule.

The muscle as a whole carries the arm forwards with the clavicular fibres elevating it while the lower sternocostal fibres are powerful flexor adductors pulling the arm downwards, i.e. an anterior equivalent of latissimus dorsi. As such these fibres can also have a powerful dislocating role on the shoulder joint which is balanced in activity by the weak flexor adductor but strong relocator, coracobrachialis.

1 Deltoid
2 Deltopectoral groove
3 Clavicular fibres of pectoralis major
4 Sternocostal fibres of pectoralis major

The large mass of muscle is very obvious on the male chest when put into activity by pressing the arms across the chest, a movement not used to any great extent in practice. Here the separate portions are readily visible with the lower fibres curving up deep to the clavicular, giving the rounded anterior wall to the axilla, with pectoralis minor lying behind them on the way to the coracoid process and with the anterior fibres of deltoid overlapping.

As will be appreciated the sternocostal and clavicular parts are often used for opposing movements, the clavicular fibres raising the arm in flexion adduction while sternocostal fibres lower it. The powerful activity of the clavicular fibres is seen in **158**.

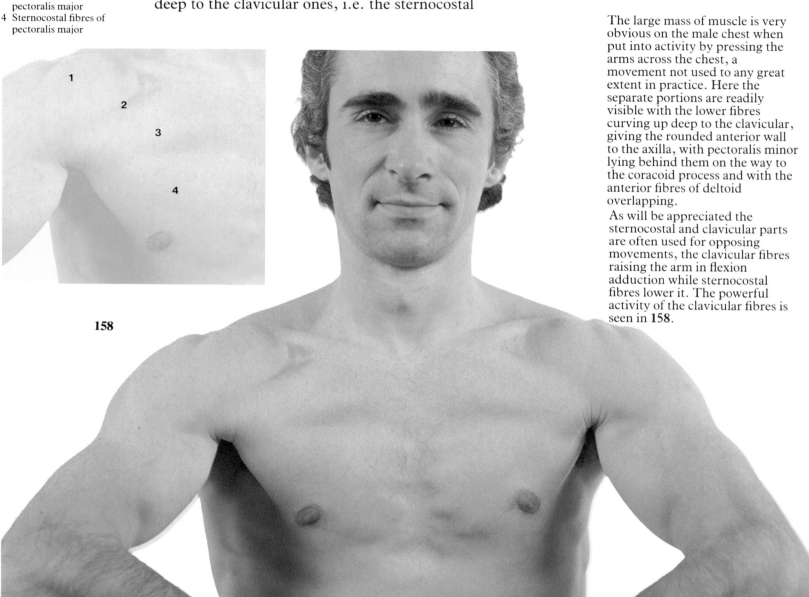

158

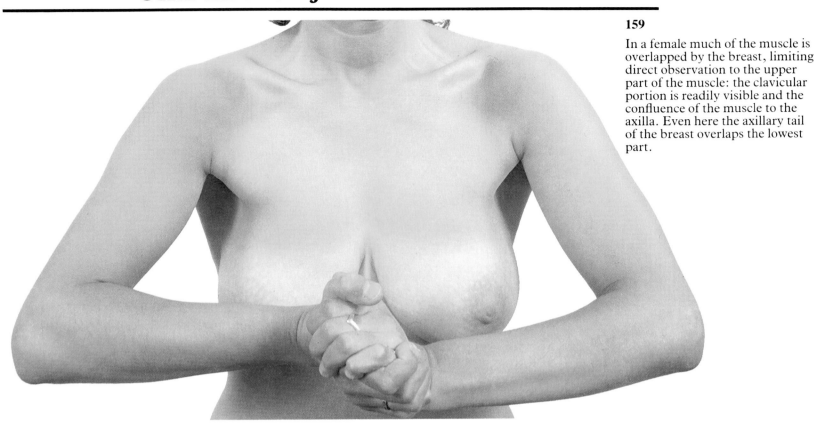

159

In a female much of the muscle is overlapped by the breast, limiting direct observation to the upper part of the muscle: the clavicular portion is readily visible and the confluence of the muscle to the axilla. Even here the axillary tail of the breast overlaps the lowest part.

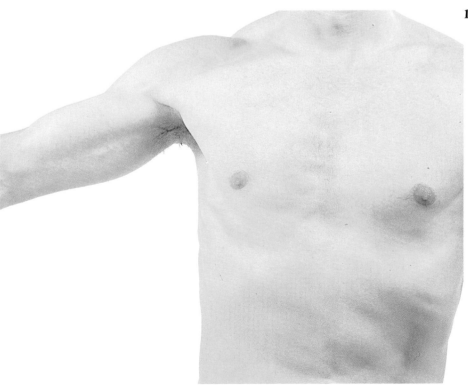

160

The sternocostal fibres are seen here pressing down hard in flexio. adduction. Coracobrachialis can be seen contracting as it runs down the arm with the short head of biceps. Note also how the external oblique muscle of the abdomen of the active side is acting with the internal oblique of the other side to control the trunk against the rotational force induced by the arm's activity.

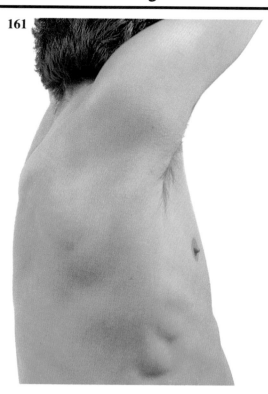

161

The sternocostal fibres of pectoralis major are put on stretch when the arm is carried above the head in flexion. This should be within the normal range of passive stretch of the muscle (**161**) so long as the shoulder girdle is in a neutral position, but not if it is retracted. This fact has been made use of in one method of artificial respiration to induce the muscle to pull up on the chest wall, though this method is no longer used to any extent due to the greater efficiency of a mouth-to-mouth technique.

If the arms are fixed, the sternocostal fibres can be used as accessory muscles of respiration, pulling the chest upwards to assist inspiration. The muscles are commonly used in this way in respiratory distress (dyspnoea) due to either disease or after severe exercise as shown in **162** where the athlete has fixed his hands on his hips. Only the sternocostal part is active.

The upper part of the muscle is innervated by the lateral pectoral nerve (C5, 6 and 7) from the lateral cord of the brachial plexus whilst the lower part receives the medial pectoral nerve (C8 and T1).

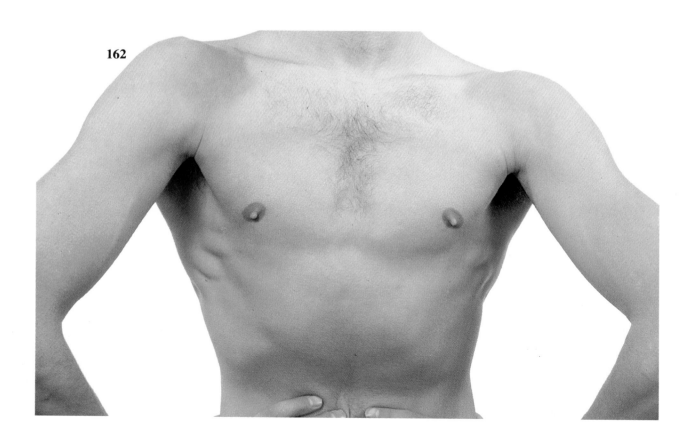

162

MUSCLES ACTING OVER THE SHOULDER GIRDLE AND JOINT

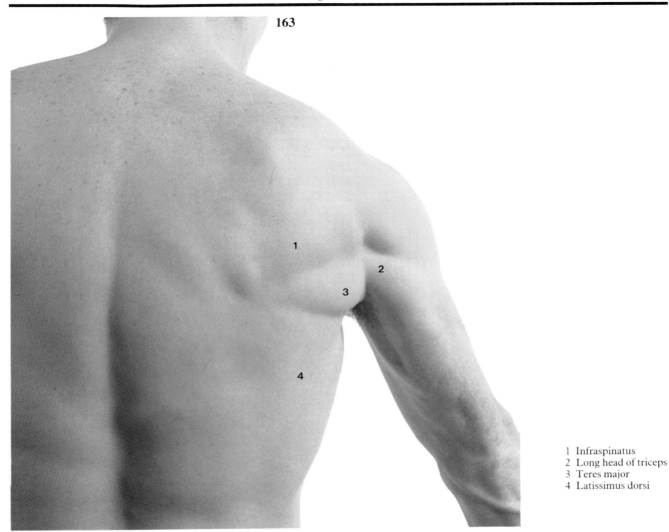

1 Infraspinatus
2 Long head of triceps
3 Teres major
4 Latissimus dorsi

Latissimus dorsi covers much of the back below trapezius. It is a large fan-shaped muscle attached to the spines of the lower six thoracic vertebrae (beneath trapezius) and of the lumbar and sacral vertebrae by an aponeurotic lumbar fascia (overlying the erector spinae muscles) and from the posterior part of the iliac crest. Its deep surface also has slips attached to the inferior angle of the scapula and the lower ribs. From this fan the muscle fibres converge on the intertubercular (bicipital) groove of the humerus, forming a thin ribbon-like tendon which is inserted into the floor of the groove immediately in front of teres major. The muscle acts as a powerful adductor-extensor of the arm at the shoulder joint and, through the scapula and humerus, depressing the shoulder girdle.

Because of its powerful downwards pull the muscle is also a potential downwards dislocator of the shoulder joint, were not that joint so essentially maintained by supportive or synergistic muscles; in this case the long head of triceps, which is a very weak adductor extensor but a strong relocator. Both muscles can be seen acting powerfully as downward pressure is exerted by the hand (**163**).

The nerve supply comes from the posterior cord of the brachial plexus (C6, 7 and 8) and, like the nerve supplying serratus anterior runs down the lateral chest wall where it is vulnerable to injury including the surgical removal of the breast, where both the axillary tail and lymph nodes may need to be excised.

MUSCLES ACTING OVER THE SHOULDER JOINT

These can be considered in two groups, the rotator cuff muscles and others. The rotator cuff muscles are muscles acting over the shoulder joint whose tendons of insertion are incorporated into the capsule of the joint on their way to the bony insertion. They thus induce movement at the joint and also act as dynamic ligaments of the joint. They are *supraspinatus* (although not a rotator), *subscapularis*, *infraspinatus* and *teres minor*. *Teres major, deltoid* and *coracobrachialis* also act over this joint but not connected to the joint capsule.

Supraspinatus arises from the supraspinous fossa and runs through the joint capsule into the uppermost part of the greater tubercle of the humerus. As it is overlaid by trapezius its examination must depend upon its function. It is an important abductor of the arm at the shoulder joint but its greatest value is in the first 15–20 degrees of abduction from the side when the other major abductor, deltoid, is ineffective (**164**). Thus loss of the muscle (or nerve supply – suprascapular nerve – C5 and 6) means that the arm can only be abducted if it can be swung out or otherwise lifted to a level at which deltoid can take over (**165**).

Attempted abduction against resistance.

164

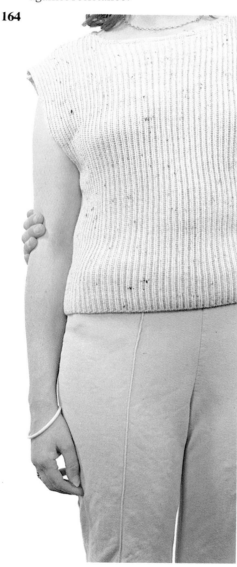

Deltoid can now abduct without supraspinatus.

165

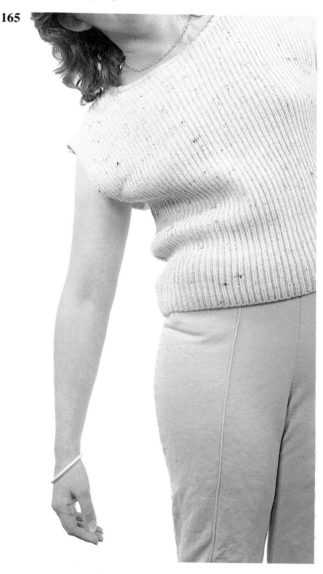

The person is asked to raise the arm from the side, keeping the body upright. This is impossible if supraspinatus is inactive. In this case resistance has been applied only to compare relative strengths of the two sides in case of reduced muscle power on one side.
Even if supraspinatus is inactive the arm can be raised by such a manoeuvre to carry the arm into deltoid's range of activity.

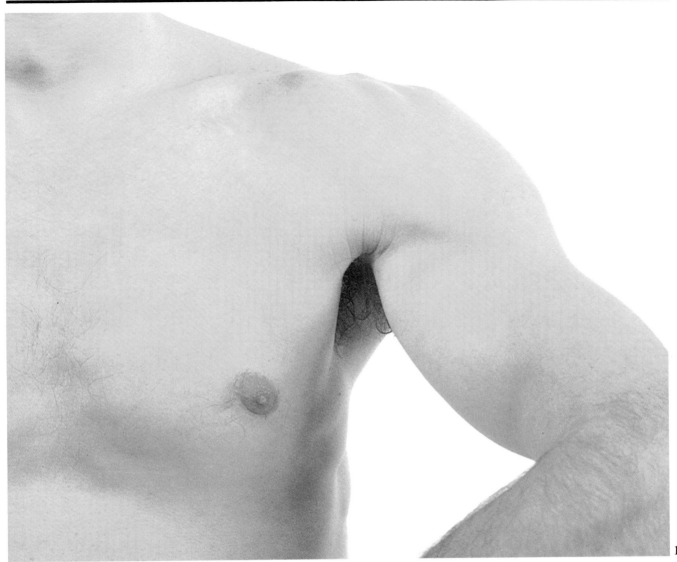

166

Deltoid is the other major abductor and though more powerful than supraspinatus is ineffective with the arm at the side. It arises from the anterior margins of the lateral third of the clavicle and the acromion and from the underside of the spine of the scapula. It is a multipennate muscle with tendinous intersections near the wide origin, from which muscle fibres converge to a rough zone about the middle of the lateral aspect of the humerus. As such it covers the shoulder joint above, in front and behind and makes the prominent rounded swelling of the shoulder. Although mainly an abductor its anterior and posterior fibres act also in flexion with medial rotation and extension with lateral rotation. It is supplied by the axillary nerve (C5 and 6) which, running round the neck of the humerus is vulnerable in fractures and dislocations of the neck and joint. As the same nerve supplies skin over the muscle towards its insertion, the safety of the nerve can be tested by sensation at that site rather than attempting to move the muscle which could be both painful and dangerous (see page 173).

Note that when the muscle is put into powerful action a ridged effect is produced due to the tendinous intersections of the multipennate muscle (**166**).

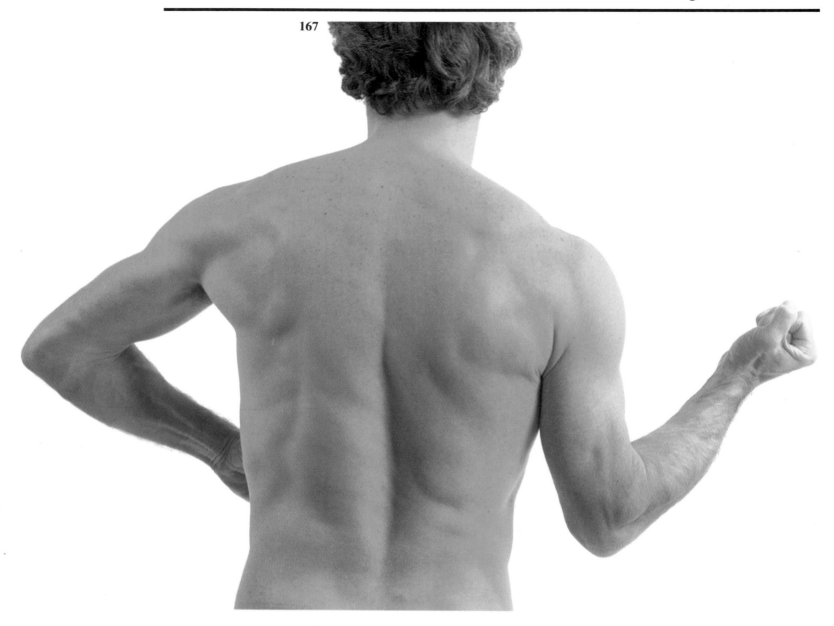

167

Subscapularis is another muscle not available for direct examination. It comes from the major part of the deep surface of the scapula and runs through the joint capsule to the lesser tubercle of the humerus. It is a powerful medial rotator of the humerus at the shoulder joint and loss of the muscle makes it difficult to take the hand to the back. In **167** the left arm is being rotated but is pressing against the abdominal wall rather than being put to the alternative test of carrying it to the back. Note: tests for rotation at the shoulder must be carried out with the elbow flexed to about 90° to prevent confusion with forearm rotation – pronation and supination. The nerve supply is from the subscapular branches of the posterior cord of the brachial plexus – C5 and 6.

Teres major acts with subscapularis as a medial rotator but, as it runs from the lower axillary border of the scapula, close to the angle, to the

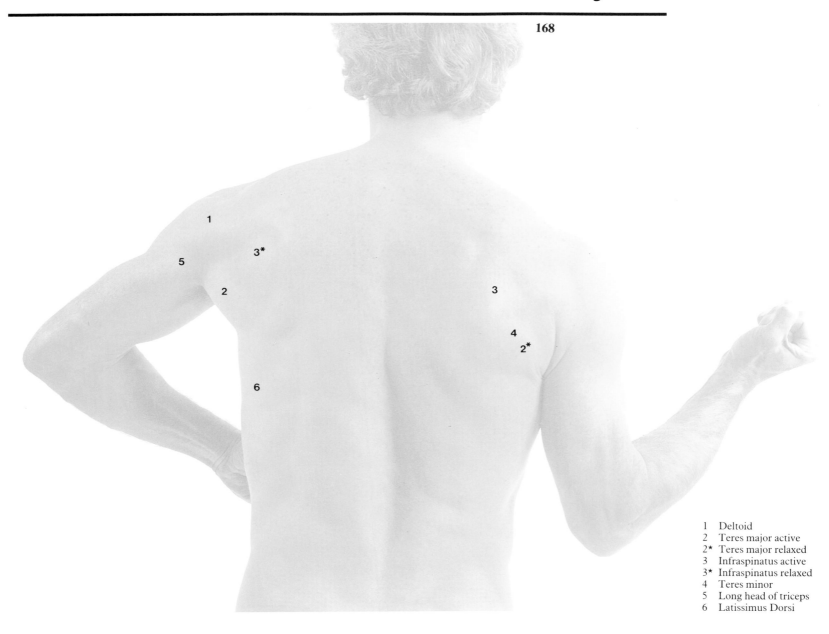

168

1 Deltoid
2 Teres major active
2★ Teres major relaxed
3 Infraspinatus active
3★ Infraspinatus relaxed
4 Teres minor
5 Long head of triceps
6 Latissimus Dorsi

crest of the lesser tubercle (medial lip of the bicipital groove) of the humerus, it is also a strong adductor with some extension. Unlike subscapularis it can readily be seen when the arm is medially rotated (**167**) where it forms the greater part of the posterior wall of the axilla.

Infraspinatus and *teres minor* are both lateral rotators. Infraspinatus comes from the infraspinous fossa of the scapula and teres minor alongside it from the axillary border. They run to the middle and inferior impressions on the greater tubercle of the humerus respectively. They can be seen forming a prominent bulge on the right side of **167**. Here the muscles are difficult to separate from the surface but sometimes a groove may show between them. They have different nerve supplies: infraspinatus from the suprascapular branch of the upper trunk of the brachial plexus (C5 and 6) and teres minor from the axillary nerve (C5 and 6).

THE AXILLA

The axilla or arm-pit is the hollow below the shoulder and is a hair-bearing area in both adult males and females. Its anterior wall is made up mainly of fibres of pectoralis major with pectoralis minor behind. The posterior wall consists of teres major with the ribbon-like tendon of latissimus dorsi immediately in front. Close to pectoralis major a bundle of muscle, made up of the short head of biceps and coracobrachialis runs down the arm with the cords of the brachial plexus surrounding the axillary artery immediately behind. The axilla is also a very important site for lymph glands draining lymphatics from the arm and, most importantly, the breast.

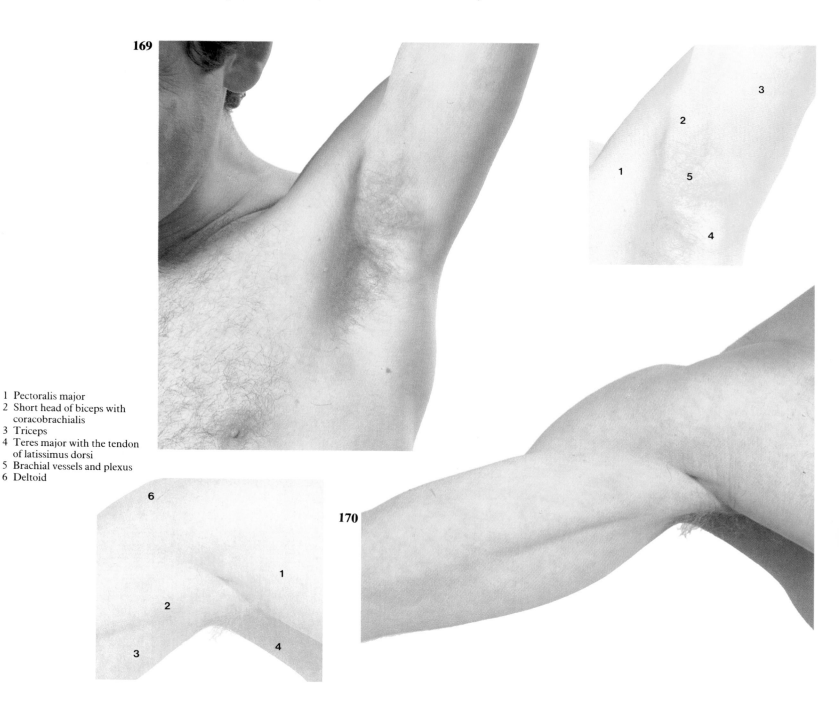

1 Pectoralis major
2 Short head of biceps with coracobrachialis
3 Triceps
4 Teres major with the tendon of latissimus dorsi
5 Brachial vessels and plexus
6 Deltoid

The axillary artery runs through the axilla where its pulsations can be felt by pressing towards the bone. The axillary artery is the continuation of the subclavian, changing its name at the lateral border of the first rib and again to brachial artery at the level of the lower border of teres major, i.e. the posterior wall of the axilla. In fact the pulsations of the artery can be felt through much of its course in the upper arm by pressing against the humerus in the groove to the medial side of biceps muscle (**171**).

The medial, lateral and posterior cords of the brachial plexus bear the relationship to the axillary artery in the axilla that their names indicate. Pressure here can induce sensations of nerve compression and the nerves are also available for brachial plexus local anaesthetic block. However as the cords are spread around the artery and its attendant vein, the local anaesthetic must be more widely spread than in the more proximal injection sites (page 72).

Examination of the axilla is often required where lymph glands may be swollen and palpable as from infection or carcinoma. The glands may be felt in relation to all parts of the axilla but, where there is possible spread from the breast, care must be taken to include the anterior wall behind pectoralis major (**172**).

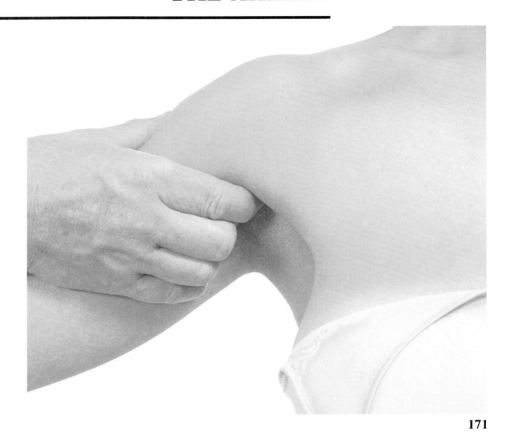

171

172

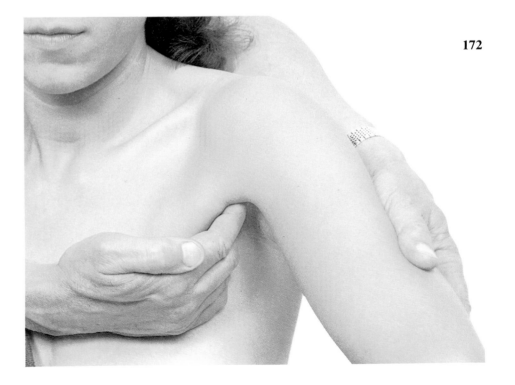

MUSCLES ON THE UPPER ARM

Biceps brachii is the most prominent muscle of the region and the characteristic isometric activity to demonstrate this muscle is probably the most universally known of any in the body (**173**).

It arises by two heads. A long one comes from the supraglenoid tubercle of the scapula and runs by a tendon, through the shoulder joint (surrounded by a synovial sleeve) and then the intertubercular sulcus (bicipital groove). The short head arises with coracobrachialis from the coracoid process of the scapula and then runs down on the medial side of the long head. The two bellies join shortly above the elbow joint and form a rounded tendon which is inserted into the posterior part of the bicipital tuberosity of the radius (**174**). It is a powerful flexor at the elbow and rotates the radius to supinate the forearm. It plays some part as a flexor at the shoulder but its role here is primarily supportive of the joint. Close to the elbow a flat sheet runs medially from the main tendon, the

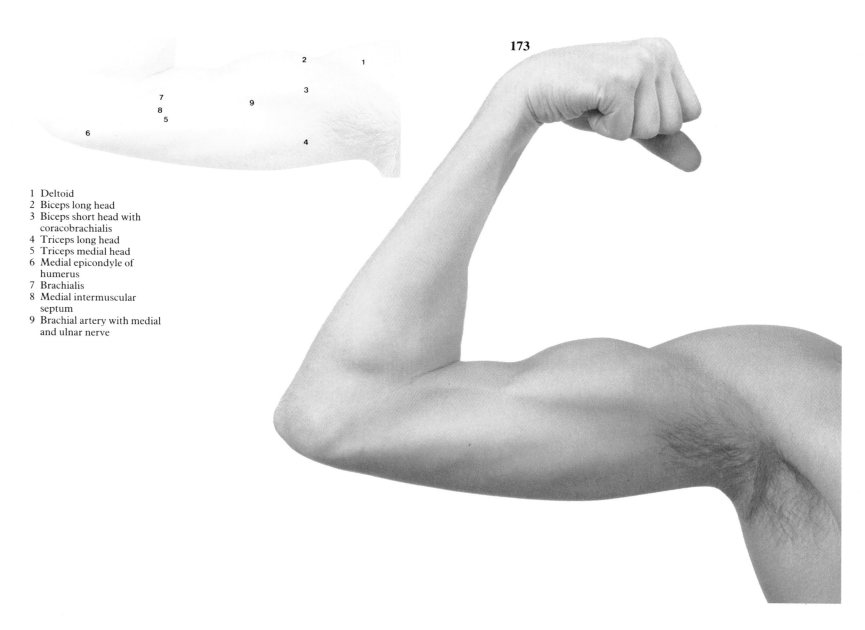

173

1 Deltoid
2 Biceps long head
3 Biceps short head with coracobrachialis
4 Triceps long head
5 Triceps medial head
6 Medial epicondyle of humerus
7 Brachialis
8 Medial intermuscular septum
9 Brachial artery with medial and ulnar nerve

bicipital aponeurosis, to be inserted through the deep fascia around the arm into the ulna. This sheet comes under tension in supination and transmits some flexor pull to the ulna. It also overlies and gives some protection to the main vessels and the median nerve at the elbow, though the basilic vein overlies it. The basilic vein then runs up the arm for a variable distance medial to biceps before piercing the deep fascia to join the brachial veins.

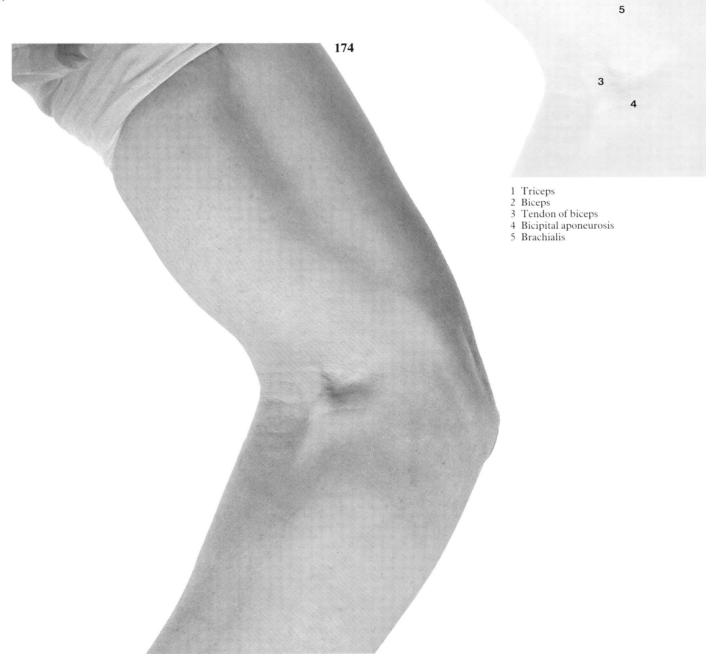

174

1 Triceps
2 Biceps
3 Tendon of biceps
4 Bicipital aponeurosis
5 Brachialis

MUSCLES ON THE UPPER ARM

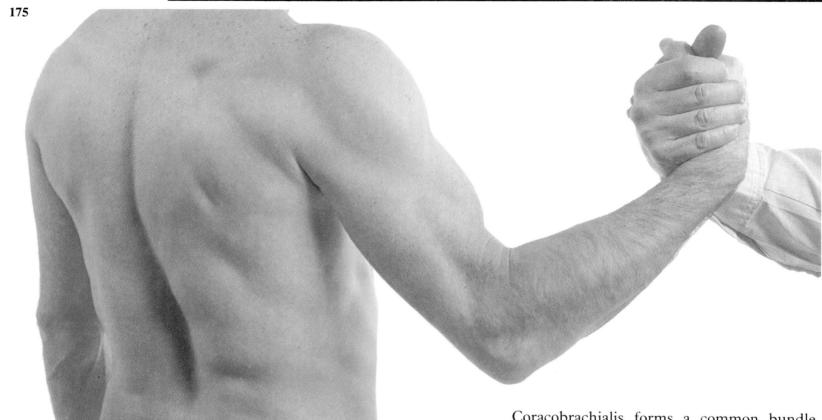

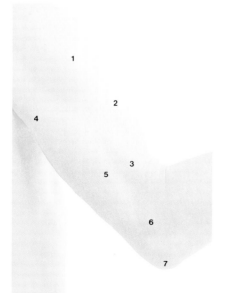

1 Deltoid
2 Biceps
3 Brachialis
4 Long head of triceps
5 Lateral head of triceps
6 Lateral epicondyle of
  humerus
7 Olecranon

Coracobrachialis forms a common bundle with biceps before running deeper, a variable distance down the arm, to run into the medial aspect of the humerus. Coracobrachialis can be separated functionally from biceps by forcibly adducting the arm in some degree of flexion (i.e. by pectoralis major) with the elbow straight and biceps therefore relaxed. See **176**.

Brachialis is the other major flexor at the elbow and is situated primarily in the upper arm. It arises from the front of the humerus and up laterally to extend around the insertion of deltoid. It runs down in front of the elbow joint to be inserted into the front of the coronoid process of the ulna thus flexing the elbow. As it mostly underlies biceps it is less obvious from the surface but due to its wide attachment to the humerus, it extends beyond the overlying muscle, particularly on the lateral side (**175**).

All the above three muscles are supplied by the musculocutaneous nerve (C5, 6 and 7) which leaves the lateral cord of the brachial plexus in or below the axilla, pierces coracobrachialis and then runs between biceps and brachialis to run down the lateral aspect of the arm, becoming superficial after passing deep to the junction between median cubital and cephalic veins to become the lateral cutaneous nerve of the forearm. Although loss of the musculocutaneous nerve leaves the front of the upper arm wasted in appearance the elbow is still capable of quite strong flexion through brachioradialis.

Triceps muscle (**176**) makes up the main bulk of the back of the upper arm though its three heads often appear separately. The long head (1) arises from the infraglenoid tubercle of the scapula and plays its main role in maintaining stability of the shoulder joint while the arm is loaded. The lateral head (2) arises from the back of the humerus above and lateral to the radial groove while the medial head (3) comes from below and medial to the groove. The lateral and long heads join together and overlie the medial head as they approach the olecranon.

Triceps brachii is the main extensor at the elbow joint. The radial nerve, the terminal branch of the posterior cord of the brachial plexus (C5, 6, 7, 8 & T1) runs around the shaft of the humerus beneath triceps and supplies the muscle. However the branches to triceps come off before the section of the nerve most vulnerable to a mid-shaft fracture of the bone, and hence the muscle would retain its nerve supply if the radial nerve were divided by the fracture.

176

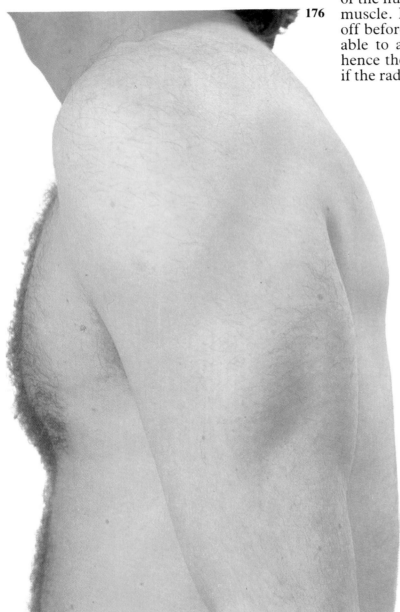

1 Deltoid
2 Biceps
3 Brachialis

177

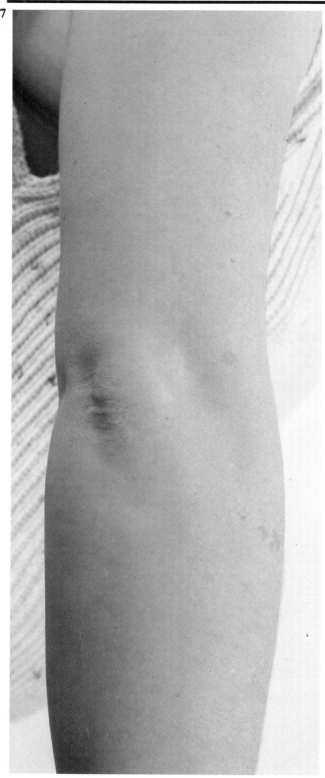

The most prominent feature of the elbow is its bony point, the olecranon of the ulna, the lever of insertion for triceps muscle. As it is an important pressure point when resting on the elbow, the skin is here separated from the bone by a bursa. No doubt because of this the overlying skin has a relatively poor blood supply in spite of the otherwise rich anastomosis around the elbow joint. The medial epicondyle of the humerus is prominent and easy to feel though masked anteriorly by the common origins of the flexor muscles. On its posterior aspect the groove for the ulnar nerve is easily palpable in a slim person and pressure here may give the sensation of nerve pressure; a blow here gives a much more unpleasant sensation which is the reason for the region being described as the 'funny bone'. Laterally the lateral epicondyle, though smaller than the medial, is readily palpable, especially from the back.

1 Triceps
2 Brachioradialis
3 Extensor carpi radialis longus
4 Lateral epicondyle of humerus
5 Anconeus
6 Extensor muscles of forearm – Common Origin
7 Olecranon with overlying bursa
8 Ulnar nerve in cubital tunnel
9 Medial epicondyle of humerus
10 Flexor carpi ulnaris (the dash indicates the position of the radio-humeral joint space)

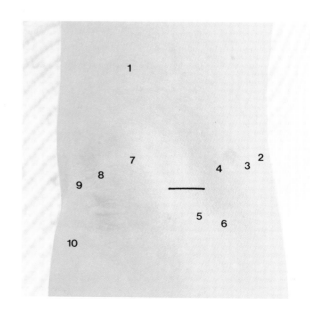

BONY POINTS OF THE ELBOW, FOREARM AND WRIST

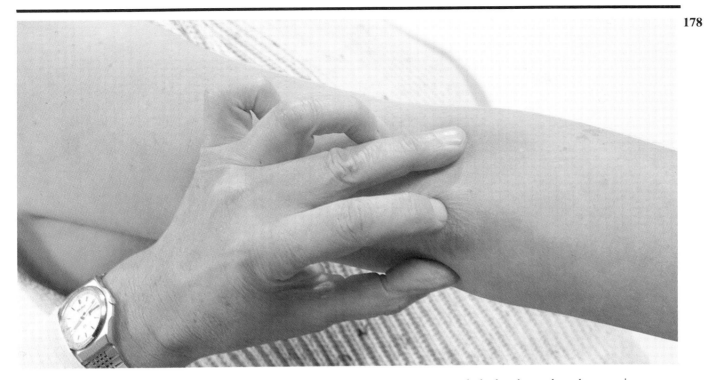

When examining the elbow it is important to remember that, with the arm extended, the above three bony points should be in a line (178), but with the arm bent they should form a triangle (179), a relationship which may be changed in fractures around the joint.

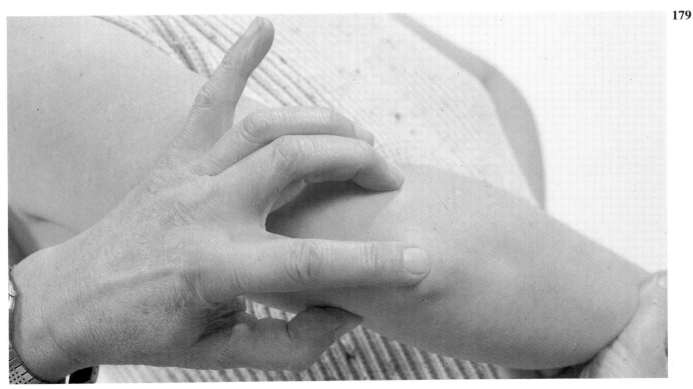

180

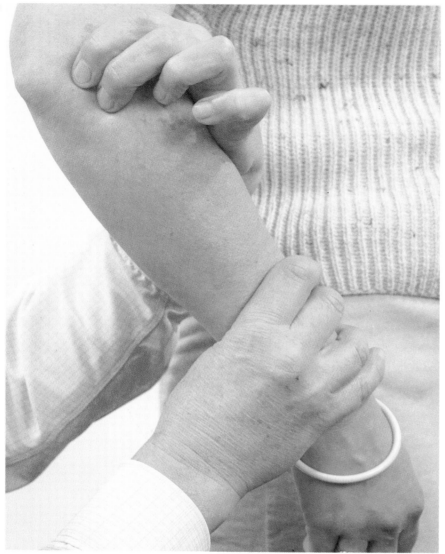

Below the lateral epicondyle, the head of the radius should be palpable and felt rotating as the forearm is pronated and supinated. The joint space should also be felt between head of radius and the capitulum of the humerus (**180**).

The whole of the posterior surface of the ulna is palpable from the olecranon to the very prominent distal end or head at the back of the wrist with the styloid process at the tip. In supination the tendon of extensor carpi ulnaris runs behind it but in pronation the tendon moves on to the ulnar border of the wrist (see **181**) and the head of the ulna becomes more prominent dorsally.

1 Ulna
2 Head of ulna
3 Tendon of extensor carpi ulnaris

181

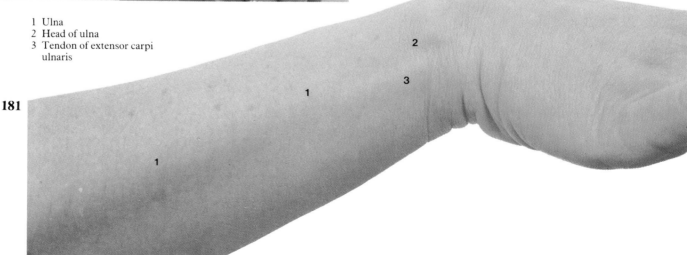

BONY POINTS OF THE ELBOW, FOREARM AND WRIST

The upper part of the radius is masked by muscle but the lower half or so gives a bony border to that side of the forearm through to the radial styloid which extends some 2 cm distal to that of the ulna. (It should be remembered that the whole load of the carpus is upon the obliquely sloping distal end of the radius with none on the normal ulna.)

The dorsal tubercle of the radius (Lister's tubercle) is a prominent feature of the back of the wrist but usually only to palpation, having tendons running to either side of it (**182**). It is important to be aware of the feel and appearance of the distal end of the radius because of the common fractures of the region. Abductor pollicis longus and extensor pollicis brevis tendons mask the tip of the radial styloid on the border of the wrist but it can be felt behind these tendons, forming the proximal wall of the anatomical snuff box, and also from the front where it produces a low swelling between the tendons of abductor pollicis longus and flexor carpi radialis (**183**).

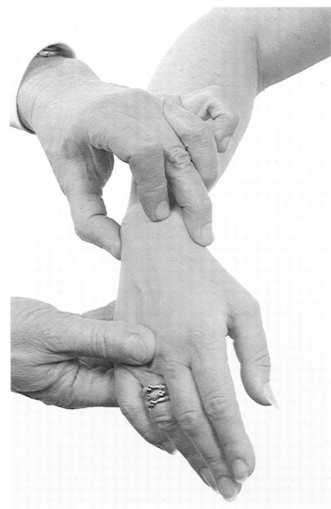

182
The examiner's thumb overlies the ulnar styloid and the middle finger the radial styloid. The index indicates the radial tubercle.

1 Tendon of extensor pollicis longus
2 Extensor pollicis brevis
3 Abductor pollicis longus
4 Radial styloid
5 Anatomical 'snuff box'
6 Lunate

183

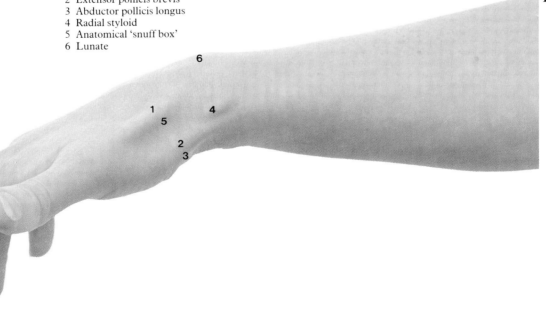

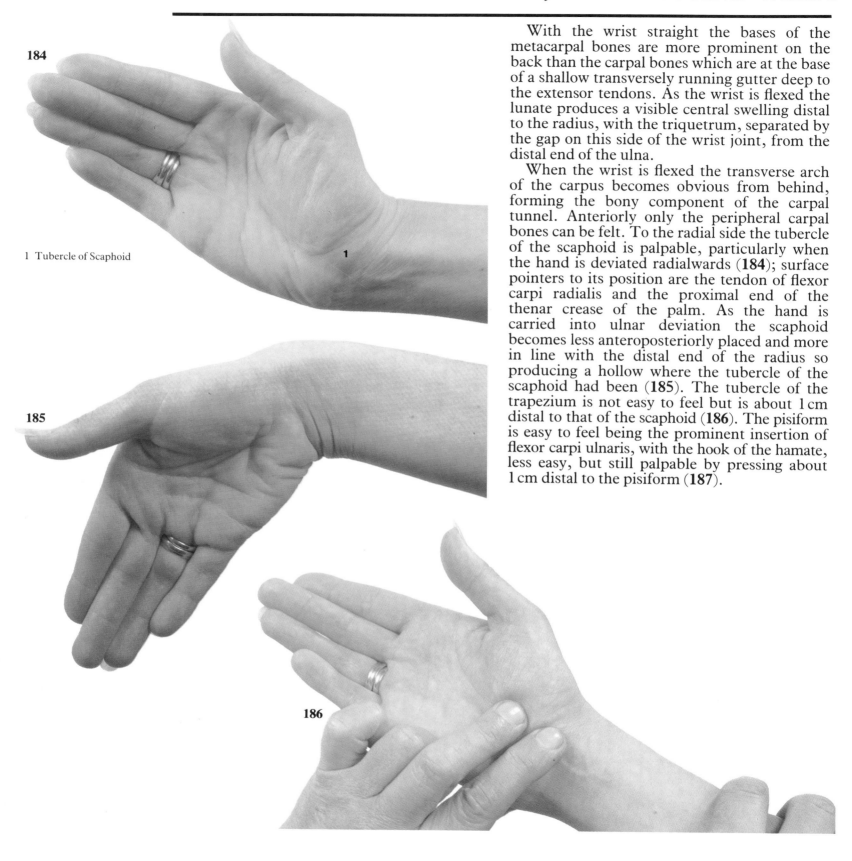

1 Tubercle of Scaphoid

With the wrist straight the bases of the metacarpal bones are more prominent on the back than the carpal bones which are at the base of a shallow transversely running gutter deep to the extensor tendons. As the wrist is flexed the lunate produces a visible central swelling distal to the radius, with the triquetrum, separated by the gap on this side of the wrist joint, from the distal end of the ulna.

When the wrist is flexed the transverse arch of the carpus becomes obvious from behind, forming the bony component of the carpal tunnel. Anteriorly only the peripheral carpal bones can be felt. To the radial side the tubercle of the scaphoid is palpable, particularly when the hand is deviated radialwards (**184**); surface pointers to its position are the tendon of flexor carpi radialis and the proximal end of the thenar crease of the palm. As the hand is carried into ulnar deviation the scaphoid becomes less anteroposteriorly placed and more in line with the distal end of the radius so producing a hollow where the tubercle of the scaphoid had been (**185**). The tubercle of the trapezium is not easy to feel but is about 1 cm distal to that of the scaphoid (**186**). The pisiform is easy to feel being the prominent insertion of flexor carpi ulnaris, with the hook of the hamate, less easy, but still palpable by pressing about 1 cm distal to the pisiform (**187**).

BONY POINTS OF THE ELBOW, FOREARM AND WRIST

The tubercle of the scaphoid and the pisiform are the bony resting points of the 'heel' of the hand; hence the scaphoid's vulnerability to fracture when falling on the compacted extended wrist. Here the scaphoid is trapped against the distal end of the radius whereas the pisiform is free to move and usually escapes injury. As the scaphoid (and the trapezium) lie in the base of the anatomical snuff box, pain on pressure here, rather than over the tubercle is characteristic of scaphoid fracture.

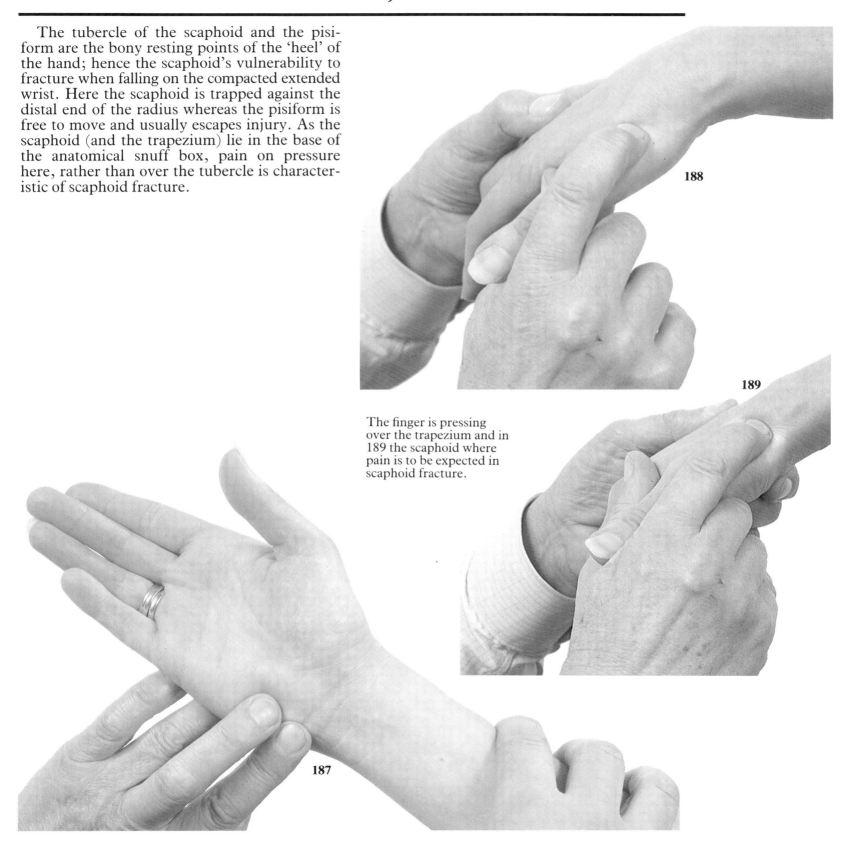

The finger is pressing over the trapezium and in 189 the scaphoid where pain is to be expected in scaphoid fracture.

190

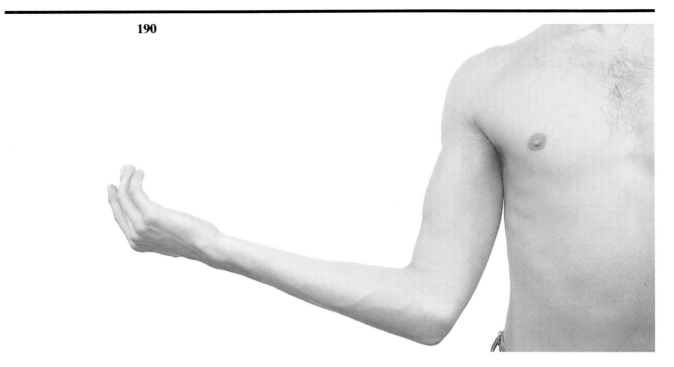

Rotation occurs at the shoulder joint and, as pronation and supination, in the forearm. Thus with the arm extended at the elbow both can be used and failure at one site may be overcome by use of the other, particularly in a patient intent on minimising the disability. With the arm flexed at the elbow, however, the two rotatory functions become separated. For this reason when examining ranges of movement at the two joint systems it is important to do so with the elbow flexed to about 90°.

At the shoulder the direction of the bent forearm can be used as the register of the angle of rotation. External rotation should carry the arm through some 90°, i.e. roughly into the plane of the trunk (**190**), while internal rotation should allow the forearm to be placed behind the back (**191**).

191

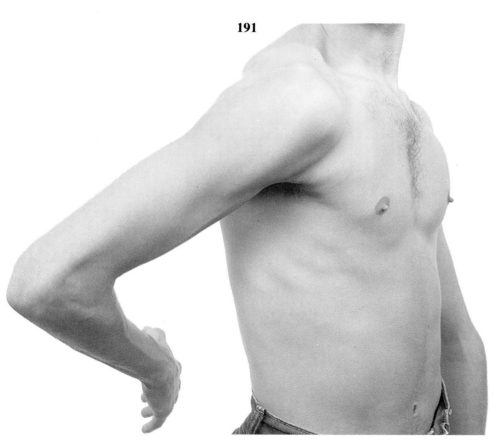

As a quick and useful clinical guide to functional rotation at the shoulder the patient can be asked if they can do their own hair and (if a woman) they can fasten brassiere straps at the back, or if a man he can touch the opposite scapula (**192, 193**).

To test pronation and supination with the elbow flexed and the elbow at the side the palm of the hand should be able to face upwards and possibly a little way outwards (supination, **194**) and be able to be placed comfortably on a flat surface (pronation, **195**).

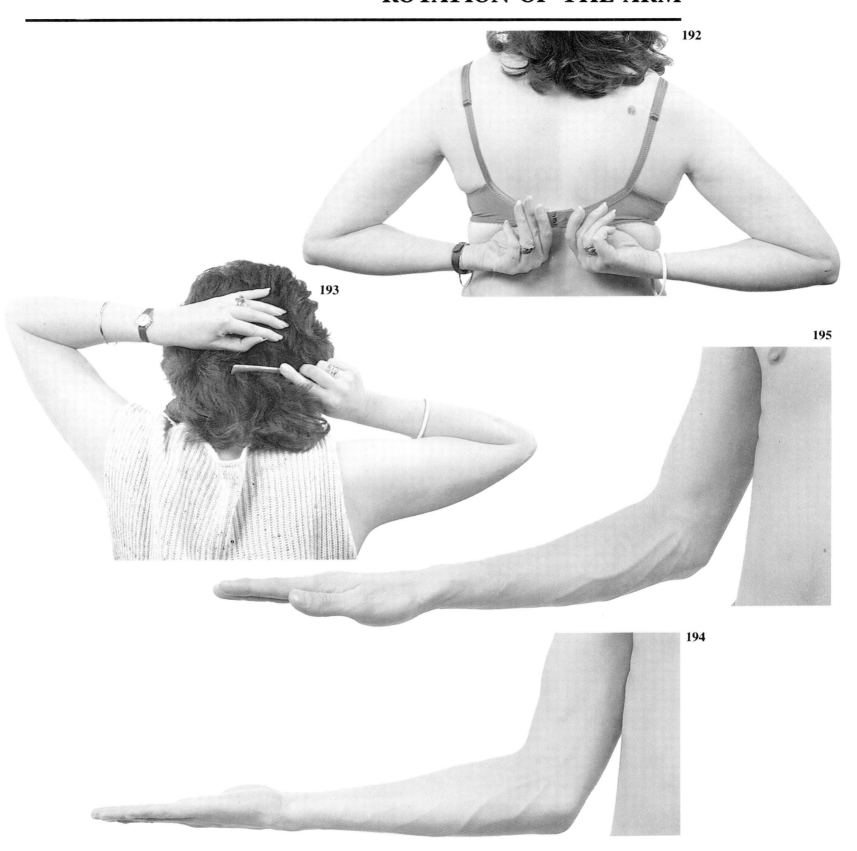

PRONATION AND SUPINATION

These are extremely valuable movements and any loss is a major disability. They are brought about by rotation of the forearm bones around an axis through the middle of the head of the radius and the attachment of the triangular fibrocartilage of the distal radio-ulnar joint to the base of the ulnar styloid. However this must not be taken to imply that the distal end of the radius moves around a fixed ulna. Were that to be the case the hand would also flap about that fixed point and would be useless for rotatory activities (**196**).

For effective hand function it is necessary for the hand to be carried on an axis through the distal end of the radius, lunate and capitate to the index and middle metacarpals and fingers.

This is achieved by the ulna being able to move laterally at the elbow and so produce a reciprocal movement to that of the radius at the distal radio-ulnar joint (**197**).

The strength of supination (biceps and supinator) is usually described as being greater than that of pronation (pronator teres and pronator quadratus), and for this reason in ergonomic design it is usual to set power rotation for right handed supination, e.g. screw threads. However it is worth stressing that maximal supinating power output is with the elbow in partial flexion and from full pronation to a little beyond the midprone position, falling off thence to full supination.

196

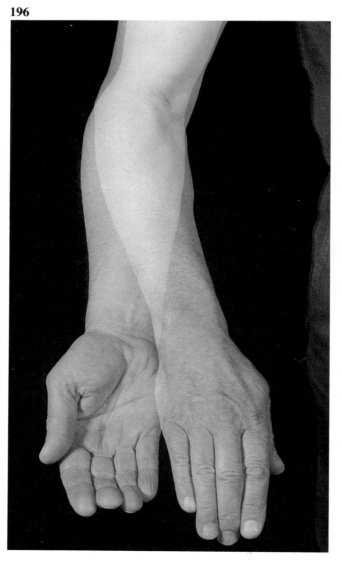

197

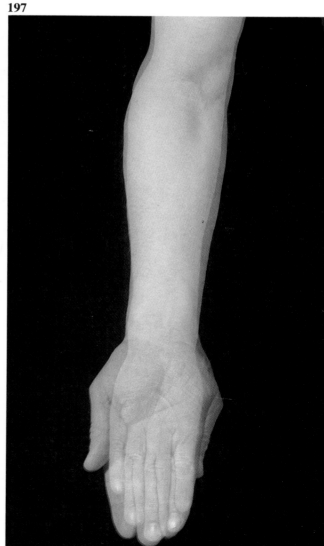

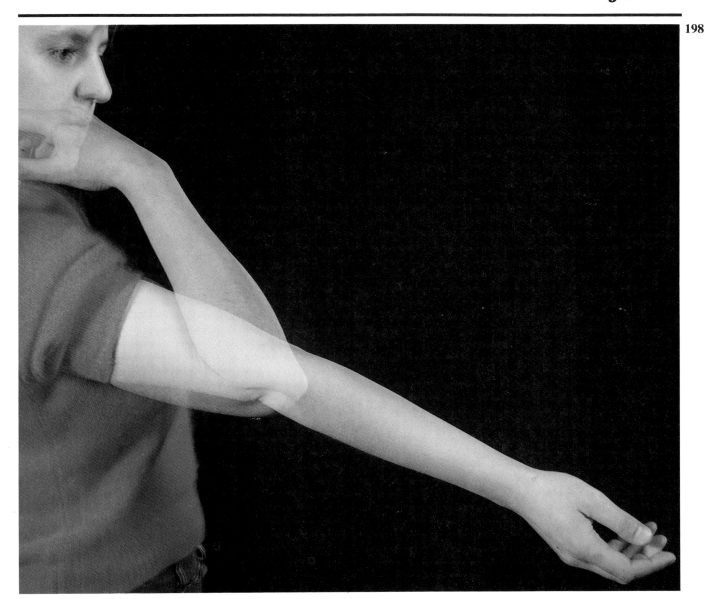

198

It is usual to consider the elbow as a pure hinge joint and certainly this is its most obvious movement (**198**). Normal flexion is limited only by contact between the soft tissues of the upper arm and forearm. Extension is to about 180° but this may be considerably greater in lax jointed individuals. Extension at the joint is limited, as in all normal joints, by the soft tissues, and in this case principally brachialis muscle, and not as so often stated, contact between olecranon and humerus. Lateral movement at the joint is minimal, limited by the collateral ligaments and supportive muscles.

This is not, however, true of the ulna during pronation and supination, where lateral movement is essential at the elbow joint (see page 118).

The line of the arm through the elbow to the forearm in the supine (anatomical) position is not straight, having a lateral angulation of some 10–20° and sometimes even more, particularly in women. This is called the carrying angle but few people would carry with the arm fully supinated in extension. In fact the carrying angle is obliterated in the normal carrying midprone position.

THE CUBITAL FOSSA

This is the hollow on the front of the elbow with the arm in the supine anatomical position, with the palm facing forward (**199**). The medial wall is made up of the common flexor muscles from the medial epicondyle and particularly pronator teres from the supracondylar ridge while the lateral wall is formed by brachioradialis. As both pronator teres and brachioradialis are inserted into the radius the fossa is triangular. Its floor is made up of the muscle and tendon of brachialis together with contributions from the capsule of the elbow joint and from supinator muscle on the radius. It is however much more than just an anatomical hollow, for a number of important structures lie within or superficial to it. The brachial artery with its attendant veins runs down in the upper arm, medial to biceps, to enter the cubital fossa before dividing into its radial and ulnar branches, usually about the level of the neck of the radius. It is at the cubital fossa that the stethoscope is placed over the artery when measuring blood pressure.

1 Biceps
2 Brachioradialis
3 Pronator Teres
4 Median Cubital Vein
5 Basilic Vein
6 Cephalic Vein

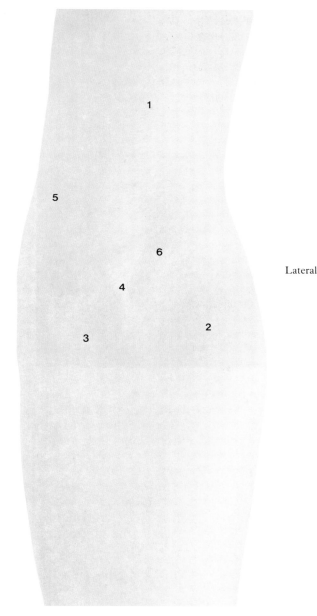

Medial

Lateral

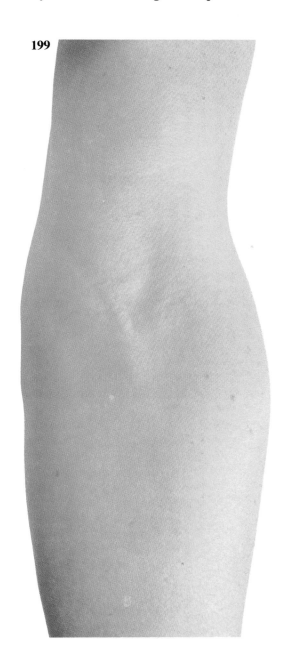

199

The median nerve runs through the fossa to the medial side of the artery before running into the forearm under the fibrous arches between the origins of pronator teres and of flexor digitorum superficialis (within whose fascial sheath the nerve runs on the deep surface of the muscle).

More superficially the median cubital vein (a vein commonly used for venepuncture) joins the medially placed basilic vein to the cephalic. It is often possible to find the median cubital vein even in a fat person whose veins may generally be hidden. However it must be remembered that it usually overlies the brachial artery.

Although the fossa faces anteriorly in the anatomical position, in relaxed carriage of the arm it faces more medially with the forearm also a little pronated so that the palm of the hand faces medially; the position also of a military 'attention' (**200**).

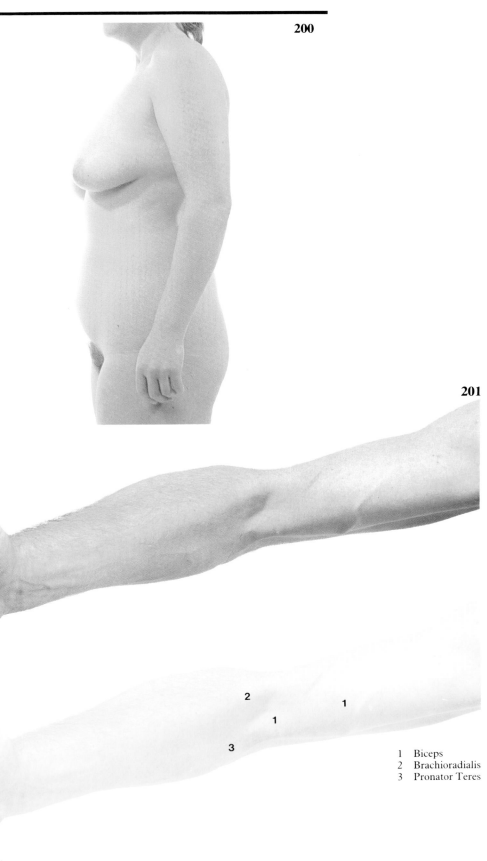

200

201

1	Biceps
2	Brachioradialis
3	Pronator Teres

THE CUBITAL FOSSA

When the arm is brought into action with a bent elbow, the humerus may be rotated by infraspinatus and teres minor into the anatomical position dependent upon the positioning of the working hands but for most manual activity the forearm is further rotated to a midprone position or to full pronation for keyboard or similar actions. The lateral wall of the cubital fossa becomes much more obvious when the arm is flexed against resistance (**201**). Brachioradialis is a powerful flexor at the elbow joint, particularly valuable in the midprone position of much hand activity. If the elbow is flexed against resistance in a supine position powerful activity will be seen in biceps, brachialis and brachioradialis.

If however the arm is similarly flexed in a prone position (**202**), biceps becomes relatively inactive and pronator teres acts as a pronator but weaker flexor. If greater power is required in flexion pronation, biceps will act only so far as not to overpower the pronator muscles.

202

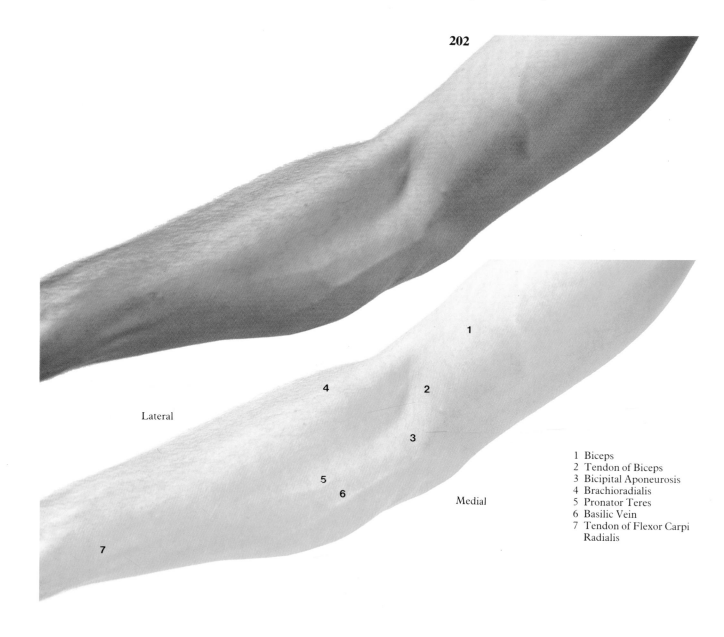

Lateral

Medial

1 Biceps
2 Tendon of Biceps
3 Bicipital Aponeurosis
4 Brachioradialis
5 Pronator Teres
6 Basilic Vein
7 Tendon of Flexor Carpi Radialis

Although the 'wrist joint' strictly means the radiocarpal joint, since it always works in conjunction with the midcarpal joints, they must be considered together functionally and clinically. In traditional anatomy teaching the wrist is capable of flexion, extension, abduction, adduction and circumduction from the essentially ineffectual anatomical position of the arm and, probably because of this viewpoint, flexion and extension seem to have become the most important movements in both standard descriptions and clinical studies. If however the arm is brought into more functional positions the situation changes and adduction (or, more practically, ulnar deviation) becomes the main functional movement with abduction (radial deviation) for recovery (**203**). Ulnar deviation at the wrist is required to bring the gripping hand

203

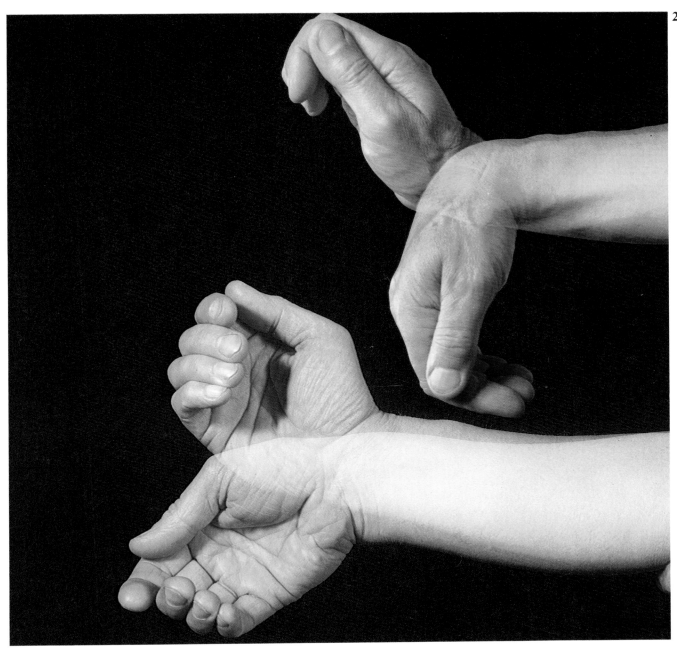

MOVEMENTS AT THE WRIST

into a position for tools and household implements, e.g. screwdrivers, door handles, knives etc., to be carried in the line of the forearm to allow their dynamic control by forearm rotation (**204–5**). This wrist movement pattern is required also in a more dynamic role for a light hammer, paint brush, controlling a chisel etc (**206**). A degree of flexion is useful, particularly for toiletry (but most can be managed on a straight wrist), whilst a little extension gives maximal power to a hand grip, but these movements are of far less general importance than adduction (ulnar deviation).

In accordance with the functional requirements, the range of ulnar deviation is far greater than that of radial deviation and so also is the precision of control (**207–212**).

204

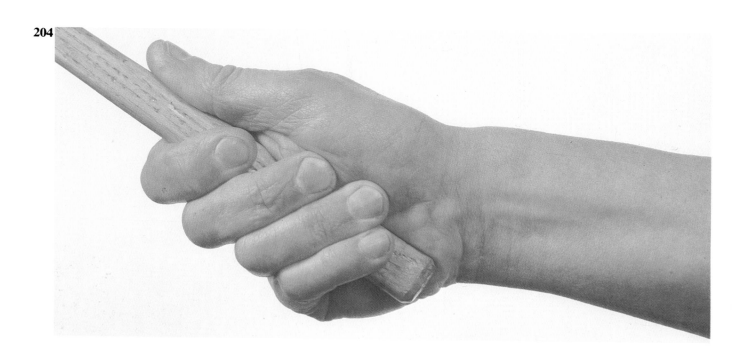

205

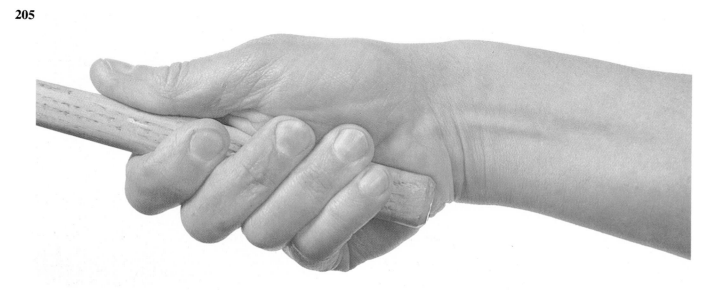

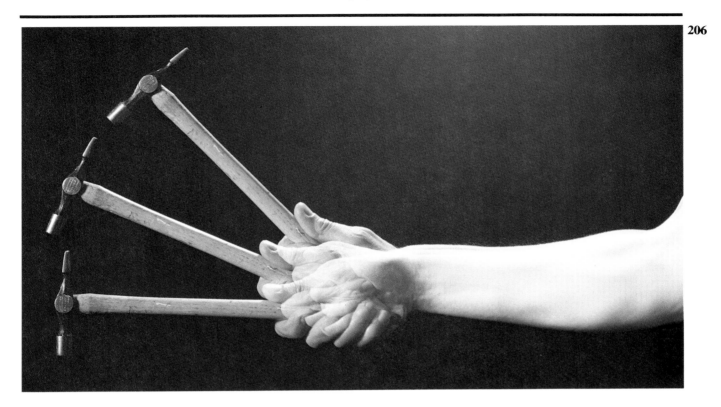

206

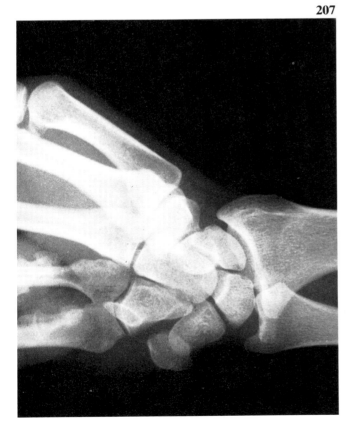

207

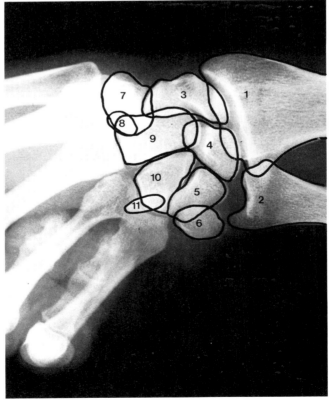

208

1 Radius
2 Ulna
3 Scaphoid
4 Lunate
5 Triquetrum
6 Pisiform
7 Trapezium
8 Trapezoid
9 Capitate
10 Hamate
11 Hook of Hamate

125

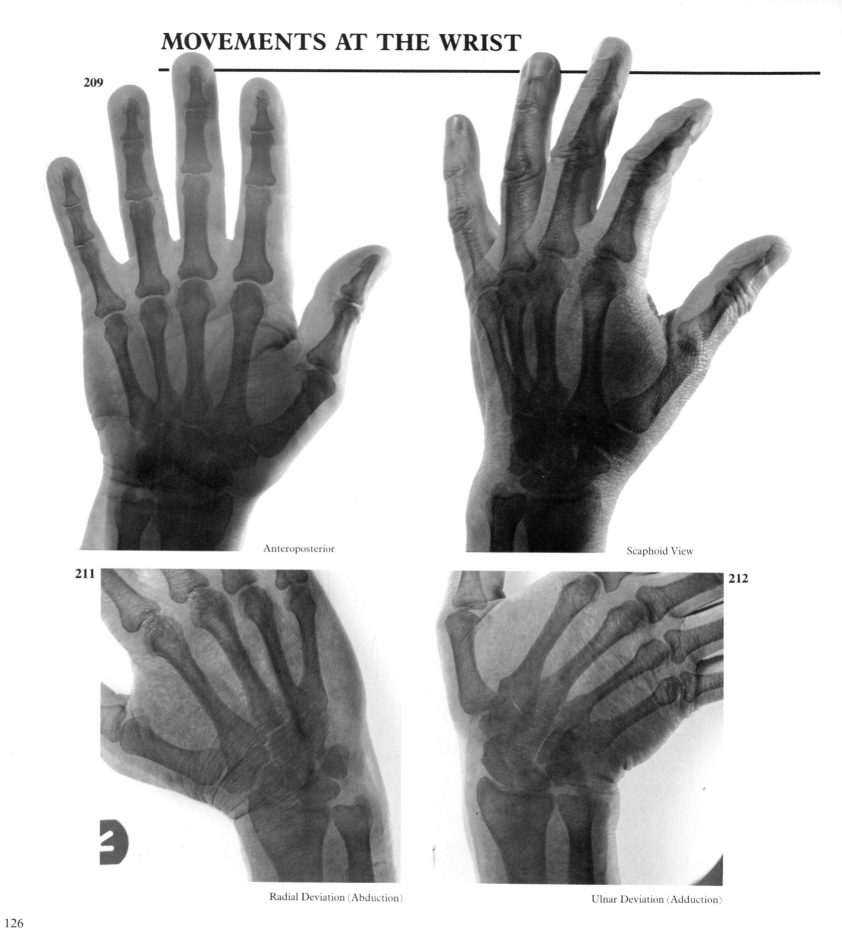

209 Anteroposterior

Scaphoid View

211 Radial Deviation (Abduction)

212 Ulnar Deviation (Adduction)

Movement at the wrist is valuable, but even more so is stability. The long muscles controlling the fingers cannot work effectively unless the wrist can be fixed (213). Conversely, if the wrist is to be moved, the fingers will almost always be fixed as in a grip or at least immobile. This is not universally true; certain keyboard and string musical instrumentalists need, on occasions, to combine wrist and finger movement but the movements are under perfect control at the wrist and commonly in a different plane from the digital activity, thus maintaining a steady base for the digital activity.

On occasions, due to disorganised joints or loss of available muscles to control both wrist and digits, it is necessary to fix the wrist by arthrodesis. Loss of wrist movement can be overcome to a great extent if the joint is fixed in some degree of ulnar deviation, to allow objects to be gripped in line with the forearm. As many actions are carried out in the midprone position, e.g. light hammering, this action can be taken over at the elbow, working as it does in the same plane. In fact the wrist is used normally for precision work with the elbow taking over for heavier activities. The differences are readily seen when using different types of hammer (see 206, 214, 215).

213

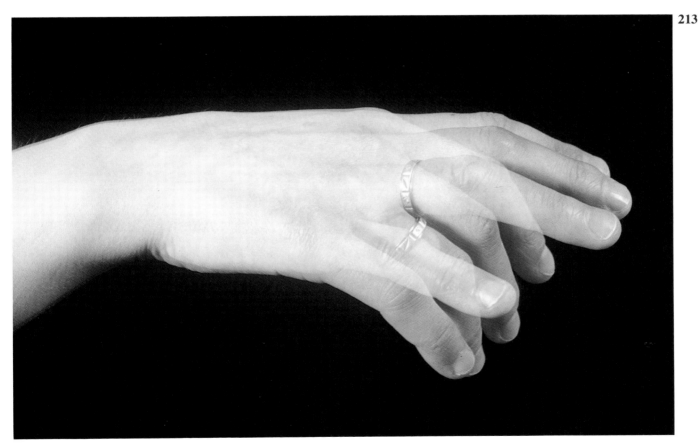

A cyclograph showing that in digital movement the wrist joint remains fixed.

MOVEMENT AT THE WRIST

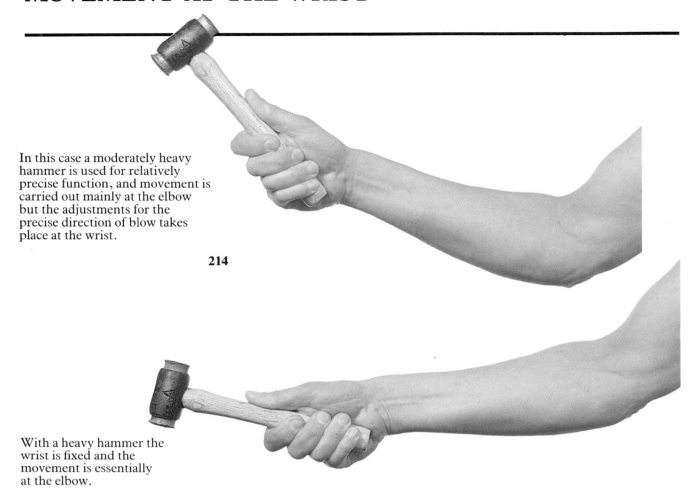

In this case a moderately heavy hammer is used for relatively precise function, and movement is carried out mainly at the elbow but the adjustments for the precise direction of blow takes place at the wrist.

214

With a heavy hammer the wrist is fixed and the movement is essentially at the elbow.

215

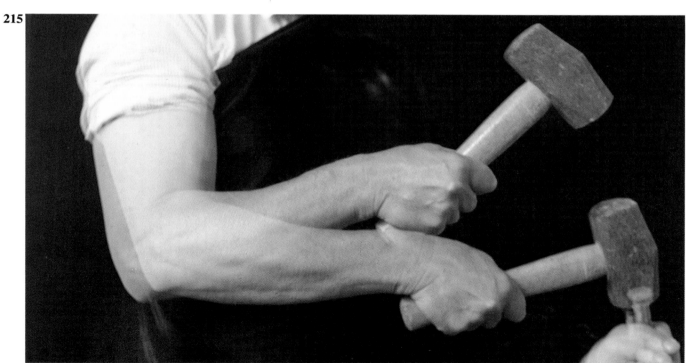

MUSCLES ON THE FRONT OF THE FOREARM

With the exception of brachioradialis, the superficial muscles on the front of the forearm (i.e. the flexor aspect, **216**) arise from the medial epicondyle of the humerus and, in the case of pronator teres, the supracondylar ridge. Of the five muscles, *flexor carpi radialis* and *palmaris longus* come only from the epicondyle and run superficially down the forearm, palmaris longus centrally and flexor carpi radialis a little more to the radial side to produce the most prominent tendons at the wrist. Palmaris longus usually has a long thin tendon which can be valuable for a tendon graft, although the muscle is very variable, and is absent in some 13% of the population.

The other three muscles have double origins. *Pronator teres*, which forms the medial border of the cubital fossa, takes a second attachment from the coronoid process of the ulna and runs obliquely across to the middle of the lateral aspect of the radius at the outermost point of its curvature.

Flexor digitorum superficialis arises also from the coronoid process of the ulna and the oblique line of the radius; it and its tendons form a fullness to the ulnar side of palmaris longus.

Flexor carpi ulnaris arises additionally from the posterior border of the ulna (arching over the ulnar nerve) to run down the medial border of the arm to the pisiform bone.

Flexor carpi ulnaris is supplied by the ulnar nerve (C7 & 8) while the other four are innervated by the median nerve.

Deep to these muscles are *flexor digitorum profundus* and *flexor pollicis longus* but they are not readily seen from the surface in the forearm, whilst, deeper still, pronator quadratus crosses between radius and ulna in the distal quarter of the region. All these three muscles are innervated by the anterior interosseous branch of the median nerve, though the part of the flexor digitorum profundus to the ring and little fingers is innervated by the ulnar nerve.

Brachioradialis appears also most prominently on the front of the forearm, though it is usually considered with the extensor group because of its radial nerve supply. It runs from the lateral supracondylar ridge down to the distal end of the radius forming the main fleshy mass on the radial border of the forearm.

The position of the superficial flexor muscles can be indicated by a hand with its heel at the medial epicondyle. The thumb – pronator teres; index – flexor carpi radialis; middle – palmaris longus; ring – flexor digitorum superficialis and the little – flexor carpi ulnaris.

216

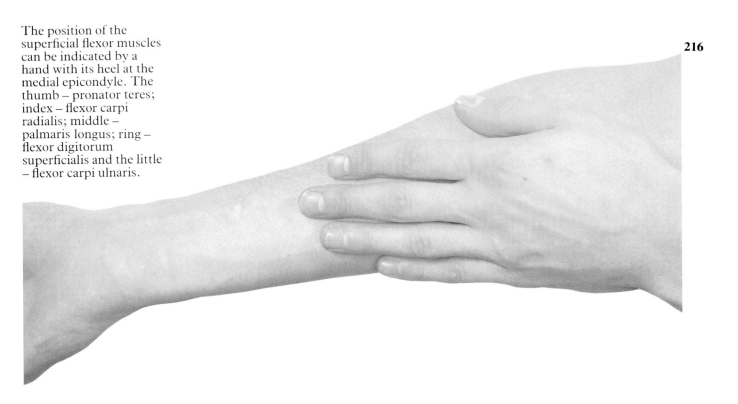

TENDONS ON THE FRONT OF THE WRIST

On firm or resisted flexion of the wrist, palmaris longus and flexor carpi radialis tendons stand out strongly (**217**). Palmaris longus is about the centre of the wrist but flexor carpi radialis lies at approximately the axis of radiocarpal movement and hence flexor control. Flexor carpi radialis has been called an abductor at the wrist but this description is no longer tenable. It is in fact a flexor which, approaching full flexion, tends to pull the hand even a little to ulnar deviation due to the slope of the distal end of the radius. Most important is its being bound in its own fibrous tunnel close to the carpus on the axis of the radiocarpal joint and thus, with its extensor counterpart, extensor carpi radialis brevis, acts as a close compactor of the wrist, so giving central stability, either for digital move-

ment on a fixed wrist or in controlling the axis of ulnar/radial deviation.

Palmaris longus, although only a small muscle is a fairly powerful flexor, since its insertion into the flexor retinaculum and thence the palmar aponeurosis gives it excellent leverage, whilst it also tenses the palmar aponeurosis, of value in a grip. It is important to be aware of its frequent absence and variability (it may even have a muscle belly near the wrist). Its tendon is sometimes removed to be used as a tendon graft. When palmaris longus is absent the tendons to the ulnar side, flexor digitorum superficialis, become more prominent, particularly that to the index finger which may be confused by the unwary for that of palmaris longus.

217

1 Flexor Carpi Radialis Tendon
2 Palmaris Longus
3 Flexor Digitorum Superficialis
4 Flexor Carpi Ulnaris

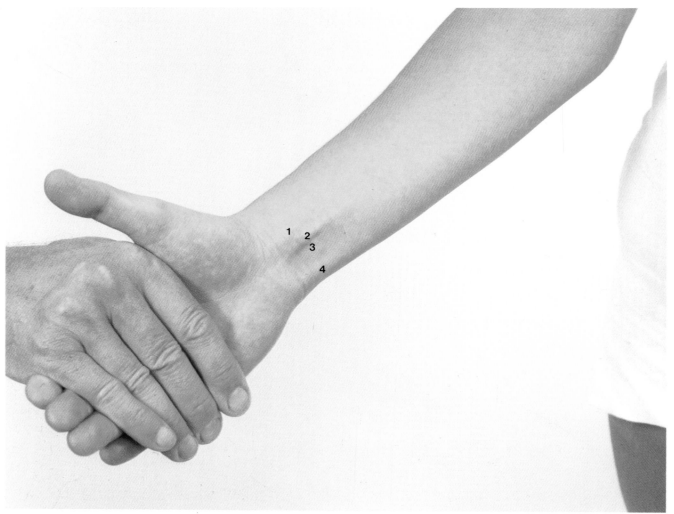

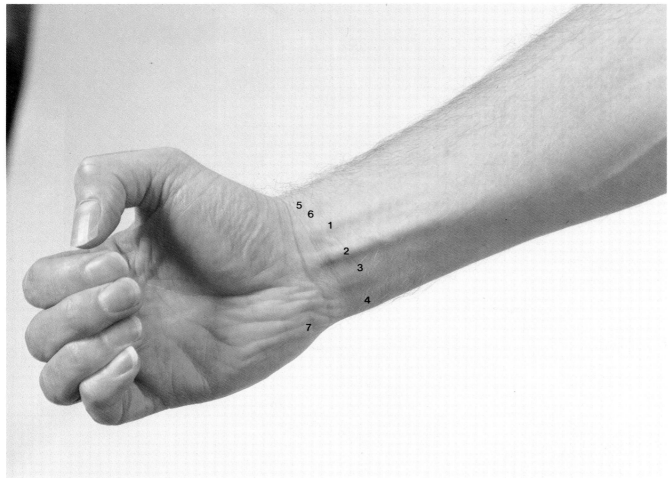

218

1 Flexor Carpi Radialis Tendon
2 Palmaris Longus
3 Flexor Digitorum Superficialis
4 Flexor Carpi Ulnaris
5 Abductor Pollicis Longus
6 Radial Styloid
7 Pisiform with Palmaris Brevis

Flexor carpi ulnaris lies to the ulnar border of the wrist. This muscle is a powerful adductor (ulnar deviator) and flexor at the wrist, working in ulnar deviation with its extensor counterpart. Its insertion to the pisiform bone and through it to the hook of the hamate and the pisometacarpal ligament gives it excellent leverage for flexion while the wide ulnar carpal separation gives the ulna carpal-sided leverage on the radiocarpal joint.

To the radial side, flexor carpi radialis is separated by the subcutaneous radial styloid from the anterior of the two abductors (radial deviators) of the wrist, abductor pollicis longus, which stands out on the radial border of the wrist outside the radial styloid (**218**).

Flexor digitorum superficialis, with the deeper flexor digitorum profundus and flexor pollicis longus run through the carpal tunnel, formed with the overlying flexor retinaculum, while flexor carpi radialis runs through its own tunnel. Palmaris longus runs superficial to the retinaculum, bound to its surface. The retinaculum is not readily palpable so its extent must be assessed from externally available features. It extends from the distal flexor crease of the wrist to level with the outstretched thumb. Medially it is attached to the pisiform bone and the hook of the hamate and, laterally, to the tubercles of the scaphoid and trapezium, the medial and lateral attachments being little more than 2.5–3 cm (1 inch) apart, so creating with the shapes of the carpal bones the quite constricting carpal tunnel.

MUSCLES ON THE BACK OF THE FOREARM

The superficial extensor muscles take a common origin from the lateral epicondyle of the humerus and the supracondylar ridge. Brachioradialis, the muscle coming from higher up the ridge, has been described with the anterior muscles in view of its flexor role. *Extensor carpi radialis longus* also comes from the supracondylar ridge below brachioradialis and, below that, *extensor carpi radialis brevis* arises from the epicondyle. These three muscles can usually be identified, quite easily, running down the radial side of the back of the forearm (**219**).

219

1 Brachioradialis
2 Extensor Carpi Radialis
  Longus
3 Extensor Carpi Radialis
  Brevis
4 Extensor Digitorum
5 Extensor Carpi Ulnaris

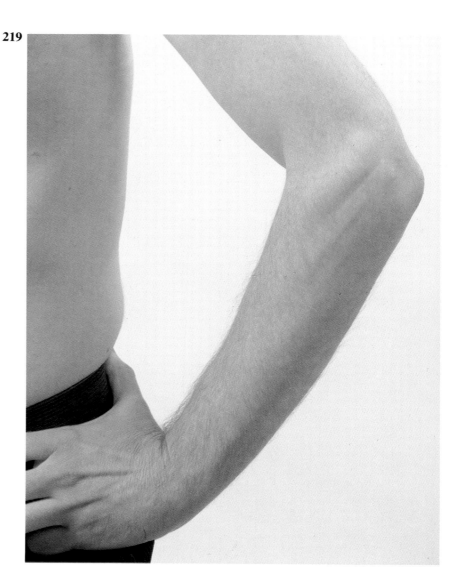

MUSCLES ON THE BACK OF THE FOREARM

Extensor digitorum (communis) comes from the common extensor origin and forms a prominent longitudinal swelling, when active, along the back of the arm parallel with extensor carpi radialis brevis and running to the centre of the back of the wrist (**220–221**).

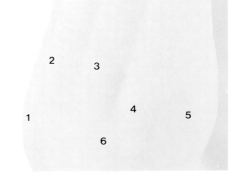

220

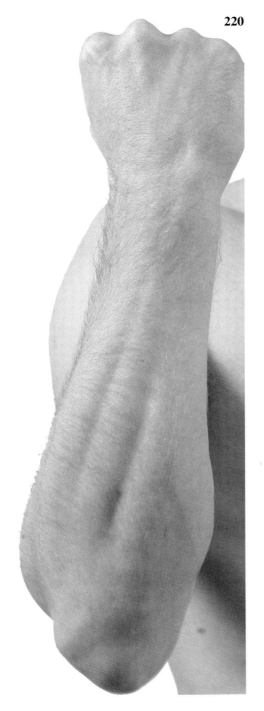

221

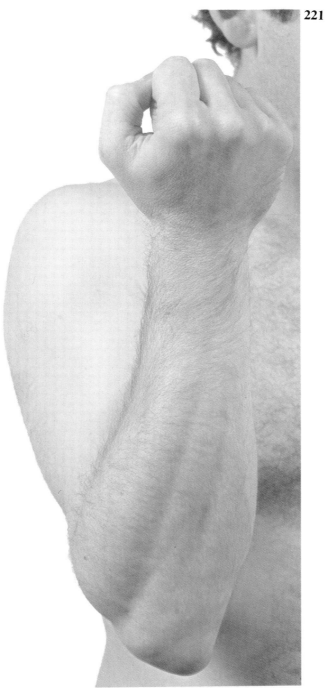

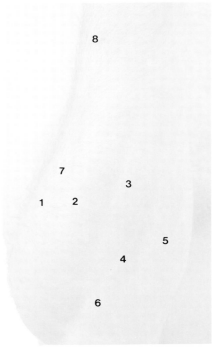

1 Extensor Carpi Radialis Longus
2 Extensor Digitorum
3 Extensor Carpi Ulnaris
4 Subcutaneous Border of Ulna
5 Flexor Carpi Ulnaris
6 Anconeus
7 Extensor Carpi Radialis Brevis
8 Abductor Pollicis Longus

MUSCLES ON THE BACK OF THE FOREARM

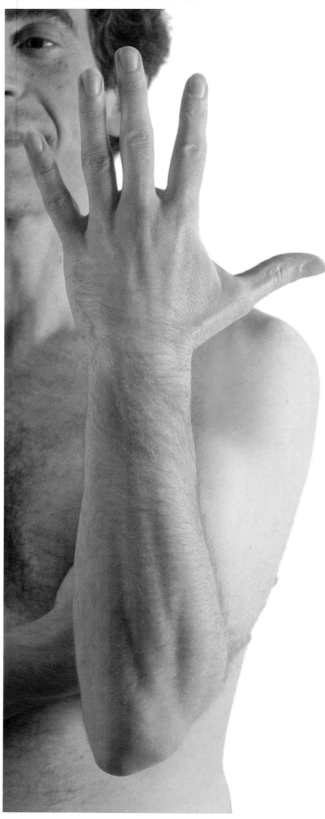

Extension of the individual fingers shows appreciable separation of the muscle into its digital components even though the tendons are commonly linked by bands on the dorsum of the hand (**222**).

Between extensor digitorum and the subcutaneous surface of the ulna, *extensor carpi ulnaris* forms a prominent swelling when the wrist is tensed or forcibly extended and particularly ulnarly deviated (see page 133). The small *extensor digiti minimi* lies between extensor digitorum and extensor carpi ulnaris but it is difficult to differentiate this, from the surface, from the component of extensor digitorum which goes to the little finger.

Anconeus is a muscle which runs from the lateral epicondyle obliquely across to the ulna. It is usually described with triceps in view of its common nerve supply with that muscle from the radial nerve. It is often said to be an extensor at the elbow but this function is of minimal value. Far more important is that it becomes active (and hence prominent from the surface) in pronation, during which it is responsible for pulling the ulna across and behind the radius.

In addition to anconeus, brachioradialis and extensor carpi radialis longus are innervated from the radial nerve. The other muscles are supplied from its posterior interosseous branch which passes through and supplies supinator, around the neck of the radius. Extensor carpi radialis brevis is commonly supplied before the nerve enters supinator whereas branches to the other muscles arise shortly after it leaves supinator.

The thick muscle mass to the medial side of the ulna is the flexor carpi ulnaris, included among the flexor muscles.

Whereas the flexor tendons, other than flexor carpi ulnaris, are concentrated centrally in relation to the carpal tunnel, those on the back of the wrist are spread around the outside of the bony arch of the tunnel. While the flexor retinaculum is attached to the carpal bones, the extensor retinaculum forms six fibro-osseous compartments over the distal parts of the radius and ulna.

Abductor pollicis longus runs over the radial styloid, usually having two tendons, and these run, together with the more dorsally placed extensor pollicis brevis, in the same fibro-osseous compartment. Extensor pollicis brevis may be absent or very small, hence the importance of knowing of the frequent duplication (some 80%) or occasionally a further thin tendon to the abductor.

The second compartment transmits the two extensor carpi radialis tendons; longus going to the base of the second metacarpal and brevis to the third. These two tendons are crossed by extensor pollicis longus which turns around the dorsal tubercle of the radius to run across to the distal phalanx of the thumb. When the thumb is extended the raised tensed thumb tendons create a hollow between them, the anatomical 'snuff box', with the scaphoid and trapezium in its base (**223**). Due to the overlying tendon, the two carpi radialis tendons are less easy to examine than the other dorsal tendons. However if the wrist is forcibly extended, preferably against resistance, with the thumb relaxed, the tendon of extensor carpi radialis longus can be felt easily just distal to the end of the radius and the brevis tendon before its insertion (**224**). As the longus muscle acts with abductor pollicis longus as the radial deviators at the wrist, this movement resisted with relaxed thumb (i.e. in flexion) will make these two tendons obvious.

The extensor digitorum and indicis tendons run together through the wide fourth compartment, still over the dorsal aspect of the radius, while the small extensor digiti minimi tendon runs in its own compartment over the radio-ulnar joint.

Extensor carpi ulnaris runs over the dorsum of the ulna only in the usually described supine position. With movement towards pronation, including the most commonly used midprone position the tendon runs on the ulnar border of the wrist, where it can be felt on forced ulnar deviation running in the gap between the ulnar styloid and the base of the fifth metacarpal. This important fact is very little appreciated and in certain conditions such as rheumatoid arthritis where there is increased dorsal movement of the distal end of the ulna, operations have been described to return the tendon to what was erroneously thought to be its correct position.

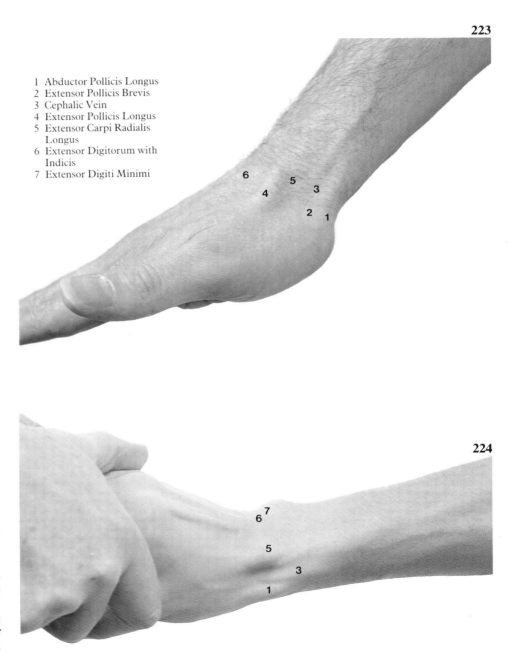

1 Abductor Pollicis Longus
2 Extensor Pollicis Brevis
3 Cephalic Vein
4 Extensor Pollicis Longus
5 Extensor Carpi Radialis Longus
6 Extensor Digitorum with Indicis
7 Extensor Digiti Minimi

THE HAND

Whereas the legs have a primary locomotor rôle, the arms can be considered to have become largely freed from this function, due to man's upright posture. It is not unreasonable to consider the arms as the versatile spacial extenders of the range of the hands' functions. Conversely it is unreasonable to consider the hands without also considering the need for the arms to position them. Thus the shoulders and elbows vary the range wherein the hands can function whilst shoulder and forearm rotation offer directional positioning to the hands.

In many anatomical and surgical texts the hands are considered only in their locomotor rôle as grasping instruments. This is an improper approach, for their ability to carry out even their grasping and gripping functions requires a very great sensory input, hence the failure to produce satisfactory mechanical replacements either as prostheses for lost hands or for other types of handling. The hand's efficiency depends upon its remarkable neurological control, with its large cortical representation in the brain.

The hand thus has two primary roles, both of which must be examined; its sensory reception and thence central perception, and its locomotor control which also depends upon fine neurological organisation, both kinaesthetic and motor.

225

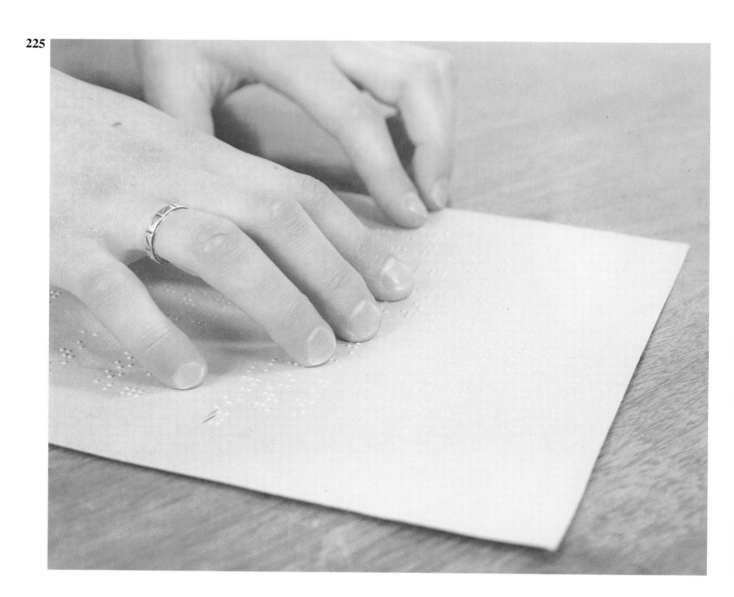

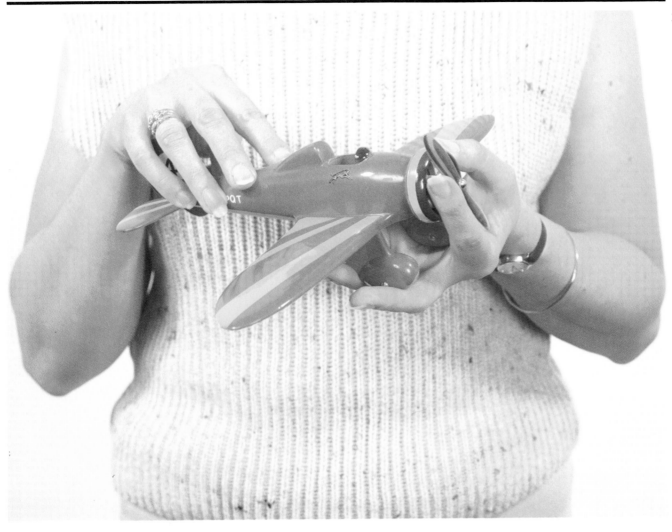

In the developing embryo, special sensory placodes are described related to the organs of sight, hearing and olfaction but far less often is mention made of a similar placode at the end of the developing limb bud. This placode is the precursor of the area of special tactile sensibility of the palm of the hand, which extends around the finger tip to include the nail bearing area. Even in a congenital 'amputation' of the limb this special tactile zone exists at the limb tip making it a much more valuable instrument than a traumatic amputation.

The hand has been described as the eyes that see in the dark and around corners. It can pick out the correct coin from pocket or bag simply by touch; it can read braille (**225**); it can assemble equipment, nuts bolts etc., in positions where direct vision is impossible. These activities could not be carried out with the normal tactile sensibility available to other parts of the body or even in the hand after median nerve injury, despite good repair, due to reduction in the available nerve fibres, though this latter problem can often be helped by perception training.

In the hand the fine epicritic sensibility is amplified by a considerable ability to recognise and appreciate shapes i.e. steriognostic sense, which combines the fine tactile sensibility with a remarkable position sense, allowing a full three dimensional appreciation (**226**). This appreciation is such as to permit the exquisite mechanical control of which the hand is capable.

THE SKIN OF THE HAND

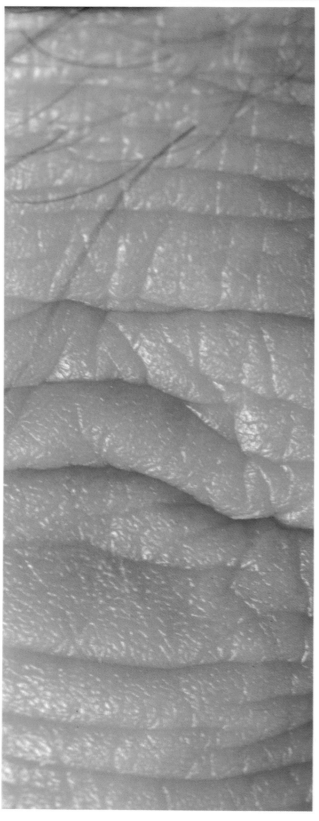

Because of the special functions of the hand, the skin and immediately subjacent tissues differ considerably from that of the rest of the body. The considerable range of movement of both whole hand and individual parts necessitates considerable freedom of movement of the skin, particularly on the back, where full flexion increases the skin distance from wrist to finger tip by some 30%. The skin thus lies loosely on the underlying tissues on the back of the hand to allow free movement, and in the fingers, although adherent over the middle and distal phalanges, surplus is provided at the joints, producing the transverse ridging (227). Over the back of the hand, also, the skin is thin and elastic and shows such pigmentation as is characteristic of the body, together with a light covering of hair which may be marked in some males (228).

On the palm the skin is quite different. Even in dark-skinned races the palm remains quite pale, only the flexion creases being markedly pigmented (230). Hair is absent and the skin thick, the surface being thrown up into papillary ridges, beneath which are large numbers of sensory end-organs. As is well known, the patterns created by the ridges, the finger and palm prints, are characteristic for the individual. Nevertheless the ridges generally run in directions best to improve grip.

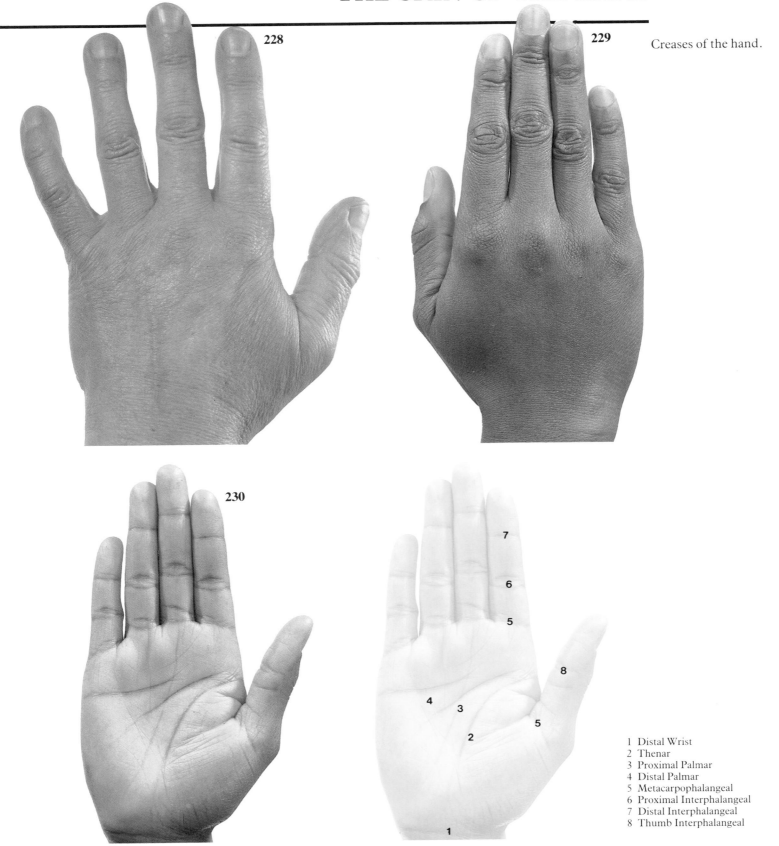

Creases of the hand.

1 Distal Wrist
2 Thenar
3 Proximal Palmar
4 Distal Palmar
5 Metacarpophalangeal
6 Proximal Interphalangeal
7 Distal Interphalangeal
8 Thumb Interphalangeal

THE SKIN OF THE HAND

The palmar skin is devoid of sebaceous glands but has large numbers of sweat glands whose ducts are coiled in the thick epidermis before opening onto the papillary ridges (231). Although the sweat glands have an important thermo-regulatory function coupled with the hand's rich vascularity, they also serve to keep the epidermis soft and supple, greatly enhancing the rôle of the papillary ridges' efficiency in grasp as well as tactile sensibility. Drying of the skin is particularly damaging to its transmission of sensory stimulae to the underlying end-organs.

In the palm (232) the skin must not be free to move, except locally, and hence is bound down to the palmar aponeurosis, fibrous flexor sheaths of the fingers and deep fascia at the flexion creases and also in the central triangle of the palm. The intervening regions have subcutaneous fibro-fatty pressure pads, important for grip. The pads at the digits' tips are further specialised in that the distal part of the pad is a firmly supported tactile zone while the more proximal part is readily deformable for grip, the firmer distal part acting as a stop pad (233–234).

231

232

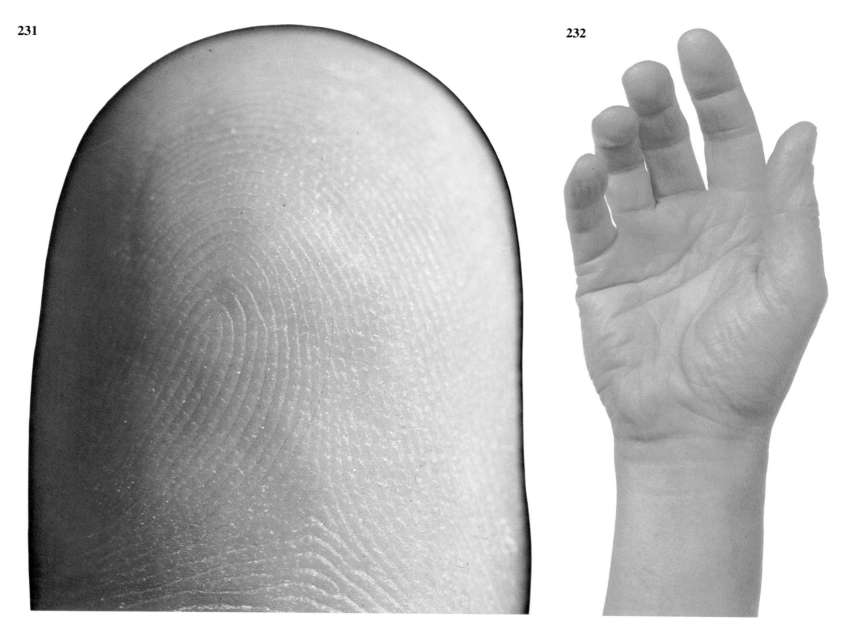

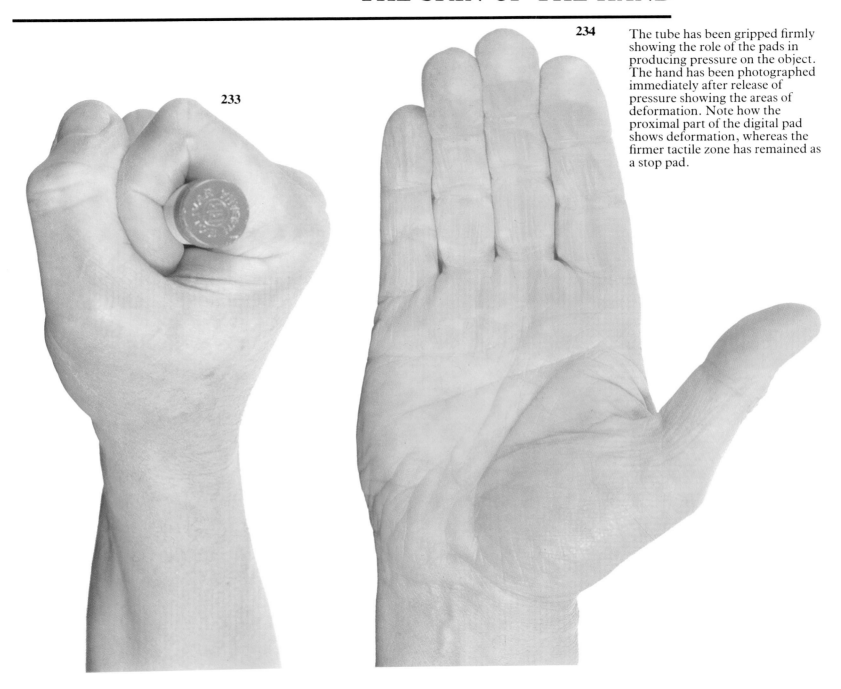

233

234 The tube has been gripped firmly showing the role of the pads in producing pressure on the object. The hand has been photographed immediately after release of pressure showing the areas of deformation. Note how the proximal part of the digital pad shows deformation, whereas the firmer tactile zone has remained as a stop pad.

The distal palmar pad and those of the proximal and middle phalanges, overlie transverse binding fasciae. The superficial transverse metacarpal ligament with its linkage with the palmar aponeurosis and by deep connections with the deep transverse metacarpal ligament forms not only a firm base for the pad but also a retinacular system for the digital tendons. The tendons are also bound down in the fingers by the fibrous flexor sheaths, vital for control of the tendons and hence digital movement, which also give a firm base for the digital pads. The distal digital pad is supported by fibrous binding to the terminal phalanx but the flattened nail also gives it considerable lateral and distal support.

THE SKIN OF THE HAND

The nail (**235**), made of hard keratin, as is the stratum corneum of the skin and the hairs, grows in what is, developmentally, part of the palmar surface and is so innervated. The skin forms a groove on either side of the nail, the nail groove, and here the nail is attached to the epidermis at the nail wall and also at its root where the eponychium overlies and is adherent to the root of the nail. Loss of adherence, both laterally and at the eponychium (often due to crude manicuring), exposes the region to infection which commonly becomes chronic and difficult to cure. The nail root lies beneath the overlying skin proximal to the eponychium. The actual growth of the nail occurs on the deeper aspect. Possibly the lunula represents a region of immature nail, but its opacity is also influenced by the thicker underlying epidermis not allowing the rich vascularity to show through, as occurs in the pinker area more distally.

235

1 Body of nail
2 Nail wall
3 Lateral nail groove
4 Lunula (Best seen on thumb and index finger)
5 Eponychium
6 Nail bed in proximal nail groove
7 Approximate extent of nail bed

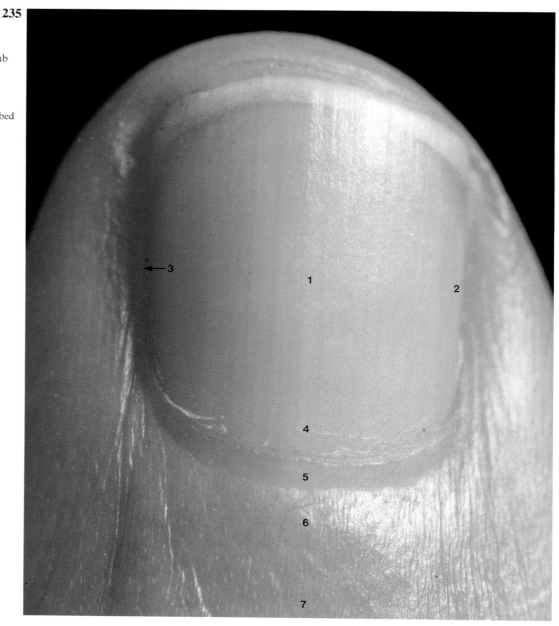

THE SKIN OF THE HAND

Between the bases of the fingers the palmar skin forms webs which slope away to the back. The webs extend some one to two centimetres beyond the metacarpophalangeal joints (236). As the proximal digital creases are level with the webs, the metacarpophalangeal joints lie well proximal to these creases (237); the distal palmar crease which lies just proximal to the joints is really the flexion crease for these joints. The proximal digital crease is thus a binding of the skin to the fibrous flexor sheath of the digit, separating the distal palmar from the proximal digital pad. However, the other two digital creases approximate quite closely to the interphalangeal joints.

As the palmar and digital creases are skin-binding creases they also represent lines of minimal tension in the skin and are thus ideal surgical incision lines. (Where sweating may be marked it is often advisable to avoid the humid gutter and cut parallel to it.)

At the ulnar side of the proximal part of the palm, the palmaris brevis muscle runs into the skin. This pulls up the skin to enhance palmar contact in a power grip but also produces a protective pad over the ulnar nerve which, although tucked in close to the pisiform bone is vulnerable to external pressure, running, as it does, superficial to the flexor retinaculum.

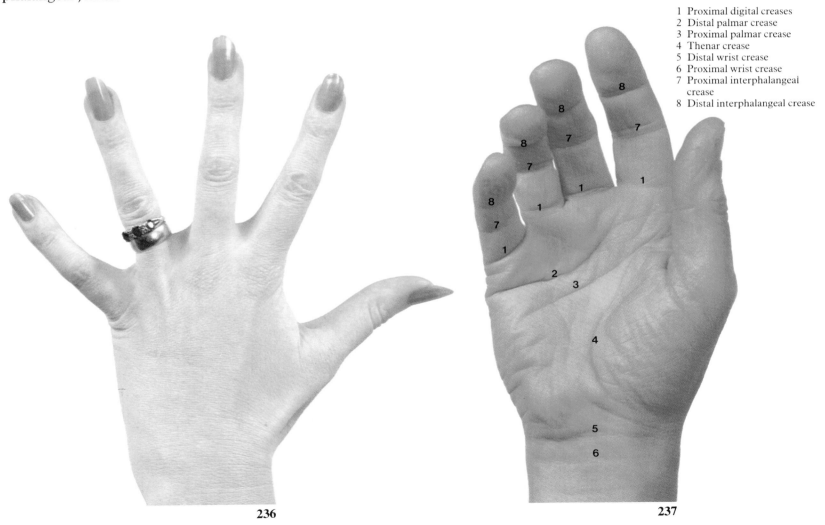

1 Proximal digital creases
2 Distal palmar crease
3 Proximal palmar crease
4 Thenar crease
5 Distal wrist crease
6 Proximal wrist crease
7 Proximal interphalangeal crease
8 Distal interphalangeal crease

236

237

HAND FUNCTIONS

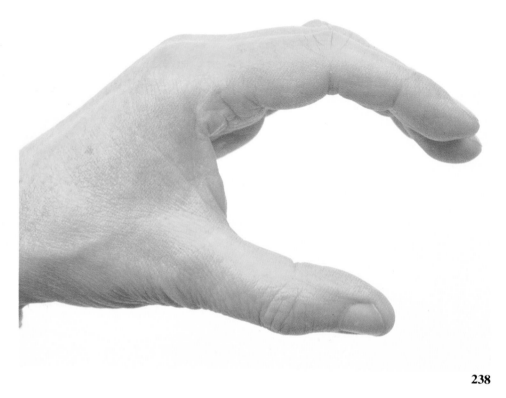

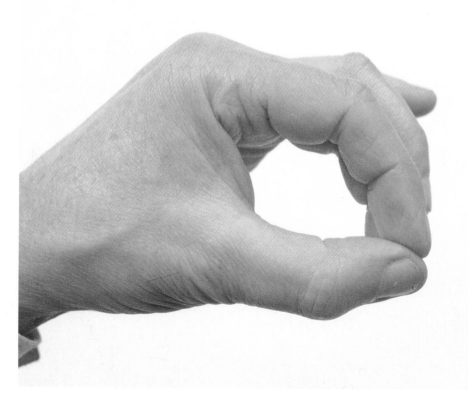

The hand is capable of many activities, often complex, which have made their analysis difficult. Knut (Canute) the Danish king of England (1016–35) gave a valuation to each of the digits in case of loss but it was really not until Napier, in 1955, saw in hand functions a series of simple basic patterns of activity, thereby facilitating analysis. In effect the hand has two major functional patterns with several lesser ones.

Precision grip and finger movement. This is essentially a fine and precise grip or digital movement which requires fine kinaesthetic control and is also usually associated with fine tactile sensibility at the finger tips. When considering such precise movement it is important to be aware that the long flexor and extensor muscles to the digits cross several joints which makes their control of all joints in the chain virtually impossible. For fine movement the ideal is that a muscle with high neuro-muscular control should move a single joint. This state is largely achieved in the hand by fixing the wrist, thus limiting movement to the digits and here to the metacarpophalangeal joints of the fingers and the carpometacarpal joint of the thumb, the more distal joints of each digit also being fixed (**238–239**). For a grip the thumb is opposed to bring it into pad to pad contact with usually the index or middle finger or, with both, to give a tripod grip (**240–241**).

238

239

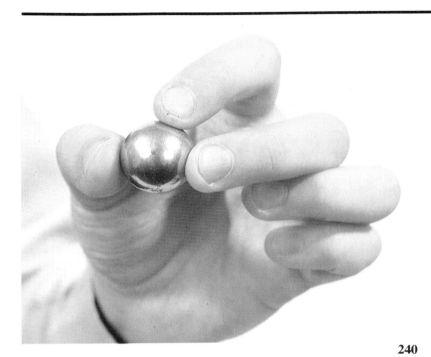

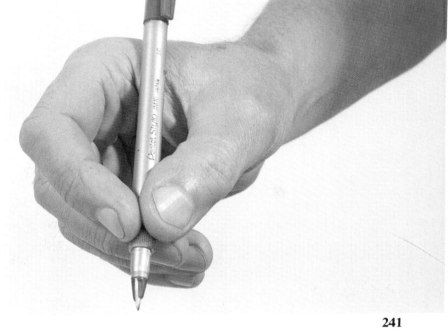

240

241

As the best tactile sensibility is derived from accurate pad to pad contact and opposition of the thumb is usually not sufficient within its precise functional range to achieve this (**242**), the finger is adjusted by slight ulnar deviation and rotation (opposition) to produce the desired contact (**243**).

The same single joint control is the ideal in carrying out many precise digital activities, such as the use of keyboards, whether computer, typing or musical. Admittedly the interphalangeal joint position may need to be changed to reach the key bank or vary from black to white keys on a piano or organ but nevertheless the prime, fine dynamic control is at the same single joint of the digit. It will be noted that for precision grip the thumb's movement and the tactile control of the three main digits all require median nerve innervation, whilst ulnar nerve innervation is required for interosseous activity. The interosseous muscles not only give the required digital deviation and rotation but the two muscles to each finger combine to give the precise flexion at the metacarpophalangeal joint, though if added power is needed the long flexors (particularly the profundus) come into play. In a similar way the thenar muscles give the one joint control of the thumb with added power, where required, from flexor pollicis longus.

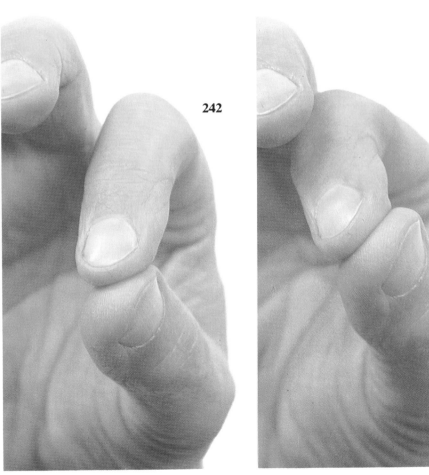

242

243

HAND FUNCTIONS

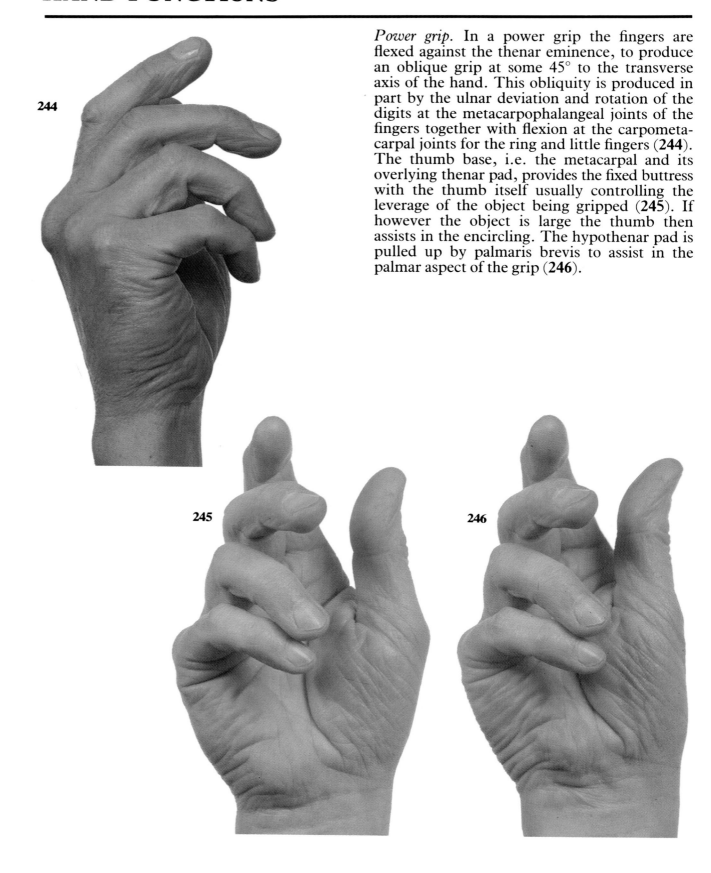

244

Power grip. In a power grip the fingers are flexed against the thenar eminence, to produce an oblique grip at some 45° to the transverse axis of the hand. This obliquity is produced in part by the ulnar deviation and rotation of the digits at the metacarpophalangeal joints of the fingers together with flexion at the carpometacarpal joints for the ring and little fingers (**244**). The thumb base, i.e. the metacarpal and its overlying thenar pad, provides the fixed buttress with the thumb itself usually controlling the leverage of the object being gripped (**245**). If however the object is large the thumb then assists in the encircling. The hypothenar pad is pulled up by palmaris brevis to assist in the palmar aspect of the grip (**246**).

245

246

With this grip, together with ulnar deviation at the wrist, the object being held can easily and comfortably be brought into line with the forearm for rotation; e.g. a screwdriver, door handle etc. or to achieve maximal effect from the wrist or elbow movement as in hammering, etc. (**247–248**).

The main power of digital flexion comes from the long flexor muscles, innervated by the median nerve, supplemented by the ulnar nerve for the flexor digitorum profundus to the ring and little fingers. The ulnar deviation and rotation of the fingers is brought about by the ulnar-sided interossei, with the hypothenar muscles for the little finger all supplied by the ulnar nerve. Flexor carpi ulnaris, the main ulnar deviator at the wrist, which is also supplied by the ulnar nerve, is also responsible with the hypothenar muscles for the flexion at the carpometacarpal joints on the ulnar border of the hand. It is the ulnar nerve which is responsible for transferring the not very useful transverse pure flexor grip of the hand (see baggage grip) into this most valuable oblique power grip, needed in so much manual activity.

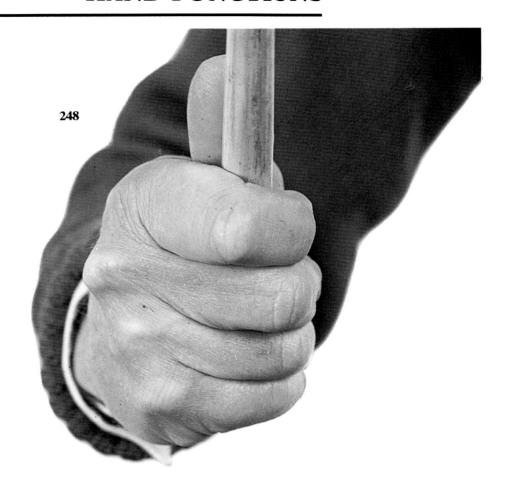

248

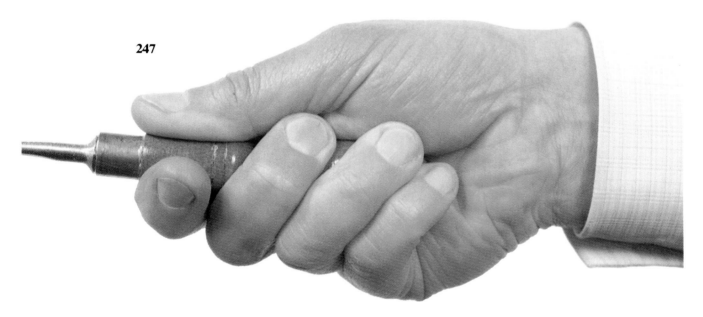

247

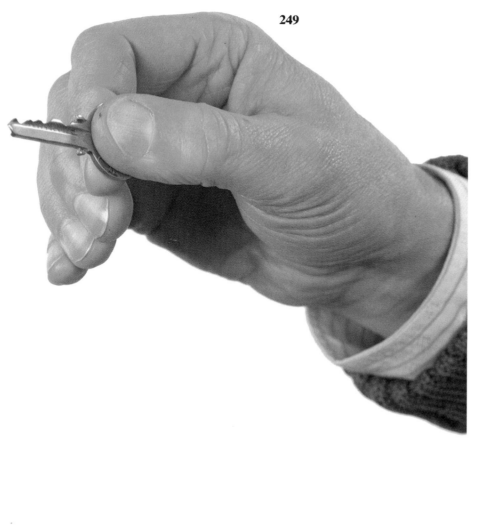

249

Key or lateral pinch grip. Here the fingers are held together in semi-flexion and packed together to form a firm buttress against which the thumb is opposed and flexed, pressing the side of the index finger (**249**). Though the fingers are close-packed and not so free to move laterally, nevertheless in order to resist the thumb the radial-sided interossei, particularly the first dorsal (**250,X**), need to be maintained in isometric contraction, while flexor pollicis longus gives power to thumb flexion once the thenar muscles have set the direction of the digit. Thus this grip requires a combination of ulnar innervation for interosseous control while the median nerve controls the thumb muscles and such digital flexion as is needed.

A similar activity of the fingers, taking counter pressure against the thumb plus the weight of an object, is seen when holding a cup or jug (**252**). In some cases the load is transferred to the middle finger and support from flexion of the index finger (**251**).

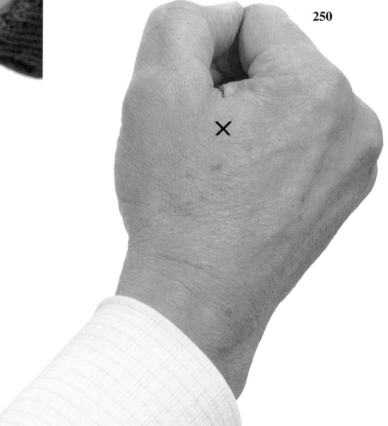

250

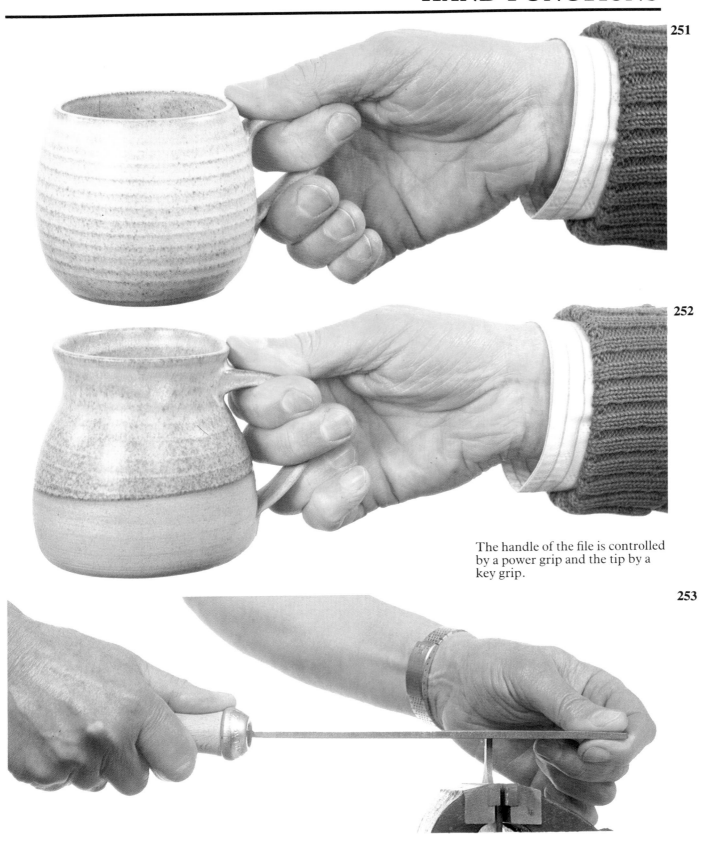

251

252

The handle of the file is controlled by a power grip and the tip by a key grip.

253

HAND FUNCTIONS

Baggage or hook grip. This is the grip developed by pure digital flexion on the axially placed hand. It is thus a transverse grip and, as the long flexor tendons responsible for its control all pull through the narrow carpal tunnel, the fingers are pulled together giving a compact strength to the hook. It should be noted that this grip is essentially an interphalangeal flexion, the metacarpophalangeal joints remaining extended. It is essentially a load bearing grip which can be sustained for long periods. As such the precise controlling interosseous muscles are not used and even the flexor digitorum profundus plays a subsidiary role. Most of the sustained power output comes from flexor digitorum superficialis which keeps the proximal interphalangeal joints at about 90°, the terminal joint being flexed (flexor profundus) as much as is necessary to complete the hook (254–255).

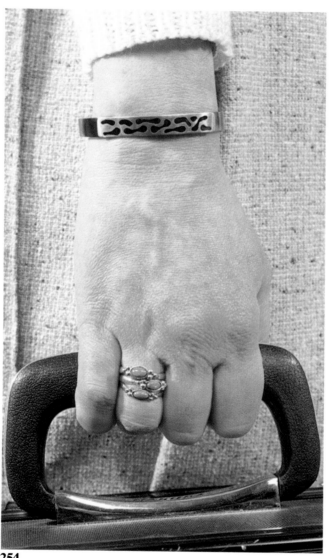

254

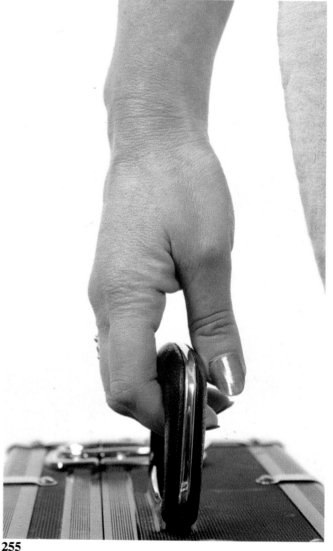

255

150

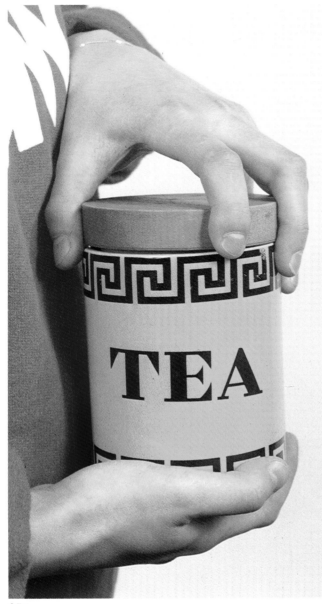

256

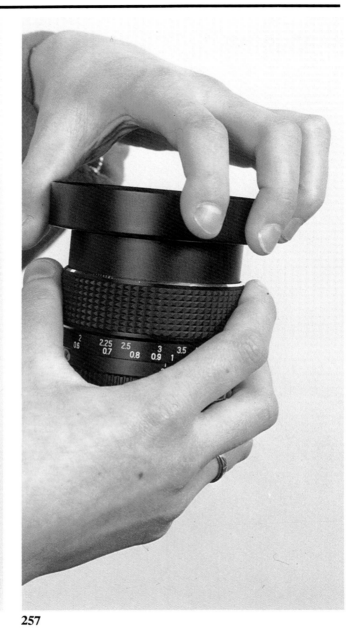

257

Power pinch is used on occasions, and is really a precision grip with added power supplied by the long flexor muscles. As the intrinsic muscles are required, unlike the baggage grip, it is fairly rapidly tiring, in spite of the main power coming from the long flexor muscles. It is valuable where a small gripping area requires greater power and directional precision than is possible from a key grip. Although relatively limited in everyday use in the normal hand it can be very valuable in a variety of conditions, including ulnar nerve palsy, where the oblique power grip becomes impossible, though here the metacarpophalangeal joints are likely to remain more extended due to loss of the interossei. It is often the major retained grip in the rheumatoid hand.

A ball-holding or centring grip is essentially digital flexion on digits abducted at the metacarpophalangeal joints of the fingers and the carpometacarpal of the thumb (**256–257**).

258

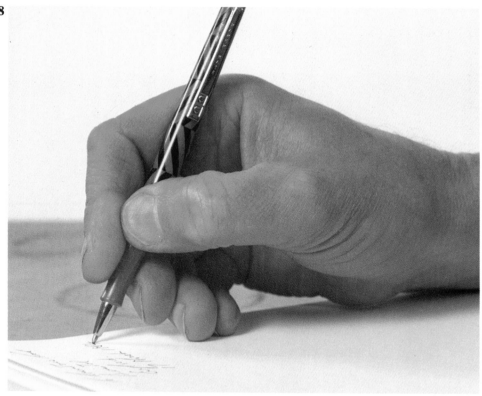

Writing is one of the more complicated activities which do not fall readily into the basic patterns. It is however not difficult to analyse if it is reduced to a series of up and down strokes together with progression controlled by radial or ulnar deviators at the wrist. The upstroke is largely of intrinsic muscle control; interosseous muscles giving metacarpophalangeal flexion with interphalangeal extension against the pen with comparable activity in the thumb (**258**), while the downstroke is controlled by the long flexors (**259**). This accounts for the finely controlled upstroke and the more dynamic downstroke, a feature of certain styles of calligraphy.

259

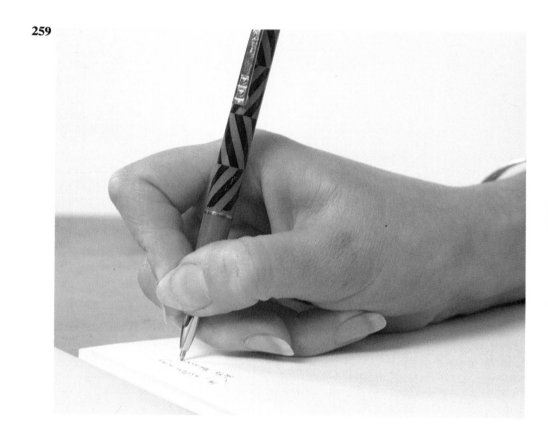

By the time a baby is born it has been practising its limb movements for a considerable time *in utero*. However these movements are relatively simple, mainly flexor-extensor in character. The hand is a very efficient grasping instrument. The fingers flex into a transverse grip which is remarkably strong but intrinsic control is as yet not developed. The thumb is also primarily controlled by the long flexor with the finer control from the thenar muscles still wanting (**260–261**). These more complicated patterns of movement and the necessary fine sensory control must await the completion of myelination during the first two years or so of life.

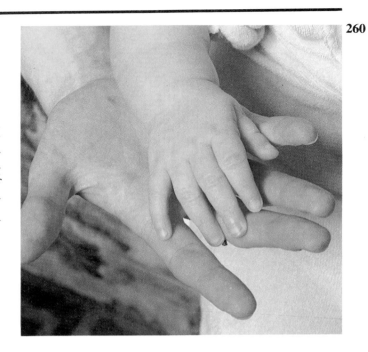

260

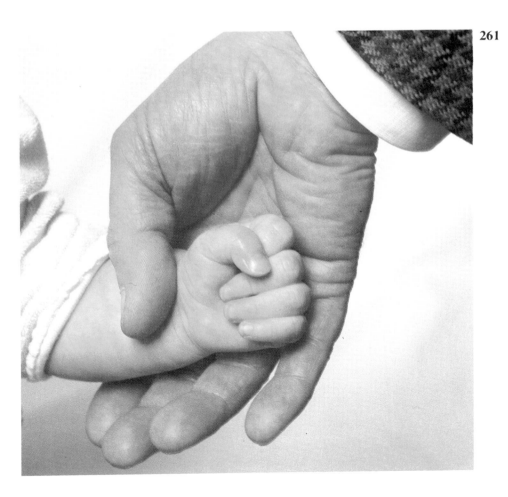

261

262

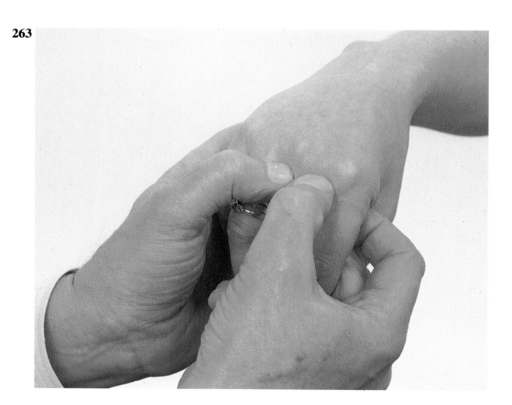

263

The fingers should be capable of flexion at the metacarpophalangeal and interphalangeal joints to the extent that the finger tips press into the palm at the level of the proximal palmar crease.

A useful clinical measurement of flexor deficiency is the distance by which the affected finger tip is separated from that crease (**262**).

Extension of the fingers should be 180° (i.e. straight) at each joint, though many people are capable of considerable amounts of hyperextension at the metacarpophalangeal joints. Again a useful measure of lack of extension is the distance the finger tip falls short of the line extended from the metacarpal. Of the individual joints, the metacarpals should be able to be flexed to 80–89°, the proximal interphalangeal to about 110° and the distal to 70–80°. In each case this brings the finger into pressure on the adjoining pads. Hence any thickening of the pads, as is common in a physically hard-working hand, may limit the ranges of flexion.

The knuckles are made up of the heads of the metacarpals and likewise in the fingers of the heads of the proximal and middle phalanges. The joints are thus distal to these prominences. The metacarpophalangeal joints are quite easy to feel from the back, particularly with the joints partially flexed; the interphalangeal joints are less easy (**263**).

Although the heads of the metacarpals are easy to palpate from the back of the hand they are less so from the palm, where they are joined by the deep transverse metacarpal ligament and overlaid by the superficial ligament and palmar pad. However as the anterior aspect of the head projects well forward of the shaft of the bone, the general swelling can be felt at the distal palmar crease (**264**).

The digital webs are some 2 cm distal to metacarpophalangeal joints.

Here the joints are identified by the examiner at the beginning of the slope to the ventrally placed webs (**265**).

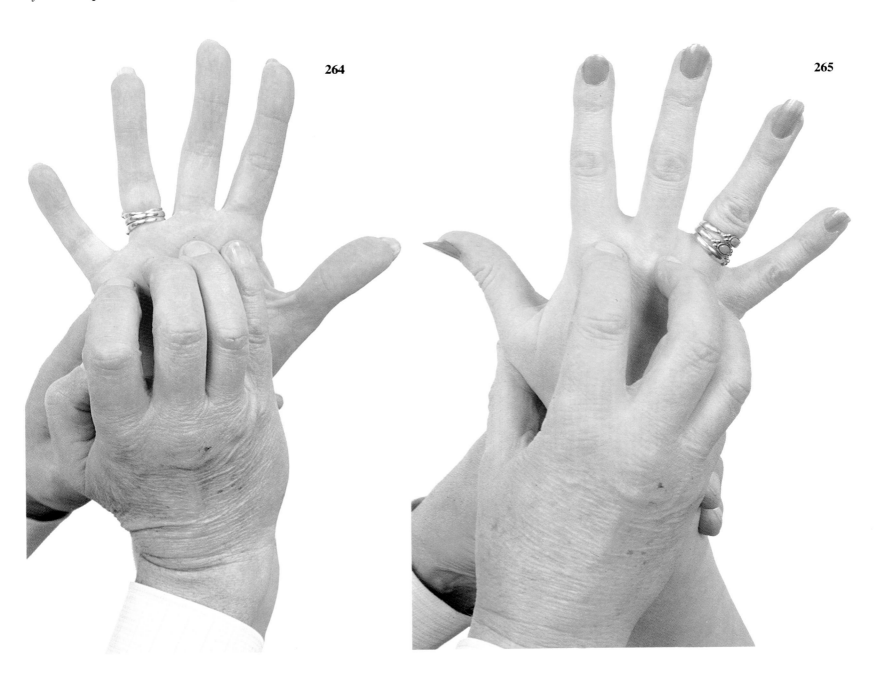

264

265

MOVEMENTS OF THE DIGITS

In considering the movements of the fingers it is important to remember the arched structure of the hand; there is a very deep transverse arch at the carpus, which, with the flexor retinaculum, produces the carpal tunnel. More shallow, though still important, is the arch at the metacarpal heads. This transverse arching is amplified by a longitudinal arch effect produced by the prominent carpus and retinaculum at the heel of the hand and the anterior projections of the metacarpal heads with the overlying tissue pad distally, giving, collectively, the hollow of the palm. Due in part to the arch of the heads of the metacarpals and the centring pull of the flexor tendons to the carpal tunnel, the natural flexion of the fingers at the metacarpal joints is to the tubercle of the scaphoid. This is added to by the curve produced by the differing lengths of the metacarpals (the knuckle curve) so that the joints are at different levels. Furthermore the curves of each of the metacarpal heads is not symmetrical nor are the collateral ligaments, so that there is a natural twist in flexion to bring the fingers thenarwards, even without muscular activity. In the power grip this is added to by flexion at the carpometacarpal joints of the ulnar two fingers and the ulnar deviator-rotatory activity of the intrinsic muscles.

266

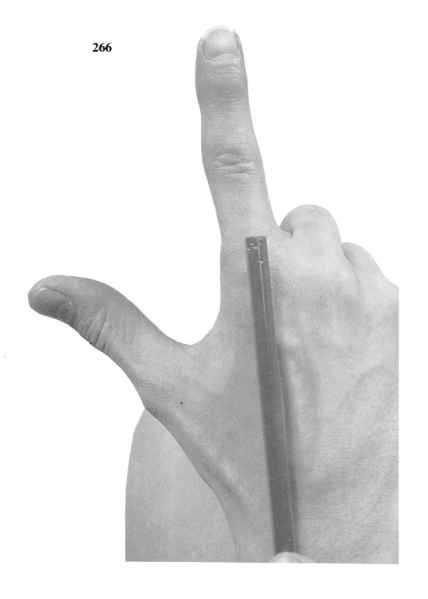

267

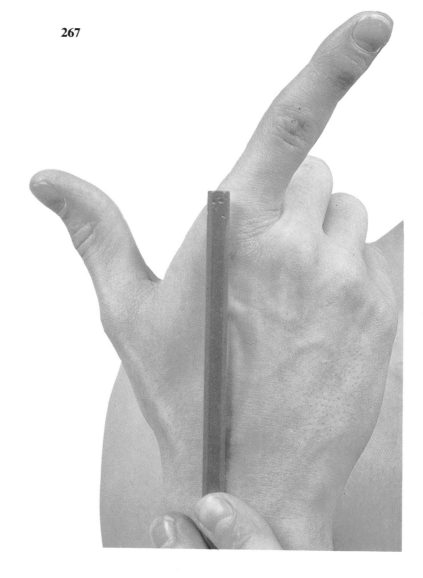

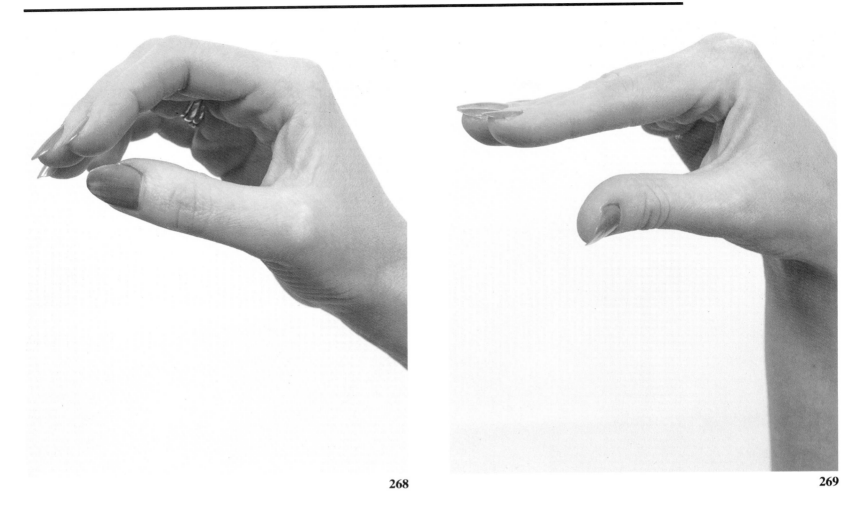

268

269

The interphalangeal joints must have lateral stability and their movements are limited to flexion and extension, but it is worthy of note that the distal interphalangeal joint is capable of a small degree of passive hyperextension which allows the pad of the finger to make maximal contact with that of the thumb, in opposition.

The metacarpophalangeal joints show lateral movements, most marked with the fingers in extension, when the collateral ligaments are slack. As the fingers are flexed, due to the shape of the head of the metacarpal, the collateral ligaments become taut so that at full flexion lateral movement is small. Thus abduction from the usually described axis of the middle finger is greatest in full extension where it is limited not by the joints but the tautness of the digital webs and the underlying ligamentous structures. Abduction in full flexion is very limited. However, as seen in the power grip, a

degree of ulnar deviation and rotation is achievable in all four digits.

In lateral movement in the individual fingers ulnar deviation is far greater than radial by some three to four times in the index and middle and twice in the ring and little fingers (**266–7**). The ulnar deviation is also more finely controlled as at the wrist.

Clinically, in an inflamed hand as after injury it has been accepted practice in the past to set the hand up in a position of rest during the healing period (**268**). Unfortunately the joints tend to fix so that metacarpal flexion and interphalangeal extension become limited. If, however, the hand is set up in a minimum of 60° flexion at the metacarpophalangeal joints with interphalangeal extension (**269**), the collateral ligaments are taut, and this gives the best chance of full finger mobility on recovery.

157

MOVEMENTS OF THE THUMB

Analysis of movements of the thumb presents some difficulty as no existing method of description is totally satisfactory and each needs some justification. Pure movements in a plane are virtually impossible at the joint. It is proposed here to use traditional anatomical terminology in spite of the difficulties. If the thumb is set at rest it will be at an angle of some 60° to the plane of the palm. Abduction carries the thumb away from, and anterior to, the palm but maintaining essentially the same angle; hence it is sometimes described as anteposition (**270**).

Adduction (or retroposition) takes it against the side of the palm. Flexion and extension takes the thumb in a plane roughly at right angles to the above (**271**). Thus flexion carries the thumb forwards on a firm axial base as when producing the key grip, or the thumb base for a power grip; it is essentially the line of direct pull of the long flexor muscle with extension of the two extensors. Opposition swings the thumb round to face into the palm and bring its pad towards those of the fingers (**272**).

270

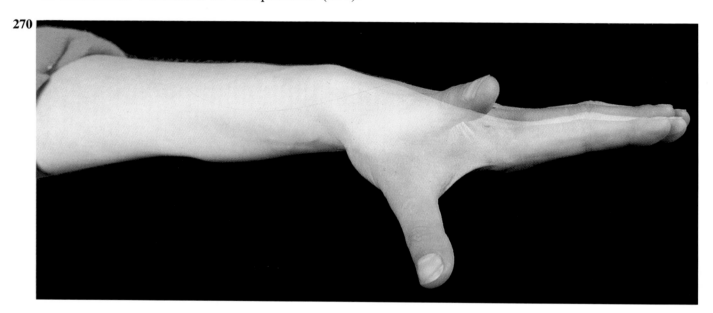

271

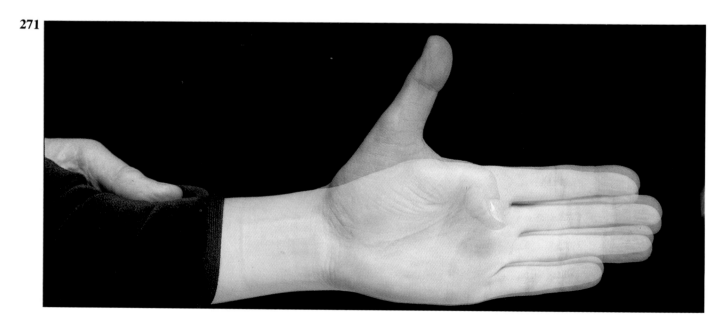

At the metacarpophalangeal joint, ranges of movement vary considerably from straight in extension to some 60° or more in flexion, though hyperextension to a considerable extent is common particularly in some Asiatic races, the well known double-jointed syndrome. Abduction and adduction occur at this joint while, as in the fingers, movement at the interphalangeal joint is limited to flexion and extension.

It is worthy of note that, under normal circumstances, flexion and extension are the prime movements at the metacarpophalangeal joint, abduction and adduction are used to bring the pad into line with that of each of the fingers (**273–274**). However, if for any reason the prime carpometacarpal joint is lost and particularly if fixed in a partially opposed position, the metacarpophalangeal joint, having good intrinsic control, can take over extremely well as the prime mobile joint.

272

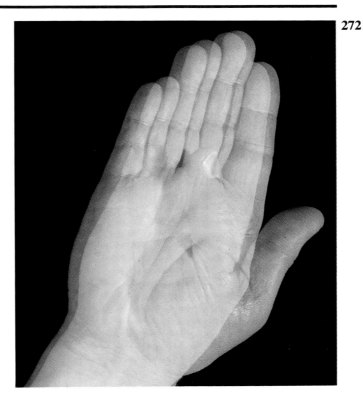

273

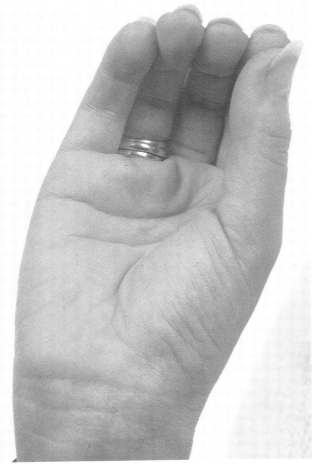

274

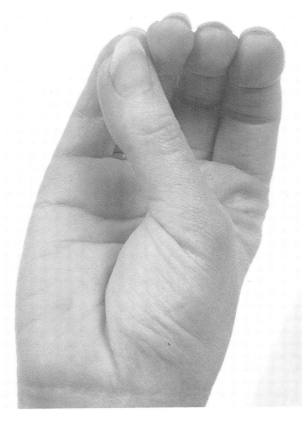

RELATIVE VALUES OF THE DIGITS

The hand is a pentadactyl (5 digital) structure of which all digits are important, although the opposable thumb is usually considered to be the prime feature. Thus the hand is sometimes described as having 5 digits or 4 fingers and a thumb so each finger may have alternative numbers. Any mistake in numbering might be disastrous if, for instance, the wrong finger were amputated. Hence digits should not be numbered but named (**275**), though it is accept-able to number the metacarpals, starting at 1 for the thumb to 5 for the little finger.

The importance of the thumb can not be underestimated, for a hand lacking an opposable thumb is grossly deficient in function. Because of this, after partial thumb loss, reconstructive surgeons will often make great efforts to rebuild a thumb-like structure of near normal length, an endeavour commonly misconceived. A good power grip requires a good thumb only as far as the metacarpophalangeal joint, the remainder merely controlling leverage. A precision grip requires an opposable thumb but the fingers can meet a shorter thumb, and if it has good tactile sensibility it is far more valuable than a larger thumb with little or no sensibility.

From a functional point of view the value of each of the fingers is by no means relative to their size: the four fingers have quite marked functional differences. The index and middle fingers are mounted on metacarpals in the axis of movement of forearm rotation and the loading region of the hand on the radius. As such they are often described as axial fingers forming a firm central base for the hand and having virtually no movement between the carpus and their metacarpals. The thumb moves around this axis on the one side and the ring and little fingers to a lesser extent on the other. All three of these peripheral digits have movement at their carpometacarpal joints to give the necessary freedom (**276**).

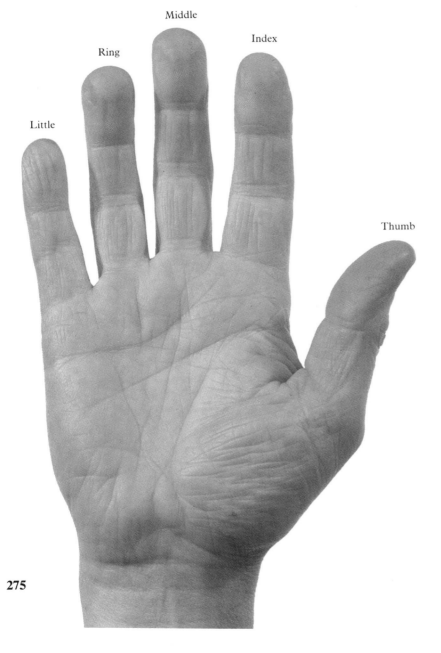

275

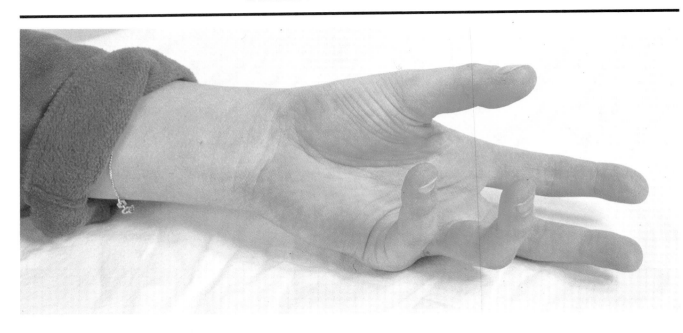

276

The index and middle fingers are the natural components of a tripod grip with the thumb having a fixed base for their single joint movement.

If the index finger is missing or injured the grip can be transferred with only moderate loss of function to the middle and ring fingers but far less acceptably to the ring and little fingers as, to achieve this, a further joint in each digit has to be brought into play, abduction at the thumb metacarpophalangeal joint and flexion at the finger carpometacarpal joints. Furthermore the little finger is too short and the flexor mobility of both fingers limited. The major dynamic rôle of the two ulnar fingers is to give width and thus valuable control to the grip and to increase the range of the hand when stretched.

Of the fingers, the index is the most mobile and independent. The belly of flexor digitorum profundus supplying it is usually separate, whereas those for the other three fingers are joined much further down the arm. The index has two extensor tendons; the extensor indicis can move independently from those of the common extensor thus giving the greater extensor freedom needed for the pointing finger. The

first dorsal interosseous muscle is the largest of these muscles and has a greater proportion of its insertion into the proximal phalanx than is usual.

The middle finger is less independently free in extension while the ring finger is far worse, a great trial to many musical instrumentalists, particularly keyboard players. The lack of freedom has been put down to cross-linkages between the extensor tendons, and this may in part be true, as the little finger with its own extensor digiti minimi has free extension. However freedom of extension is also limited by freedom of independent movement of the flexors. In the little finger there is poor independent flexion in spite of the free extension. This is not easy to explain for the lack is particularly in the flexor superficialis muscle, which although usually present and of adequate size is rarely suitable for good digital flexion if the profundus tendon to the finger is lost.

In cases of loss of the thumb, pollicisation of one of the fingers can be extremely valuable. The index can be moved quite easily but, from a practical point of view, the ring finger is the least useful in the hand and therefore often the best choice, though technically rather more difficult. Just as in mechanical activity not all the digits are equal, so also is it true of their sensory rôle. As a precision grip makes use of the thumb, index and middle fingers, fine sensory perception is required particularly in the pads of these digits. The index is the finger of prime importance in reading braille. Thus the thumb and index finger need overall sensory control in the pads whilst reduction on the ulnar border of the middle finger is less serious than on the radial side. Here also the ring finger is the least important and, for this reason, if there is sensory loss of the thumb or index finger, a portion of skin from the ulnar side of the ring finger may be transferred on a neurovascular pedicle to the area of loss. As the ulnar border of the little finger takes the surface bearing contact for the hand in many activities, the sensory control is most valuable here.

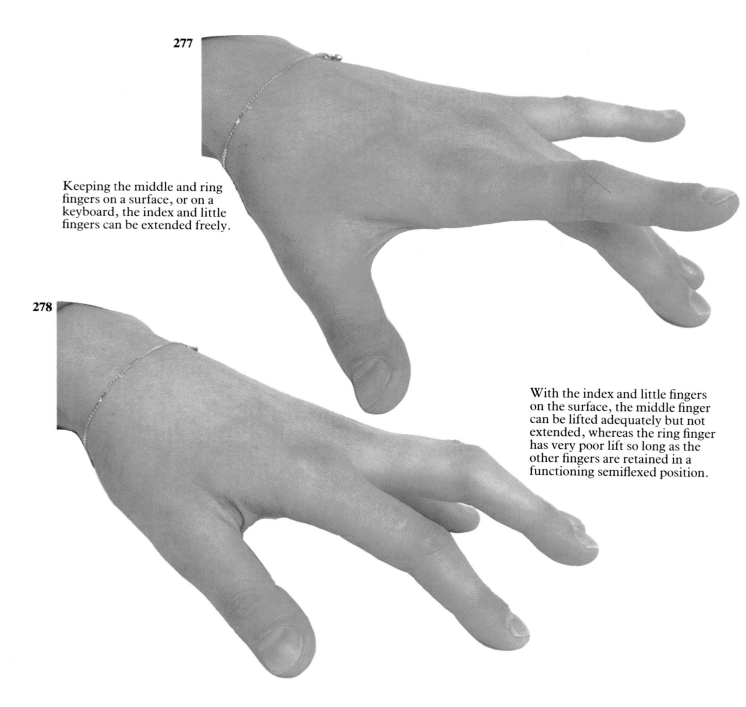

277

Keeping the middle and ring fingers on a surface, or on a keyboard, the index and little fingers can be extended freely.

278

With the index and little fingers on the surface, the middle finger can be lifted adequately but not extended, whereas the ring finger has very poor lift so long as the other fingers are retained in a functioning semiflexed position.

The little finger is often dismissed as being the least important of all the digits. It is often amputated after injury or when grossly contracted in Dupuytren's disease, whereas a greater effort may be made to save other digits. However, its loss, or even just the loss of sensation on its outer border is a serious disability in many people.

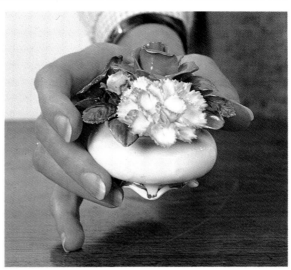

279

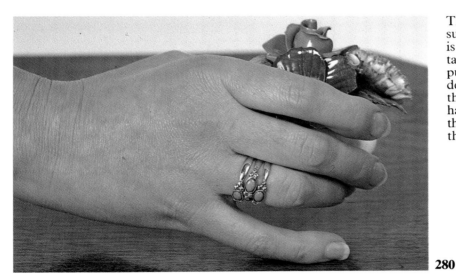

280

The little finger is used to feel the surface on which a delicate object is being placed. With this fine tactile control the object can be put down with considerable delicacy, even without the use of the eyes. Many valuable objects have been broken due to loss of this fine tactile control of the hand through the little finger.

Note how the little fingers are used to control both hands in relation to the surface and to stabilise both objects being held for fine examination.

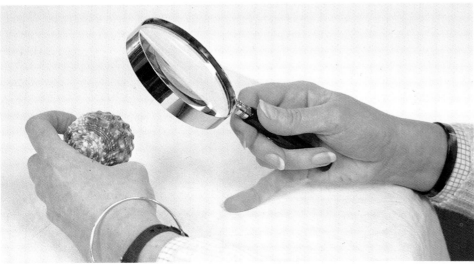

281

282

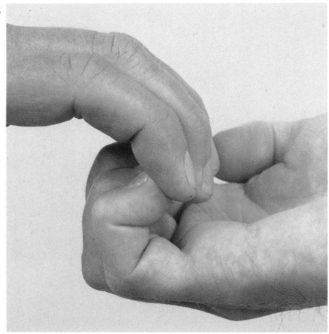

Extrinsic muscles to the fingers. Each finger has two long flexor tendons; that from flexor digitorum superficialis to the base of the middle phalanx and the one from flexor digitorum profundus to the distal phalanx. Flexor digitorum profundus is therefore capable of flexion of all the digital joints and its function can be tested by asking the subject to hook the finger. The strength of the muscle can be estimated by the examiner pulling against the hook (**282**).

As the profundus muscle produces flexion at the proximal as well as the distal interphalangeal joint, absence of function of flexor digitorum superficialis may pass unnoticed except for some loss of power, and particularly sustaining power as in a baggage grip. In fact when flexor tendons are damaged in the finger, unless conditions are ideal, it is common practice to remove the superficialis tendon, so as to achieve the best functional result from the repaired or grafted profundus tendon. The superficialis muscle flexes the proximal interphalangeal joint and, although it is possible to contract this muscle in isolation from the profundus, it is difficult to explain to a patient how, and even more difficult to achieve. However, the individual components of the superficialis muscle can be isolated far more than can those of the profundus, which work more closely together. Thus if all the fingers except one are held in full extension by the examiner, and the patient asked to bend that finger, the superficialis will be the only muscle to flex the finger effectively at the interphalangeal joint. Each finger can be left free in turn (Apley's test). It will be noted that the distal interphalangeal joint is lax without effective flexor or extensor control (**283**).

In the little finger, control from the superficialis may be less free, with flexion weak and not characteristic of superficialis action as in the other fingers.

Flexor pollicis longus is the power flexor of the thumb and particularly of the interphalangeal joint. Thus its function can be tested by hooking the thumb, as the digitorum profundus is tested in the fingers. However a very useful test of several muscles is provided by asking the subject to press the thumb pad against that of the little finger. For this to be done correctly requires long muscle activity as well as opposition and short flexor activity in both digits. In fact it will be seen that flexor carpi ulnaris also contracts to

283

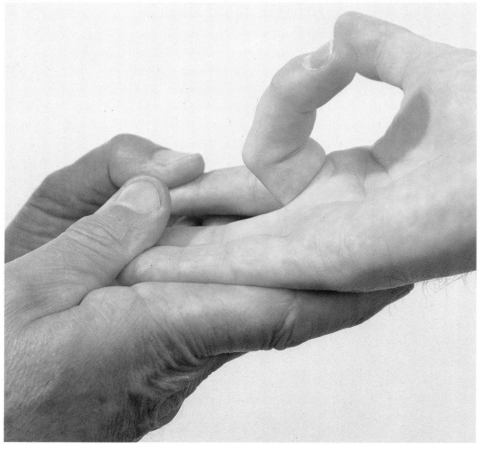

produce flexion at the ulnar side carpometacarpal joint and to stabilise the hypothenar muscle origin. To test for power the subject is asked to prevent the examiner's finger pulling the two apart (**284**).

Extensor digitorum communis sends tendons to all fingers, these being joined on the dorsum of the hand by the intertendinous connections, which play some part in limiting individual freedom of movement, though this is provided for in the index finger by extensor indicis and in the little finger by extensor digiti minimi. Although the extensor tendons do not contribute a true tendon to the proximal phalanx, nevertheless their main pull is to the metacarpophalangeal joint, unless this can be limited, to allow extension also to be transmitted to the interphalangeal joints. This is the situation seen in the claw finger of ulnar nerve palsy, where, due to the loss of the intrinsic muscles, the metacarpophalangeal joint becomes hyperextended but the interphalangeal joints remain partially flexed on contraction of the extensor muscles. If however the hyperextension is prevented in such a case, as by holding the proximal phalanx, then the interphalangeal joints can be extended. Under normal circumstances the interossei and also the lumbricals, to a lesser extent, act as flexors at the metacarpophalangeal joints and interphalangeal extensors. Thus even without the long extensors it is usually still possible to extend the interphalangeal joints as long as the metacarpophalangeal joints can be flexed. The important factor in testing for the long extensor muscles is the ability to extend the metacarpophalangeal joints (**285**).

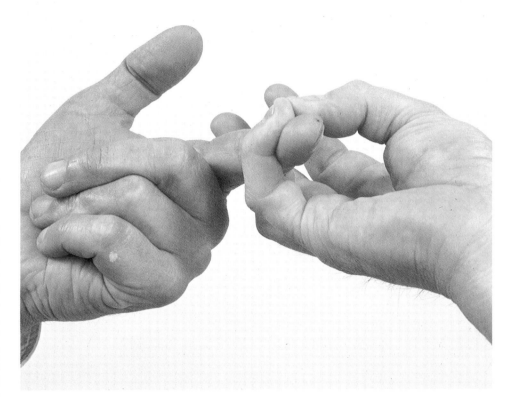

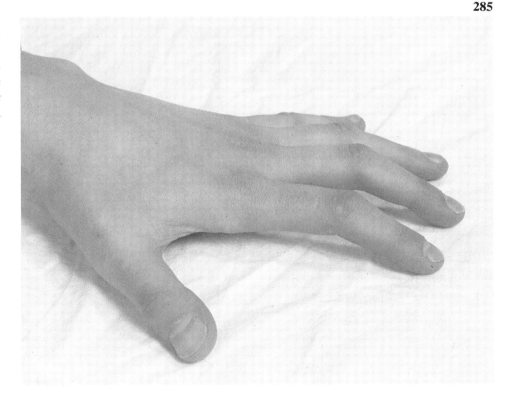

MUSCLES CONTROLLING THE DIGITS

The thumb has a muscle controlling extension in each of its joints as well as the abductor pollicis longus, though this latter muscle should also be considered as an important controller of the wrist complex.

Extensor pollicis brevis acts over the meta-carpophalangeal joint while extensor pollicis longus runs onwards over the interphalangeal joint. On examination it should be noted that brevis is frequently missing or of very small size. The two muscles can be seen in contraction by their tendons standing out and producing the anatomical 'snuff-box' when the thumb is firmly extended (286). If only the brevis muscle is missing the closely related abductor pollicis longus will be seen overlying the radial styloid. However it should be noted that extensor brevis also has an abductor pull on the thumb and therefore does not show if the thumb is extended in adduction, which is the most obvious line of pull for the long extensor.

As in the case of the fingers, the intrinsic (here the thenar) muscles contribute to the expansion controlling interphalangeal extension. Hence if the metacarpophalangeal joint is allowed to flex then the interphalangeal joint can be extended even in the absence of the long extensor (286). The main pull comes then from adductor pollicis brevis and if the interphalangeal joint is extended with the metacarpophalangeal joint flexed, the distal part of the long extensor tendon remains taut and pulling to the medial side of the flexed metacarpophalangeal joint. See Froment's sign, page 168.

286

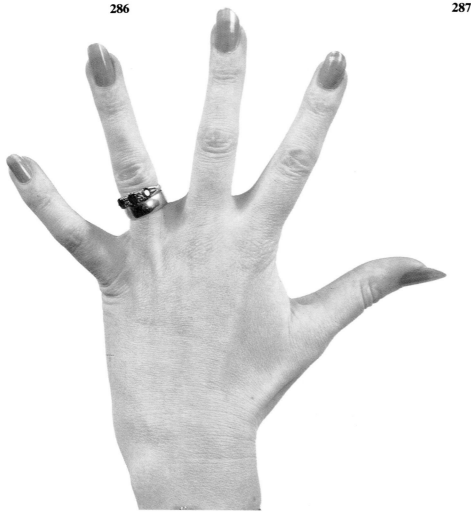

287

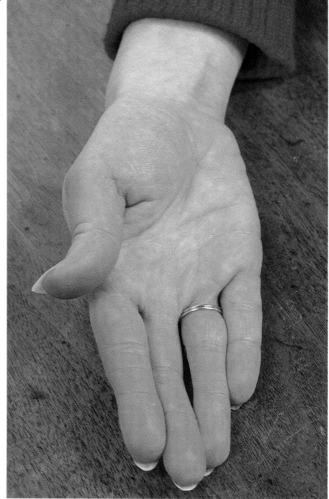

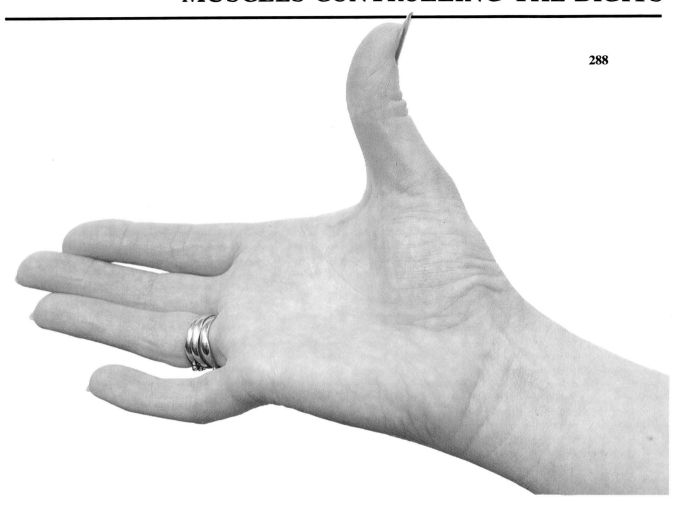

288

Intrinsic muscles. The intrinsic muscles to the fingers are the interossei and the lumbricals, with the support of the hypothenar muscles to the little finger, while the thenar muscles similarly subserve the thumb. In testing, the thenar muscles are difficult to isolate from each other, and this is complicated in clinical practice by their having both ulnar and median nerve innervation. Adductor pollicis is innervated by the ulnar nerve, which commonly supplies the deep head of the flexor pollicis brevis and may send contributions to opponens. The median nerve supplies abductor pollicis brevis, opponens and the superficial head of flexor pollicis brevis. Hence opposition is a function of median nerve innervated muscle but because of possible ulnar nerve overlap into opponens and the deep head of the flexor commonly so supplied, some degree of opposition is sometimes possible even in a median nerve palsy.

Abductor pollicis brevis is best tested by firm abduction of the thumb, preferably against pressure (**288**, see also page 179). As loss of bulk and power is a feature of the common carpal tunnel compression of the median nerve, test for this muscle is important, when its strength should be compared with that of the other side for evidence of small loss of power. However as the condition should be treated if possible before loss of power if good results are to be obtained, electrodiagnostic tests are more reliable in the early stages.

Flexor digitorum brevis activity can be shown by flexing at the metacarpophalangeal joint into the palm whilst it also acts with opponens in forced opposition as shown in **284**. It also acts powerfully with the abductor in forced abduction.

MUSCLES CONTROLLING THE DIGITS

Adductor pollicis brevis can be tested in a similar way to the adductor actions of the interossei, forcing the thumb against the side of the palm (see **291**), but it should be noted that extensor pollicis longus has an adductor pull in extension. Froment's sign is one usually described as a test for the adductor muscle (**289**). A thin object, such as a strip of paper, is gripped between the pad of the thumb and the side of the proximal phalanx of the index finger, keeping the interphalangeal joints of the thumbs extended. The grip is then maintained as the hands are pulled apart. As the thumb metacarpophalangeal joint is flexed the long extensor is ineffective, and the adductor is required to maintain interphalangeal extension. If this muscle is inactive, the thumb flexes at the interphalangeal joint due to the unopposed pull of flexor pollicis longus.

The *interosseous muscles* are the primary flexors at the metacarpophalangeal joints of the fingers, through their attachments to the bases of the proximal phalanges and by the transverse fibres into the extensor expansion (see Extensor digitorum). By virtue of their wing tendons they contribute to interphalangeal extension. In fine precision grip this extensor component balances out the elastic pull of the two long flexor muscles against the extensor, leaving the two interossei to each finger to combine for the metacarpophalangeal flexor role, each giving such ulnar or radial deviation and rotation as is required (**240**). However, traditionally, the interossei have been divided morphologically into palmar adductor and dorsal abductors on the axis of the middle finger. From the point of view of testing their flexor role, this can be carried out by asking the subject to flex the metacarpophalangeal joint with the interphalangeal extended (**290**). Their abductor power can be shown by forced abduction of the fingers (including here the abductor digiti minimi, **286**), while their adductor power can be estimated by slipping a piece of paper between each finger in turn, with all the digital joints extended, the paper being pulled out by the examiner against the adductor action (**291**).

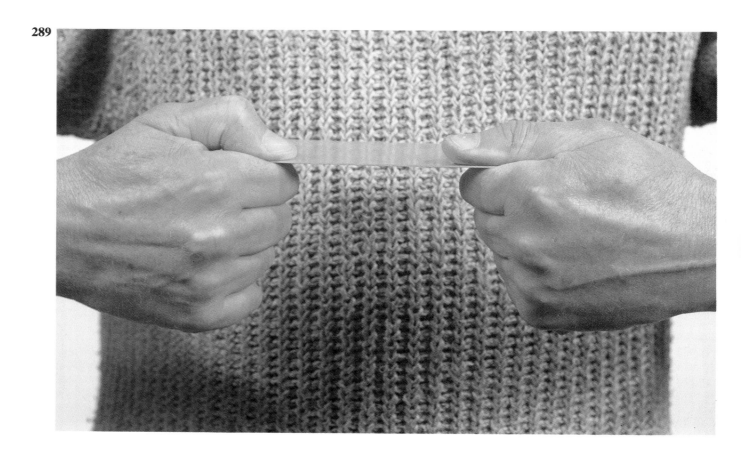

289

The *lumbricals* are difficult to test. They act dynamically only in firm interphalangeal extension and only then can they flex the metacarpophalangeal joints. They can be seen in this role to limit the clawing of the index and middle fingers in ulnar nerve palsy when they are the only remaining intrinsic muscles to the fingers. But in the normal hand this function can be carried out by the interossei. It is now usually accepted that the lumbricals are of little dynamic importance in the normal hand but, because of their rich sensory innervation, act as a potentially dynamic proprioceptive bridge between the flexor and extensor muscles. The *hypothenar* muscles act on the little finger much as the interossei, but supplemented by the opponens to give a more positive opposition to the outside finger. However, in addition, as these muscles are attached to the pisiform and the medial part of the flexor retinaculum, they form a dynamic continuum with flexor carpi ulnaris, which stabilises their origin and also acts as the carpometacarpal flexor. Their combined action other than the abductor, is seen in **245**, page 146.

290

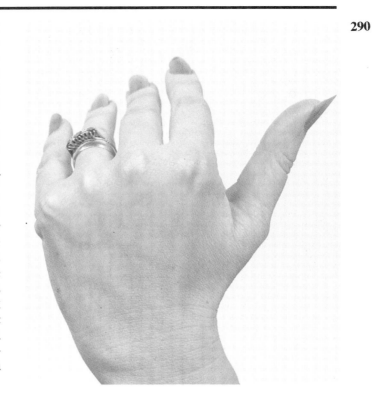

291

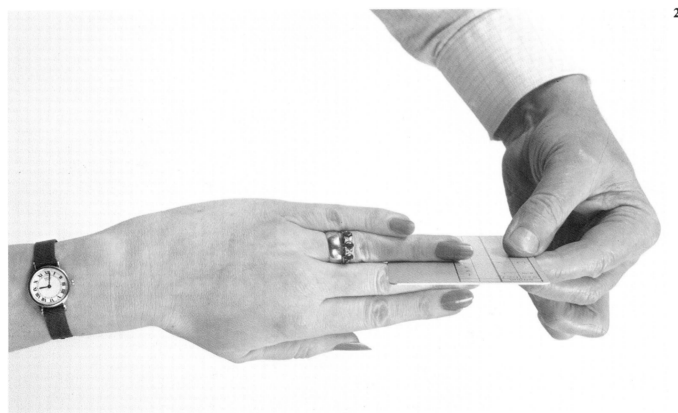

NERVES OF THE ARM AND HAND

1   Supraclavicular nerves
C(3),4
2   Intercostobrachial T2
3   Upper lateral cutaneous
(axillary) C5,6
4   Medial cutaneous of arm
(C8) T1
5   Lower lateral cutaneous
(radial) C5,6
6   Medial cutaneous of
forearm C8,T1
7   Lateral cutaneous of
forearm C5,6
8   Ulnar C7,8
8★   palmar branch
8★★   posterior branch
9   Median C6,7
9★   palmar branch
10   Superficial radial C6,7,8
11   Posterior cutaneous of
arm (radial) C5,6,7,8
12   Posterior cutaneous of
forearm (radial) C5,6,7,8

N.B. The root values given are
those of the skin supply.

The upper limb is supplied through the brachial plexus whose roots are C(4), 5, 6, 7, 8 and T1 and any neurological examination must consider not only the peripheral nerve of supply but also the roots involved. In the limbs the formation of plexuses complicates the more simple pattern of segmental supply of the trunk. However as far as the sensory supply is concerned the dermatomes of root supply remain fairly simple. The area supplied by the central root contributing to the plexus (C7), remains centrally placed, supplying the hand, but cut off more proximally, as are C6 (lateral) and C8 (medial), which supply the forearm. C5 (lateral) and T1 (medial) supply the upper arm. Thus in the upper arm there is a jump of four segments from medial to lateral and a jump of two segments in the forearm. The separation zones are quite narrow here with relatively little overlap and are known as the anterior and posterior axial lines. This is a marked distinction from the very variable overlap to be expected between adjoining segmental regions.

Diagrams of the dermatomes vary enormously, depending upon their derivation; whether from sensory loss after nerve root lesion or from stimulation or pain as in a post-herpetic syndrome. In view of this variability it is perhaps better to work to a simple pattern and remember that any map can only be an approximation to that found in a particular person.

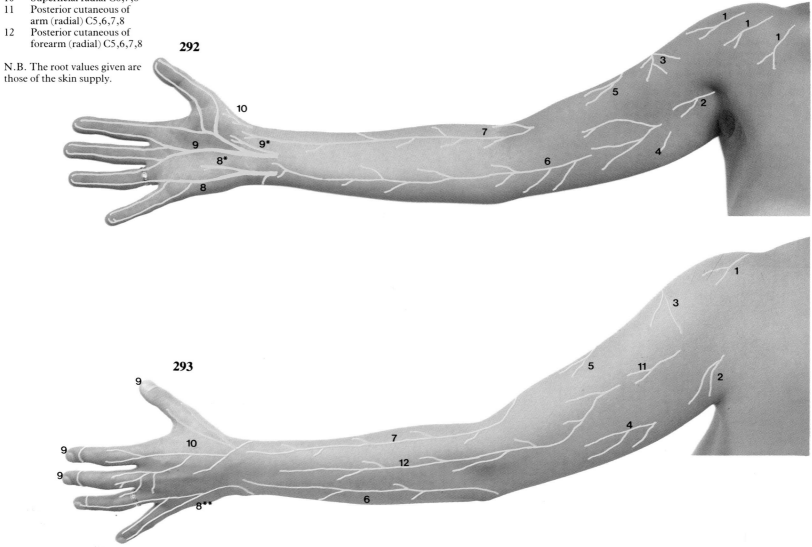

292

293

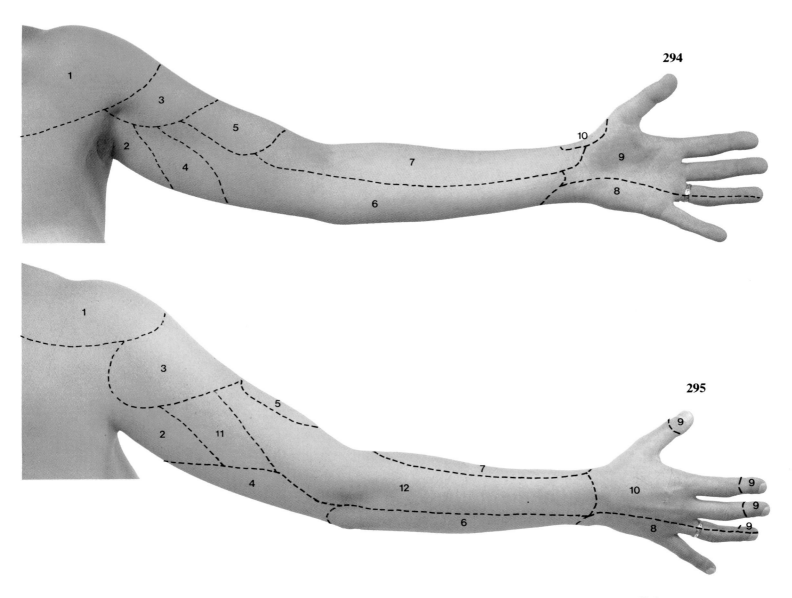

The actual nerves supplying areas of skin (**292–293**) usually have more than one root of supply and therefore the root value of a particular nerve may seem at variance with the dermatomal map (**294–295**). However it should be remembered that although a nerve may carry neurones from several roots, they do not all supply the whole area supplied by the nerve. Furthermore although the map of areas of supply looks clear this is an average and overall picture in which there is enormous variation and particularly overlap. For instance medial or lateral cutaneous nerves of the forearm may be taken for nerve grafts to repair a much more important nerve, such as the median. After removal of the sensory nerve there may be an area of total sensory loss (rarely approaching that shown on the map), whereas in others there may be virtually no area of total loss, most of the skin retaining some protective sensibility due to overlap of supply from adjoining nerves.

NERVES OF THE ARM AND HAND

As the *medial and lateral cutaneous nerves of the forearm* are used on occasions for grafts it is useful to be able to find them easily. The medial nerve is a direct branch from the medial cord of the brachial plexus and runs down the arm in the groove between biceps and triceps, and to the medial side of the brachial artery in company with the ulnar nerve. It becomes superficial usually by passing through the same fascial opening through which the basilic vein runs deep, a site which may be visible in a slim person with good veins. The lateral cutaneous nerve of the forearm is the continuation of the musculocutaneous nerve, running from between biceps and brachialis to become superficial at about the same level as the median nerve (about two-thirds of the way down the arm) and then crosses deep to the median cubital vein close to its junction with the cephalic vein.

Whereas the sensory dermatomes remain relatively simple in the limbs, the motor supply is more complicated. However, as a general rule it can be said that most muscles receive innervation from more than one root; usually two and sometimes three. In the arm the proximal muscles are innervated by the upper roots of the brachial plexus with the lower roots running distally. Thus deltoid is supplied by C5 and 6 whilst the small muscles of the hand are innervated by T1 with some contribution from C8.

The nerves given off from the roots and trunks of the brachial plexus have been noted when considering their muscles of supply. The *axillary nerve* (C5 and 6) has been noted in relation to deltoid, its major muscle of supply (with teres minor). This nerve runs from the posterior cord of the brachial plexus behind the neck of the humerus some four fingers' breadths below the acromion. Here it is vulnerable from fractures of the neck of the humerus and sometimes from dislocation of the shoulder joint. As it would be most undesirable to ask the patient to abduct the arm to test for activity in deltoid, in such an injury, an examination of the sensory area of supply over the lower part of deltoid can give satisfactory evidence of the nerve's functioning (**297**).

1 Radial
2 Median
3 Ulnar
3* Posterior branch of ulnar

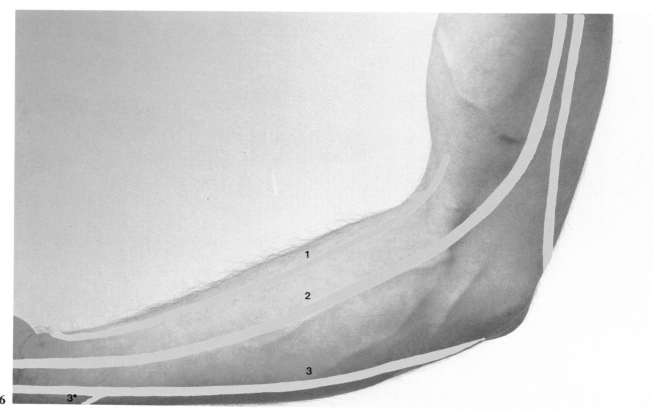

296

The *musculocutaneous nerve* (C5–7) leaves the lateral cord of the brachial plexus usually in the axilla to enter coracobrachialis and supply this muscle and then biceps and brachialis, as it runs between them, before continuing as the lateral cutaneous nerve of the forearm. Loss of the nerve will mean loss of all the three muscles, two of which are powerful elbow flexors. However the movement can still be maintained quite strongly through brachioradialis with help from pronator teres. Loss of the cutaneous supply may only be obvious from a narrow strip along the radial border of the forearm as far as the radial styloid (though the nerve may replace the radial nerve over the thumb metacarpal) (**296**).

The radial nerve, C(5), 6, 7, 8 and (T1), is the continuation of the posterior cord of the brachial plexus. It runs around behind the radius in the spiral radial groove, where, being close to the bone it is vulnerable in fractures of the middle of the shaft of the bone. If the nerve is cut at this site the supply to triceps (and anconeus) should remain intact as their branches leave the trunk above this level. However brachioradialis as well as all the extensors of the wrist and the long extensors of the fingers will lose their innervation, with dropping of the wrist when the hand is held in a pronated position (**298**).

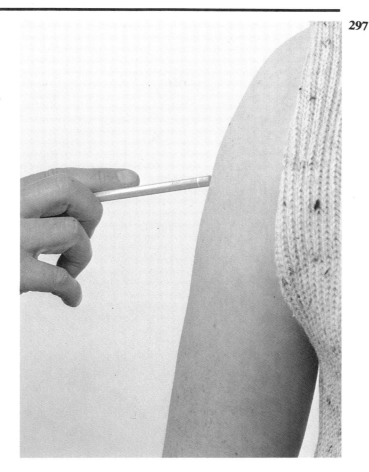

297

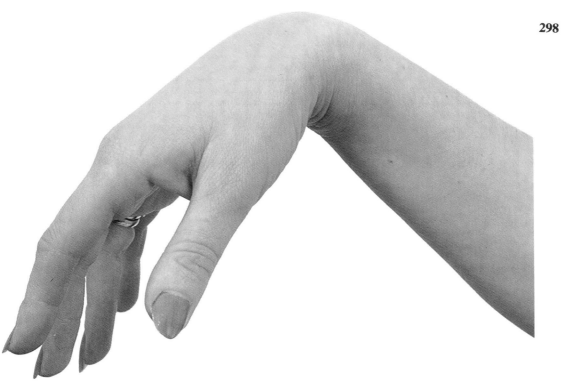

298

NERVES OF THE ARM AND HAND

The posterior cutaneous nerve of the forearm is given off before the radial nerve enters the groove in about half the cases and in the groove in the others. Thus loss of this nerve will depend on its origin. The radial nerve runs anteriorly through the lateral intermuscular septum into the anterior compartment about a third of the distance above the elbow. Here it enters the space between brachioradialis and brachialis before running deep to brachioradialis and extensor carpi radialis longus, both of which it supplies, then dividing into its two main branches.

The posterior interosseous nerve carries the motor fibres from the radial nerve and runs through supinator (which it supplies) and around the radius to supply all the remaining extensor muscles.

In 60% of cases the nerve lies on the radius after leaving supinator, where it may be vulnerable to fracture of the bone. In such a case there will be a wrist drop as in a more proximal radial nerve lesion, but brachioradialis and extensor carpi radialis longus will be intact. The superficial radial nerve is purely sensory and continues distally under cover of brachioradialis before winding onto the back of the radius (where it may be damaged in fractures). It then runs over the tendons of abductor pollicis longus and extensor pollicis brevis (where again it may be damaged or caught up in scars) to supply the back of the hand. However, due to overlap in innervation, loss of the nerve may leave only a small area of total sensory loss between the first and second metacarpals, i.e. over the first dorsal interosseous muscle.

The ulnar nerve leaves the medial cord of the brachial plexus containing C8 and T1 fibres but picks up some C7 fibres, usually by a connecting branch from the lateral cord, to go mainly to flexor carpi ulnaris. It runs down the arm fairly superficially, and is therefore somewhat vulnerable to external injury and compression. Here it lies initially between coracobrachialis and triceps and then medial to biceps, with the brachial artery, before going backwards through the medial intermuscular septum, distal to the insertion of coracobrachialis, to lie on the medial head of triceps from whence it runs behind the medial epicondyle of the humerus. Here it lies in a tunnel (cubital) created by the bone and the overlying heads of flexor carpi ulnaris, where it can be damaged by fractures of the bone, direct injury against the bone (the funny-bone) or compression by the overlying fibrous arch of flexor carpi ulnaris (cubital tunnel syndrome). Occasionally these overlying fibres are deficient, allowing the nerve to flick around the prominent epicondyle, which can produce the same unpleasant sensation as hitting the 'funny-bone' but here only on movement of the elbow.

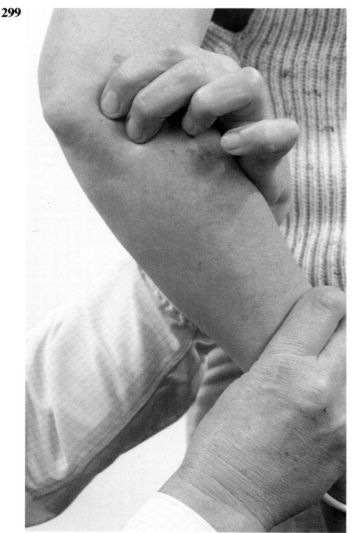

299

The head of the radius lies between the index and middle fingers. If the other two fingers were placed alongside, the little finger would overlie the posterior interosseous nerve. This is also an excellent site for electrical stimulation of the nerve.

300

At the elbow the ulnar nerve can often be palpated as it lies above and in the cubital tunnel.

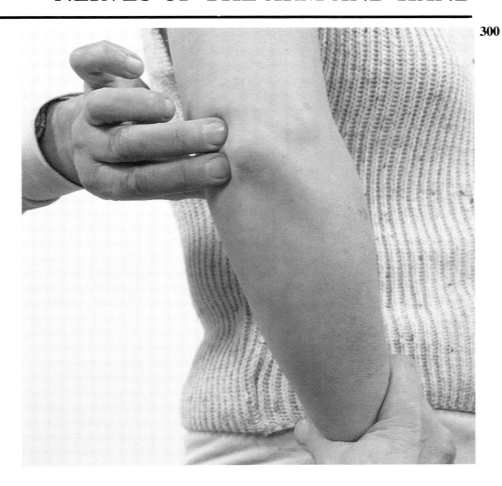

Just above the elbow the ulnar nerve is readily accessible for anaesthetic nerve block if required, or for electrical stimulation.

301

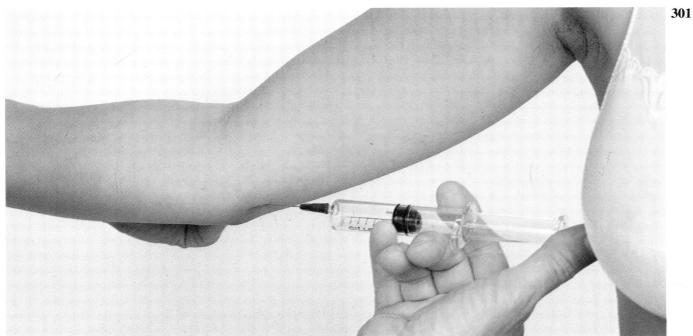

NERVES OF THE ARM AND HAND

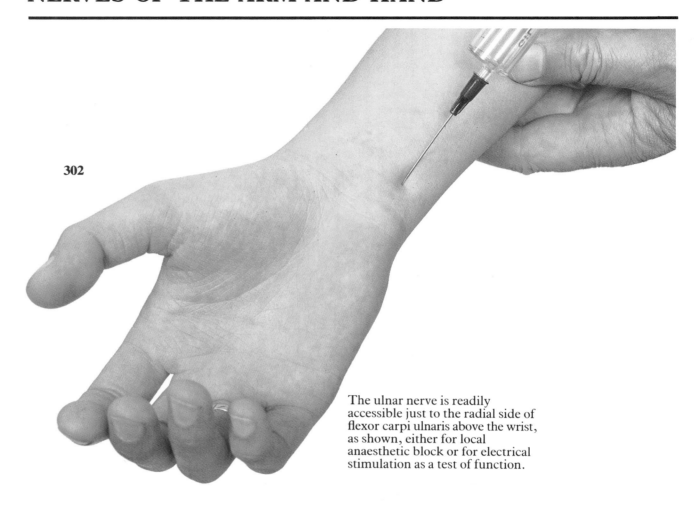

302

The ulnar nerve is readily accessible just to the radial side of flexor carpi ulnaris above the wrist, as shown, either for local anaesthetic block or for electrical stimulation as a test of function.

It should be noted that the branches to the forearm muscles (flexor carpi ulnaris and the ulnar half of flexor digitorum profundus) all leave the nerve in the upper quarter of the forearm while a branch to the elbow joint and sometimes one to flexor carpi ulnaris can arise above the joint. The nerve then runs on deep to flexor carpi ulnaris and on the surface of flexor digitorum profundus. It gives off a dorsal branch which winds around the ulna about 2–3 in above its styloid, to give sensory supply to the back of the ulnar one and a half digits (as far as the distal interphalangeal joint).

The ulnar nerve then runs to the radial side of the tendon of flexor carpi ulnaris and superficial to the flexor retinaculum where it is tucked in close to the radial side of the pisiform bone, though covered by a fascial arch and, most importantly, palmaris brevis, which gives it protection from external pressure, particularly

in a power grip (see page 146). The ulnar artery is to the radial side of the nerve.

Just beyond the pisiform, it divides into superficial and deep branches. The superficial branch runs on after supplying palmaris brevis, dividing to send the important sensory branch to the ulnar border of the little finger and a branch to the adjoining sides of the ring and little fingers, including the nail-bearing areas of the dorsum.

The deep branch runs close to the hook of the hamate (where it can be compressed, see **208**), supplying the hypothenar muscles, all the interossei and the adductor pollicis brevis and commonly the deep head of flexor pollicis brevis. The ulnar nerve also supplies the two lumbricals arising from the tendons of flexor digitorum profundus to the ring and little fingers which it also supplies.

Loss of the ulnar nerve can readily be tested by sensory examination of the area of supply in the hand, which unlike other sensory nerves in the arm has a fairly sharp separation from the area supplied by the median. Sometimes the ulnar nerve supplies rather more of the hand – two or two and a half fingers at the expense of the median nerve but this is usually due to a local crossover from one nerve to the other in the forearm or the hand. The characteristic appearance of loss of the ulnar nerve is clawing of the ring and little fingers and sometimes to a smaller extent of the index and middle (**303**). This is due to total loss of the intrinsic muscles of the ulnar two fingers but the lumbricals remain to balance the long muscles of the other fingers and give interphalangeal extension.

If the hyperextension at the metacarpophalangeal joints of the clawed fingers is prevented, as shown, the long extensors can then pull through to extend the interphalangeal joints (**304**).

Tests for the ulnar nerve can be directed to the individual muscles supplied but the most usual is to test the interossei as shown in **291**, page 169. However the thumb to little finger test is a good and rapid routine test for both ulnar and median nerves. This tests not only the ulnar innervated hypothenar muscles but also flexor carpi ulnaris.

It should be appreciated that loss of the ulnar nerve makes the oblique power grip impossible, the obliquity of action being due entirely to ulnar innervated muscle.

303

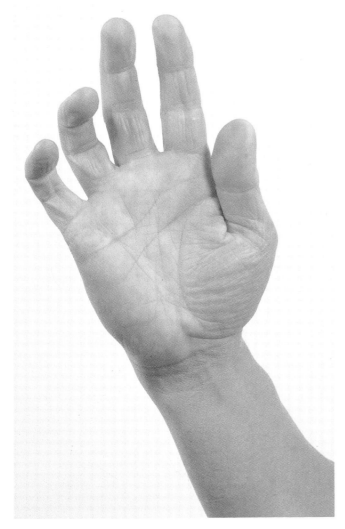

304

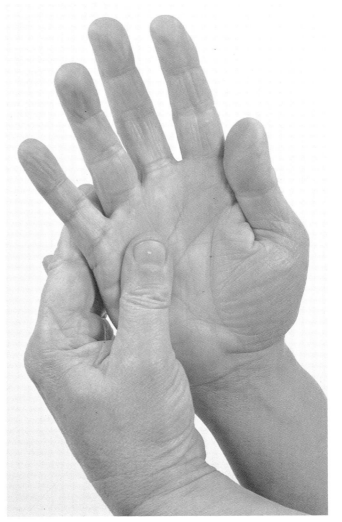

NERVES OF THE ARM AND HAND

The median nerve (C5, 6, 7, 8 and T1) is the joined termination of the lateral and medial cords of the brachial plexus in, or a little below, the axilla, and forming on the front of the brachial artery. The nerve and artery run down medial to coracobrachialis and then biceps to the elbow. Passing under the bicipital aponeurosis, it then runs under the arch of the two heads of pronator teres and then flexor digitorum superficialis (both possible compression sites), supplying both muscles. The nerve is readily accessible for electrical stimulation, either in the upper arm medial to biceps, or in the cubital fossa, before running deep.

Within the forearm, the median nerve gives off the anterior interosseous nerve, some 2–3 cm (1 in) distal to the medial epicondyle, to supply flexor pollicis longus, flexor digitorum profundus (to the index and middle fingers) and pronator quadratus. Branches of supply to palmaris longus and flexor carpi radialis come from the main nerve.

In the forearm the median nerve is bound to the deep surface of flexor digitorum superficialis by its investing fascia and then runs laterally to lie between, and deep to, the tendons of palmaris longus and flexor carpi radialis at the wrist. Here it is readily accessible for local anaesthetic block or electrical stimulation (**305**).

The nerve then runs under the flexor retinaculum in the line of the proximal part of the thenar crease.

Here it can become compressed, the carpal tunnel syndrome, usually by thickening of the synovial sheaths of the underlying tendons, particularly flexors pollicis longus and digitorum profundus, pushing the nerve against the firmly resistant flexor retinaculum.

A clinically important branch in the forearm is the small palmar branch, which leaves the main nerve about 5–6 cm (2–2½ in) above the wrist, and following the line of flexor carpi radialis runs superficially over the heel of the hand into the palm (**306**). Here it is vulnerable and if cut, although the sensory loss is insignificant, the pain if a neuroma forms at this point can be intolerable.

305

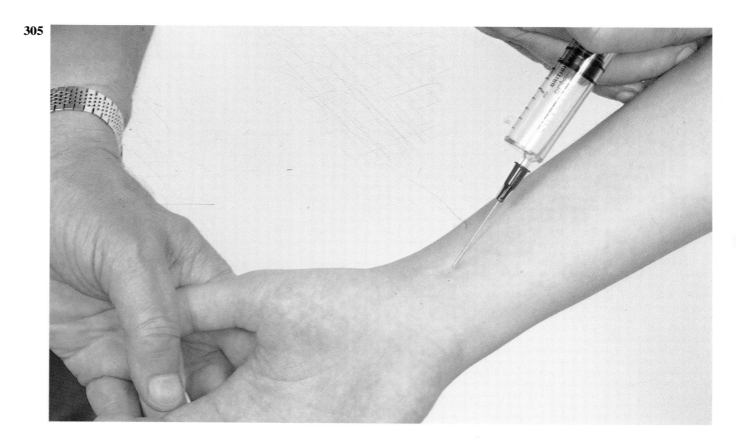

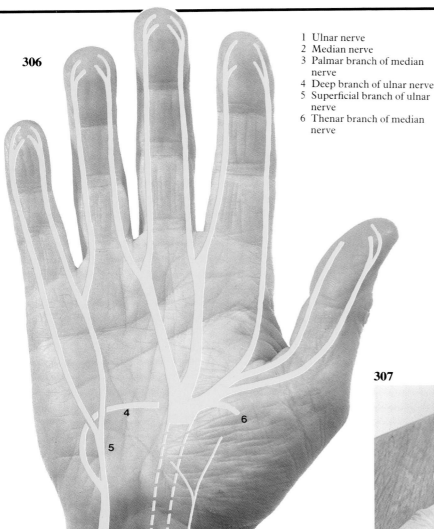

306

1 Ulnar nerve
2 Median nerve
3 Palmar branch of median nerve
4 Deep branch of ulnar nerve
5 Superficial branch of ulnar nerve
6 Thenar branch of median nerve

common 'trigger' thumb, where it is vulnerable at surgery or from open wounds. As in the case of the ulnar nerve the palmar sensory branches also supply the nail-bearing area on the dorsum of the fingers.

Loss of the median nerve is the most serious of any in the arm, for it supplies two wrist flexors, the main digital flexion and opposition of the thumb together with the necessary sensory supply of the precision acting and main sensory digits. For this reason in severe injury with only the ulnar nerve remaining this could well be transferred to link with the median where possible. Loss of the whole median nerve is obvious but partial loss can be assessed by examining for reduced sensibility in the median nerve area and for reduction in power of abduction of the thumb (**307**). These tests can be particularly useful in clinical assessment of nerve compression though electrodiagnostic techniques are more reliable.

307

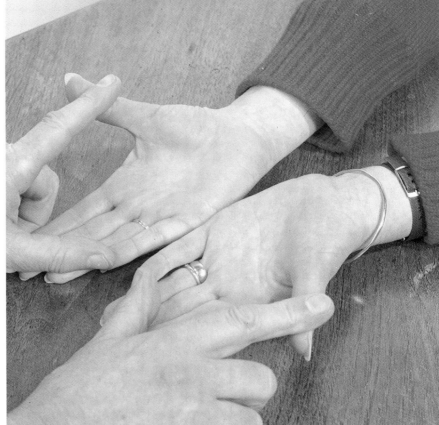

Towards the end of the carpal tunnel the thenar branch leaves the front of the nerve (unusually from the radial side as commonly described) to supply the thenar muscles. This branch usually leaves the tunnel to run back into the thenar region but often runs through the retinaculum. Then the median nerve divides into its terminal four branches; one to the radial side of the thumb and one each to the adjoining sides of the thumb and index, index and middle and middle and ring digits. It is worthy of note that the branch to the radial side of the thumb runs across the flexion crease of the metacarpophalangeal joint directly over the site of the

308

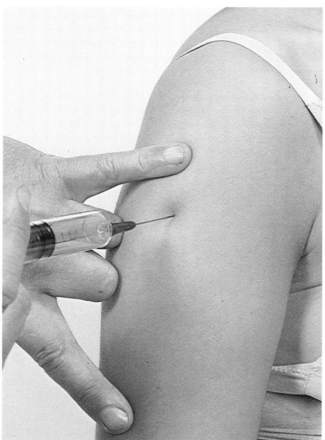

On occasions it is necessary to give injections while avoiding nerves. One site commonly used for intermuscular injection is deltoid. On the lateral side of the arm major nerves are easy to avoid (**308**).

Injections of steroids are commonly given to reduce inflammatory reaction in cases of carpal tunnel compression. Here it is vital to avoid both the median and ulnar nerves (and also not to inject the material into tendons). The injection can be given in the region of flexor digitorum superficialis, not more than 1 cm medial to palmaris longus (if present). Here it will be between the two nerves, and the injecting needle can then be eased deep to the median nerve for the maximal effect of the injection on the underlying synovial membranes (**309**).

The axillary nerve runs four fingers' breadths below the acromion but only its terminal branches reach the lateral side while the radial nerve comes to the lateral side two thirds of the way to the elbow. These sites are marked by the fingers and so the injection can be safely given into deltoid as shown.

309

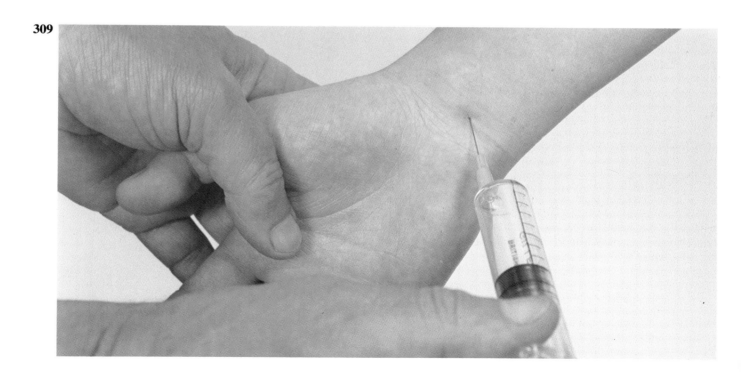

THE ARTERIES OF THE ARM AND HAND

The main arterial supply to the arm comes from the single axial axillary and later named brachial artery (**310**). This may make the arm appear vulnerable to accidental loss or disease of this artery but fortunately a good anastomosis around the shoulder region (and around other joints) usually gives a good enough supply for survival of the limb under good conditions. Fortunately, good vascular graft techniques now are available to improve the chances of good function as well as survival in many cases.

As described in the section describing the axilla (page 105) the artery runs down in the groove between triceps and coracobrachialis and then biceps to reach the antecubital fossa. In the arm, it can be felt pulsating, if it is pressed against the humerus and this manoeuvre also permits control of arterial bleeding in an emergency.

As the biceps narrows to its tendon the artery stays close to its medial border and passes under the bicipital aponeurosis, which separates it from the more superficial median cubital vein. Here about the centre of the forearm, the stethoscope can be placed over the artery when measuring blood pressure by a sphygmomanometer.

About the level of the neck of the radius, the artery divides into its radial and ulnar branches. The radial artery continues across the insertion of the tendon of biceps, to curve down under the cover of brachioradialis, to become superficial again to the medial side of its tendon in the lower third of the forearm. Here it lies between the tendon of flexor carpi radialis and brachioradialis and then the radial styloid, on the surface of pronator quadratus, and then the radius itself. Here the radial pulse is readily palpable (**311**).

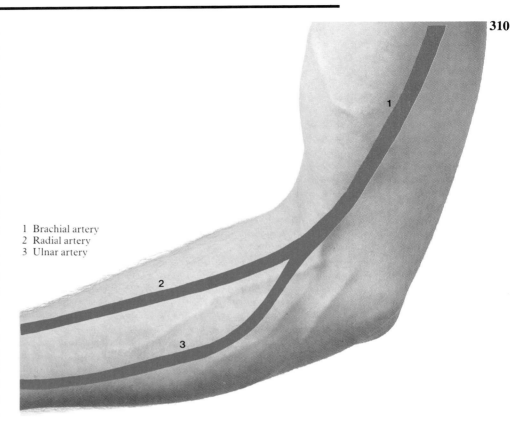

310

1 Brachial artery
2 Radial artery
3 Ulnar artery

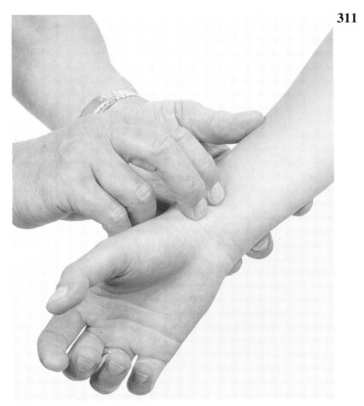

311

312

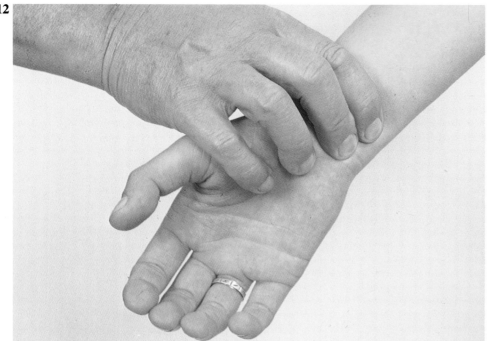

the radial artery which runs through or superficial to the thenar muscles. The superficial arch gives the major supply to the fingers via the digital arteries. Although a superficial arch between the two arteries is a standard anatomical description, it is important clinically to realise that the full arch occurs in only some 36% of cases and that the ulnar artery is the prime artery of supply to the superficial tissues of the hand in most cases. Anastomosis occurs between the deep and superficial systems but this is variable, and through this anastomosis the radial artery can sometimes play a major role in supply.

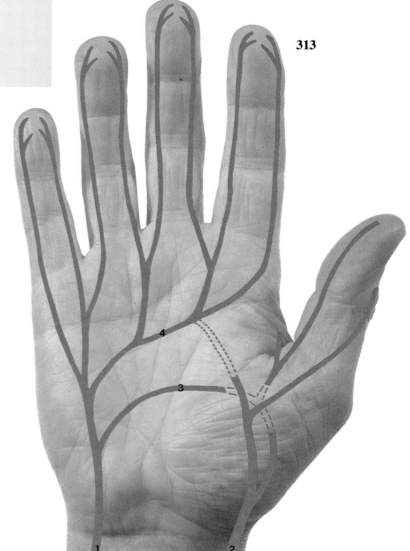

313

The artery then runs round under abductor pollicis longus and extensor pollicis brevis, in the floor of the anatomical 'snuffbox', on the surface of the scaphoid and trapezium. Then, running under extensor pollicis longus, it winds around the thumb base between the two heads of the first dorsal interosseous muscle and adductor pollicis, to enter the deep part of the palm, where it joins the deep branch of the ulna, to form the deep palmar arch.

The ulnar artery runs distally more deeply placed, under the cover of the superficial flexor muscles, which it supplies, together with its interosseous branches. It comes superficial again in the distal quarter of the forearm between the tendons of flexor carpi ulnaris and flexor digitorum superficialis, where its pulse can be felt (**312**).

The artery then runs with the ulnar nerve close to the radial side of the pisiform bone, before dividing into superficial and deep branches (**313**). The deep branch runs with the deep branch of the ulnar nerve to join the radial artery in the deep palmar arch, which lies at the level of the forcibly outstretched thumb and with the distal edge of the flexor retinaculum. The superficial branch runs on to arch across the palm just proximal to the proximal palmar crease. Here it may join a superficial branch of

THE ARTERIES OF THE ARM AND HAND

Allen's test has been devised to give a quick clinical indication of relative values in supply (**314–316**). The fingers are compressed into the palm as firmly as possible to drive the blood out of the superficial tissues. Firm pressure is then exerted over each artery in turn at the wrist so as to stop blood flow through that artery. The response in the palm is then noted when the hand is opened. Rapid flushing occurs if the free artery gives the major blood supply but the palm will remain white if the still compressed artery is of prime importance. In this case the radial artery gives an important supply to the superficial tissues.

As a general, but by no means reliable, rule the ulnar artery is the prime one for supply to the hand. With the advent of microsurgical techniques an area of full thickness skin and subcutaneous tissues with its axial blood supply may be valuable for an area of tissue loss. If then the radial artery is found to be subsidiary in a person in need of such a graft, then the artery, its venae commitantes and the overlying skin, which is supplied by several branches from the artery, can be taken for a free graft. If need be, the superficial radial nerve and even part of the radius can be incorporated into the graft, all supported on the section of radial vessels which are anastomosed with vessels of the new site. The radial area can then be covered by a split skin graft.

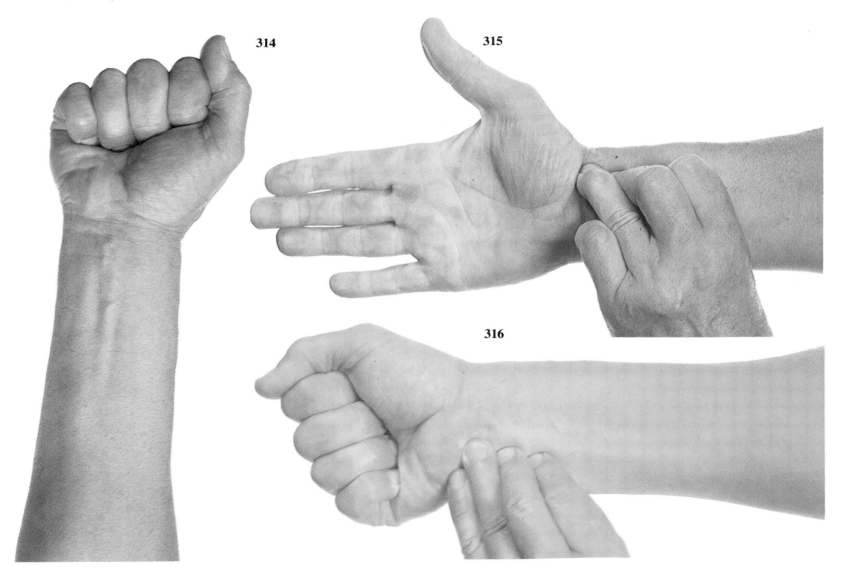

314

315

316

THE VEINS OF THE ARM AND HAND

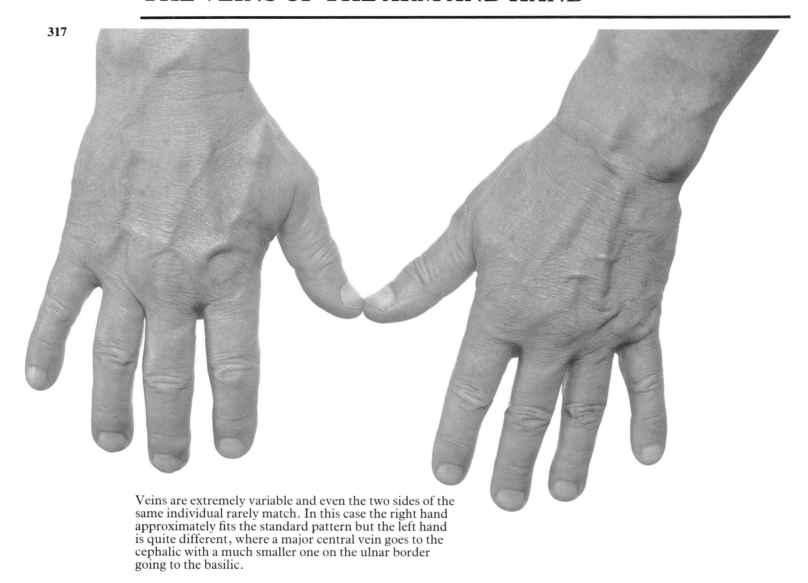

Veins are extremely variable and even the two sides of the same individual rarely match. In this case the right hand approximately fits the standard pattern but the left hand is quite different, where a major central vein goes to the cephalic with a much smaller one on the ulnar border going to the basilic.

Whereas the limbs are supplied initially by single axial arteries, major venous drainage in both arms and legs is taken superficially through two veins. In the arm these are the cephalic (i.e. to the head side if the arm is put out to the side) and the basilic veins. Also, as the veins run superficially, they are often readily visible from the surface in a slim person.

The arteries in the forearm and hand run with small venae commitantes in the palmar aspect but the major veins, with the lymphatics, leave the hand on the back. A venous plexus forms around the back of each digital joint forming into digital veins on each side of the

digit. Those of adjoining fingers unite to run in the gutter between the metacarpal heads onto the back of the hand where they most commonly join a dorsal venous arch, whose two limbs run to each side of the forearm to form the cephalic and basilic veins (317).

The basilic vein usually runs around the ulnar border of the arm and up anterior to the medial epicondyle, where it is joined by the median cubital vein from the cephalic. It then runs in the medial bicipital groove before running deep through the fascia where it links with the venae commitantes of the brachial artery to form, collectively, the axillary vein. The cephalic

THE VEINS OF THE ARM AND HAND

vein runs over the anatomical 'snuff box' and up the radial side of the arm to the cubital fossa where the median cubital vein links it with the basilic (**318**). It then continues over the lateral side of biceps to reach the groove between deltoid and pectoralis major, the deltopectoral groove, before piercing the clavipectoral fascia of the infraclavicular fossa to enter the axillary vein.

Traditionally the median cubital vein has been the one of choice for venepuncture as it is usually large, easy to find, even in a fat person, and fairly fixed in position (**318–319**). However, in modern practice the veins on the back of the hand offer many advantages for anaesthesia and infusions, without risk to the brachial artery.

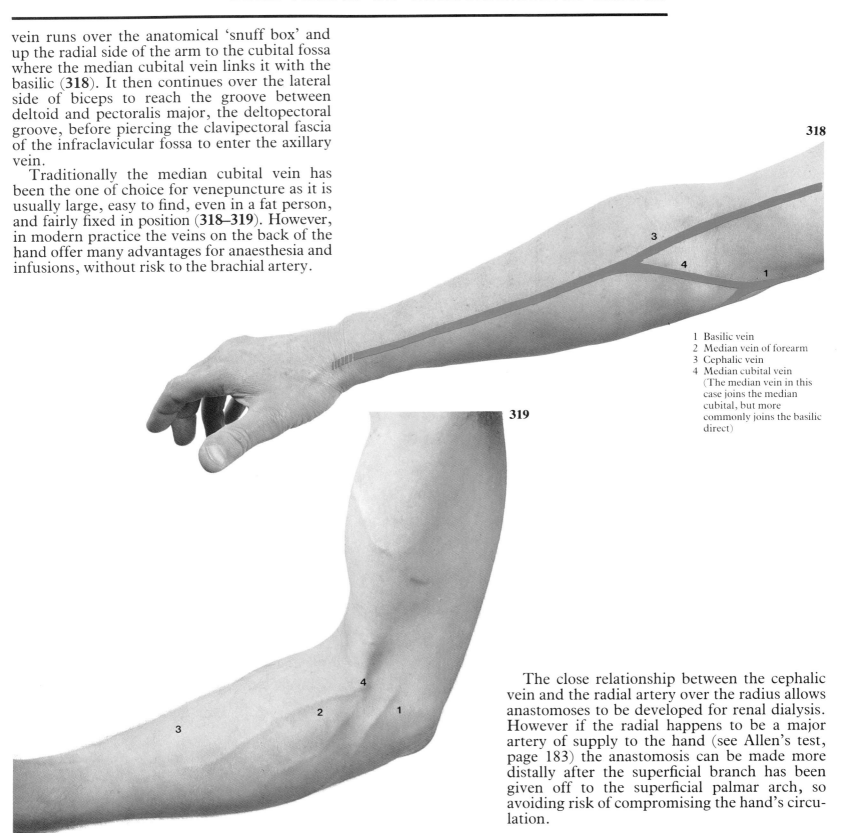

318

1 Basilic vein
2 Median vein of forearm
3 Cephalic vein
4 Median cubital vein
(The median vein in this case joins the median cubital, but more commonly joins the basilic direct)

319

The close relationship between the cephalic vein and the radial artery over the radius allows anastomoses to be developed for renal dialysis. However if the radial happens to be a major artery of supply to the hand (see Allen's test, page 183) the anastomosis can be made more distally after the superficial branch has been given off to the superficial palmar arch, so avoiding risk of compromising the hand's circulation.

THE RETINACULA AND SYNOVIAL SHEATHS OF THE HAND

The tendons in the hand must operate around angles, sometimes quite sharp, as in the fully flexed finger. They therefore need retaining in the form of the hand to prevent 'bow-stringing'. This is particularly important in the fingers, for only a few millimetres of stretch in the retaining bands will reduce the range of digital flexion enormously. As the tendons run around retaining bands they are subject to friction and therefore synovial sheaths are provided for their lubrication (**320**).

At the wrist, the flexor retinaculum is attached to the four carpal bones, pisiform and hook of hamate on the ulnar side and the tubercles of the scaphoid and trapezium on the radial (see page 125), some 3 cm in length and in width from the distal wrist crease to the extent of the thenar muscles (arising from it) and the forcibly outstretched thumb, i.e. some 4 cm (1½ in). The distal edge is roughly level with the deep transverse arterial arch and the deep branch of the ulna artery (see page 182).

The flexor tendons in the fingers run through fibrous flexor sheaths, strong over the bones but thin, for freedom at the joints. The proximal band, derived from the superficial transverse metacarpal ligament, is at the metacarpal heads, at the distal palmar crease, whilst other bands are related to the proximal and middle phalanges.

Whereas the flexor retinaculum is bound to

320

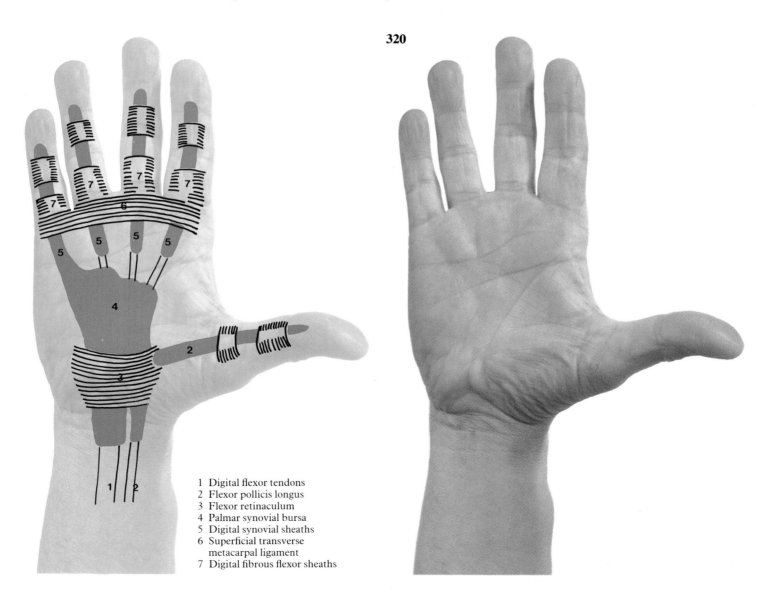

1 Digital flexor tendons
2 Flexor pollicis longus
3 Flexor retinaculum
4 Palmar synovial bursa
5 Digital synovial sheaths
6 Superficial transverse
  metacarpal ligament
7 Digital fibrous flexor sheaths

THE RETINACULA AND SYNOVIAL SHEATHS OF THE HAND

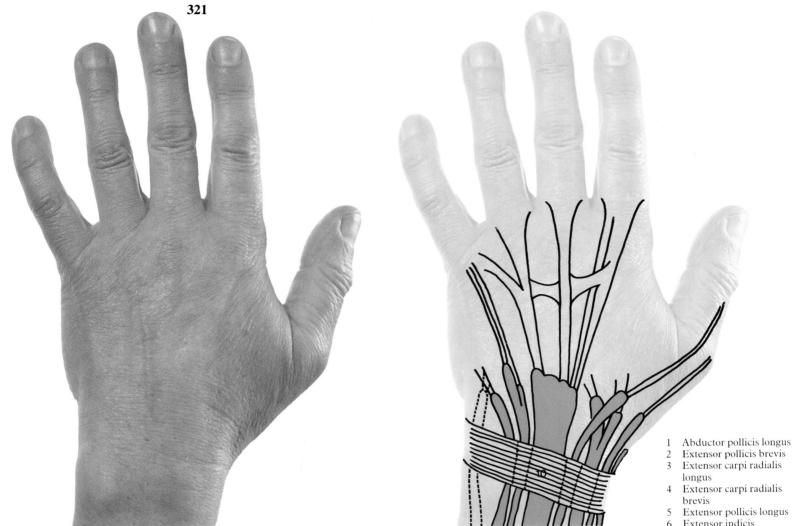

321

1	Abductor pollicis longus
2	Extensor pollicis brevis
3	Extensor carpi radialis longus
4	Extensor carpi radialis brevis
5	Extensor pollicis longus
6	Extensor indicis
7	Extensor digitorum communis
8	Extensor digiti minimi
9	Extensor carpi ulnaris in supination
9*	Extensor carpi ulnaris in pronation
10	Extensor retinaculum

the carpal bones, to form a single tunnel plus a separate deep one for flexor carpi radialis, the extensor retinaculum consists of separate fibro-osseous tunnels over the distal 3 cm (1 in) or so of the radius plus a sling around and beyond the ulna for extensor carpi ulnaris.

The synovial sheaths are designed to lubricate the tendons as they run under the retinacular system and extend as far as is needed for the tendon's range of movement. The descriptions normally given are for the hand in the extended state and therefore will vary with movement. Thus the sheaths on the flexor tendons will move proximally on flexion while those on the extensor tendons will move distally.

Under the flexor retinaculum, the synovial sheaths extend from the proximal wrist crease. Flexor carpi radialis has its own sheath extending to its insertion. Flexor pollicis longus likewise has a separate sheath through to its insertion. The digital tendons are usually said to be enclosed in a single bursa extending approximately to the proximal palmar crease, but the tendons to the little finger have an extension from this to their insertion. Those to the other fingers have separate digital sheaths which run distally from the distal palmar crease.

The dorsal sheaths extend to about a third of the way along the metacarpals from some 3–4 cm (1½ in) proximal to the wrist joint (**321**).

THE BACK

The axial skeleton is an important feature of the back, in that the spines of the vertebrae lie in a relatively superficial position. However, for all the axial role of the vertebral column, the vertebrae only lie in a relatively axial position in the neck and lumbar regions. The body of L3 is about the centre of the trunk in a reasonably slim person. In the thorax the vertebrae are placed dorsally to allow space for the heart and lungs and in the sacral region for the birth canal of the female. Thus the vertebral column shows its characteristic curves; kyphoses, that is concave anteriorly in the thoracic and sacral regions and lordoses, concave posteriorly, in the cervical and lumbar regions. As the kyphotic curve is that of the fetus in the uterus, these are known as primary curves while a lordosis is a reactive or secondary curve, to allow for straightening of the trunk after birth. It will be evident that the curved nature of the spine reduces its efficiency as an axial skeleton, as in certain places the vertebrae must be lying obliquely to the vertebral axis of the body. This is particularly important in the lower lumbar region where in the change over from the lumbar lordosis to the sacrum the body of L5 rests through its intervertebral disc on the sacrum at an angle of some 45°; a slope of 1 in 1.

Lateral curves are often seen to a very minor degree (**322**), probably due to muscular dominance of one side over the other. This type of curve is mobile and easily correctable, whereas a more fixed and less correctable curve is pathological and called a scoliosis.

It should be noted that the curves are more noticeable in the vertebral column than in the soft tissues of the trunk, which in part bridge the curve in the lumbar and cervical regions.

Of the seven cervical vertebrae, the spines are not generally easily felt. C2 (the axis) has a large palpable spine but as those of the lower vertebrae are shorter and linked by the ligamentum nuchae, the next prominent one is that of C7 the so-called vertebra prominens. It should be noted however that it is only the most prominent cervical vertebra, as the first thoracic spine is more prominent still (**323**).

322

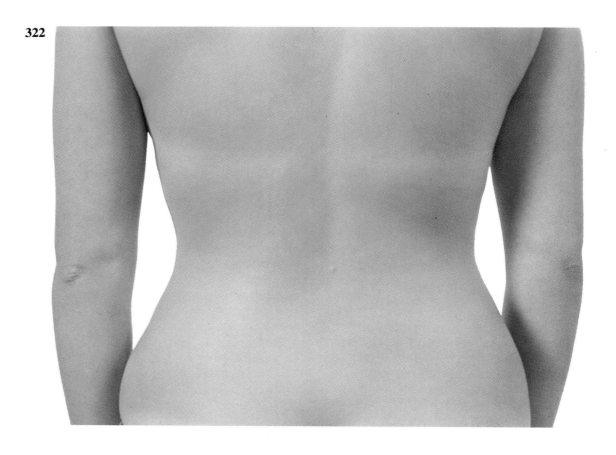

The examining finger can be run down the neck to the vertebra prominens, thence to T1 when it is possible to count down to L4.

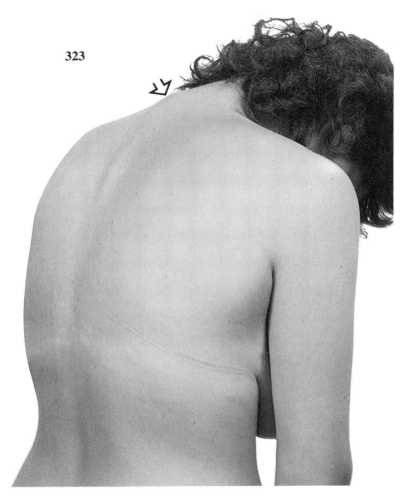

323

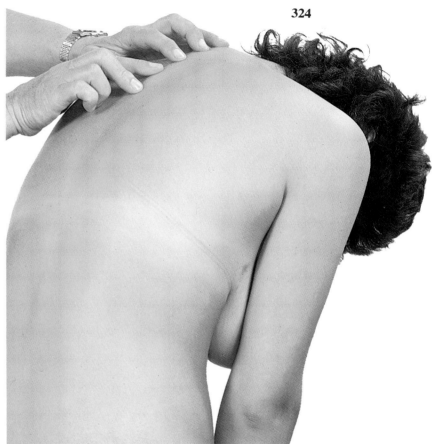

324

Of the twelve thoracic vertebrae, those after T1 have long spines which point downwards, so that the spine of a typical thoracic vertebra is level with the body of the one below. So marked is this that if an epidural or spinal needle is to be inserted into the thoracic region, it has to be pointed upwards at an angle of some 45–60°. The eleventh and twelfth spines become heavier and point more directly backwards as do the 5 heavy lumbar spines.

In upright posture most vertebral spines are not obvious, being sunk between the erector spinae muscles in the cervical and lumbar regions, though more prominent in the thoracic and sacral regions.

As the thoracic spines run downwards, are joined by thick supraspinous ligaments and covered by fairly thick skin, they are not easy to examine individually. If, however, the person is asked to bend forwards the spines project much more and can be counted down from C7 (**324**).

An alternative is to count from below, as a line joining the iliac crests crosses the spine of L4. This fact also helps to establish the site of a lumbar puncture should this be needed (**325**).

THE BACK

Lumbar puncture – From time to time it is important to examine the cerebrospinal fluid or administer a spinal anaesthetic. As the spinal cord only reaches to the level of the lower border of L1 and even in a newborn child to L3, whilst the subarachnoid space extends to about S2 it is possible to pass a needle into the space with relative safety. The patient must have the spine fully flexed to open the intervertebral space and be either lying on the side or sitting (**325**).

In the thoracic region the scapulae overlie the posterior chest wall, covering the 1–7 ribs. The spine of the scapula should be readily palpable level with the 3rd vertebral spine (body of T4), with the scapula in the resting state. The inferior angle likewise should be palpable level with T8 spine (T9 body). Below the scapula, the ribs should be palpable but not close to the vertebrae where they are covered by the thick erector spinae muscles. In view of this the twelfth rib may be impalpable if short.

The fifth lumbar vertebra and sacrum lie somewhat deep with the posterior part of the ilium projecting behind the sacrum on each side. The posterior iliac spines are usually easily found, even in an obese person, being commonly overlaid by a dimple in the skin (**326**).

325

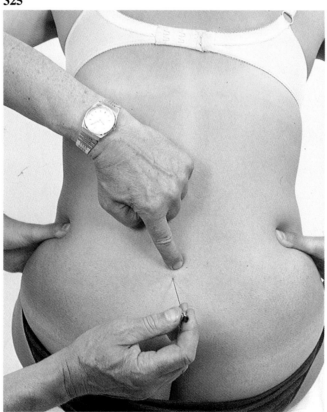

326

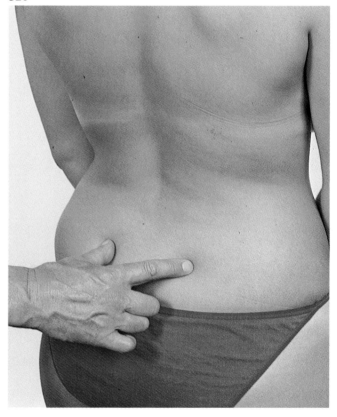

The subject's hands are pressing down above the iliac crests to identify them and from a line drawn across, the spine of L4 has been marked, the examiner's finger resting on its lower edge. The needle can be passed either above or below this spine (below in this case). After local anaesthetising of the skin, the needle goes in the mid-line at right angles to the surface, through the supraspinous and interspinous ligaments and the ligamentum flavum and dura, when a release of resistance indicates entry of the space. If the stylus is withdrawn from the needle a clear fluid should drip out (if normal) confirming the tip is within the space.

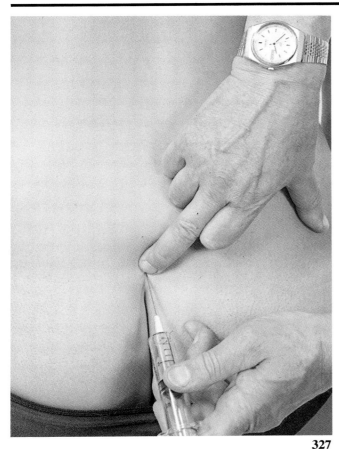

327

The finger has identified the hiatus and the anaesthetic needle is pointed upwards and forwards at about 45°.

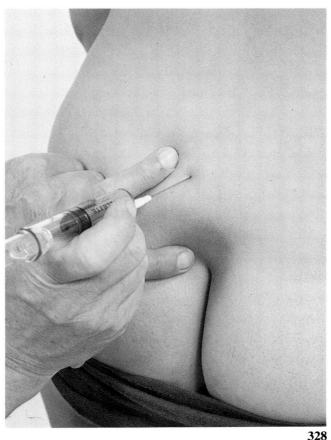

328

The two fingers mark the posterior superior iliac spine and the sacral cornua with the needle directed to S2 foramen.

The tip of the coccyx will be found in the upper part of the natal cleft. Above the coccyx the sacral hiatus should be felt at about the upper margin of the natal cleft. If the finger is moved up from the coccyx, the depression of the hiatus becomes apparent, in a slim person but is less easy to feel with increase in fat. It is important to find the hiatus for caudal or sacral anaesthesia, where the needle is passed up through the hiatus into the extradural space below the spinal cord (**327**).

The hiatus lies between the two sacral cornua where the neural arch is deficient over the fifth sacral piece. (It may extend higher in spina bifida.) As the dural space ends about S2, anaesthetic injected into the extradural space via the hiatus will anaesthetise the sacral and coccygeal nerves after they have left the dural sac.

Although extradural caudal anaesthesia is preferable and easier, occasionally block of the individual sacral nerves is carried out. The posterior superior iliac spine is level with the second sacral spine. The first sacral foramen is about 3 cms (1–1½ in) above the midpoint between these two spines and the second foramen the same distance below (**328**). The lower foramina are on a line sloping inwards from this, with the fourth level with the sacral cornua (i.e. lateral to the hiatus).

MOVEMENTS OF THE BACK

The neck is the most mobile component of the trunk and is responsible for the motility of the head on the trunk. Movements of the trunk itself are much more limited and to a large extent offer a basic positioning for activities of the arms, in standing and sitting. As such, the movements may be under considerable load, as in heavy lifting, and therefore the greater the range of movement the less the effective stability in control. Strength, rather than mobility, of the trunk is also important in movements of the leg due to the leverage and weight stresses imposed by the limb.

Note the considerable range of movement at the hip joints in flexion and permitted by the relatively long hamstring muscles. The back shows flexion in the upper lumbar and lower thoracic regions. In the lower part of the lumbar spine there is flexion from the basic standing position but not enough to obliterate the lumbosacral angle.

329

Movement in the thoracic spine must be directed primarily to thoracic function i.e. respiration and the provision of a firm base for muscle attachment for the arms. Thus in the upper part of the thorax, although the patterns of the intervertebral joints may give the impression of a wide range of movement, this is in effect limited by the ribs and sternum to a small amount of flexion and extension with little lateral flexion; essentially the amount commensurate with the respiratory role. In the lower thoracic region, the arrangement of the more flexible costal cartilages and their joints, together with the free lower 'floating' ribs, allow for greater freedom in the above movements, together with rotation.

The lumbar region allows for a very variable amount of flexion or bending forwards and extension. The movements obviously must start from a basic extended curve of the spine, the lumbar lordosis, and a continuation of this at the lumbosacral joint before the reverse curve takes over in the sacrum. Movement is facilitated by the thick intervertebral discs in the region which act as gelatinous cushions between the vertebrae, but their nature is such to make them vulnerable to rupture, particularly in the two lowest spaces, unless movement is under good control. Flexion is likely to be limited by the abdominal bulk and therefore is usually freer in slimmer individuals. On flexion abdominal bulk tends to push up the diaphragm and reduce respiratory range. Thus in bending forwards, as in touching the toes, the greatest amount of movement takes place at the hip joints with only a small amount in the lumbar (and lower thoracic) spine (**329**).

In extension the freest zone is the lower lumbar region and this can in certain circumstances be aggravated by pelvic leverage. Thus in view of the heavy loading on an already extended (lordotic) spine, this region is especially vulnerable to injury, unless good muscle control is maintained, particularly in the abdominal muscles.

Lateral flexion occurs mainly in the lumbar and lower thoracic regions. The range varies considerably between individuals, particularly in relation to body form. As the limiting factor is the approximation of the rib cage to the iliac crest, the taller slimmer person will have a greater range than a broad stocky individual.

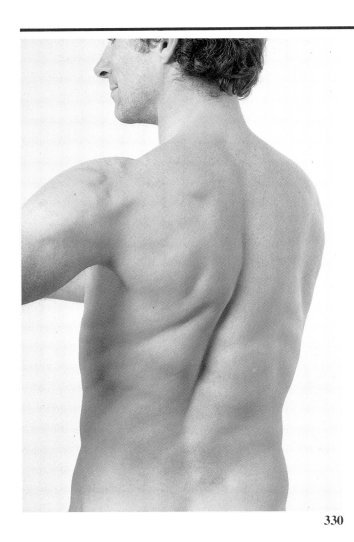

330

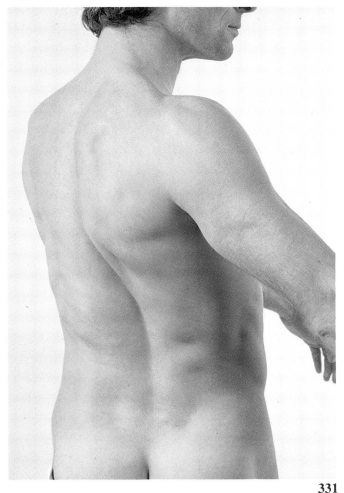

331

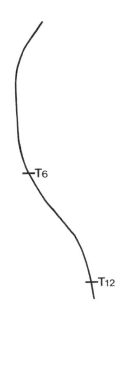

Rotation in the spine can occur in the neck and thoracic regions. The joints of the neural arches largely prevent any rotation in the lumbar region (**330–331**). In the thoracic region, although the vertebral joints theoretically allow rotation throughout, this is limited by the thoracic cage. The sternum acts as a splint for the upper half of the chest. Thus rotation is only possible in the lower half with the maximum in the region of the floating ribs (ie. the last two).

Note, as the trunk is turned to the left and right, an S bend appears in the lower thoracic region. The upper thorax remains without rotation as does the lumbar region. Vertebral levels are shown on the diagram alongside.

Although the fine control of the individual vertebrae comes from the small intervertebral muscles the main power output in trunk rotation comes from the internal and external oblique muscles of the abdomen, the internal oblique of one side acting with the external oblique of the other.

THE THORACIC WALL

The bony skeleton of the thorax is made up of the twelve ribs running around each side of the chest wall, linked at the back to the thoracic vertebrae and the upper ones at the front to the sternum. The thorax is quite narrow superiorly, widening below but the narrowness above is masked by the overlying shoulder girdle and controlling muscles. Thus posteriorly the scapulae and anteriorly the clavicles are, with related muscles, the obvious features from the surface, while the shoulders give the breadth to the chest region.

Anteriorly the clavicle overlies the short flattened but highly curved first rib, so that this rib is normally impalpable. Its costal cartilage links it directly to the upper and outer angle of the manubrium sterni just below the sternoclavicular joint. If the clavicle is raised at the shoulder, the first rib becomes palpable just below its medial third.

The sternum consists of two bony components; the broader, shorter manubrium above and the longer narrower body below. Extending a short way below that, in the divergence of the costal cartilages, is the short, usually cartilaginous xiphisternum.

The upper edge of the manubrium forms the lower border of the suprasternal notch of the neck. The lower border, having a secondary cartilaginous joint with the sternum, can be felt as a transverse ridge, some 4 cms (1½ in) below. Since the manubrium slopes somewhat compared with the more vertical sternum, the joint between the two is described as the sternal angle (of Louis, **332**).

The second costal cartilage articulates with both manubrium and sternum, by synovial joints, at the manubriosternal joint. However, as the ribs run downwards around the chest wall, from back to front, the level of the sternal angle is at the lower border of the fourth thoracic vertebra (4–5 intervertebral disc) i.e. the posterior attachment of the fifth rib.

Although the ribs articulate with the bodies and transverse processes of the vertebrae of the same number, all except the first two and last

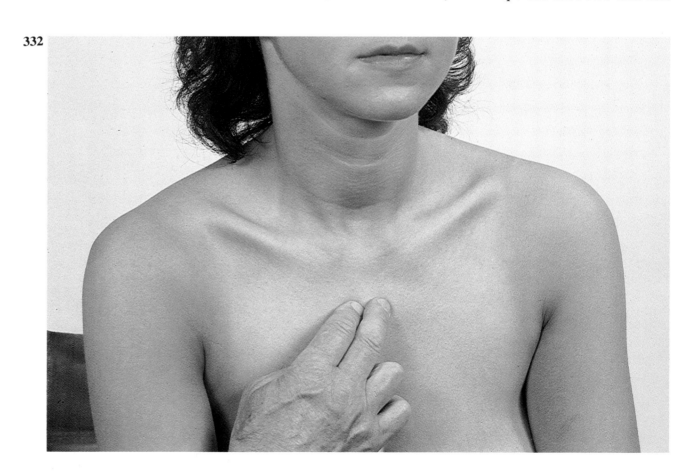

332

194

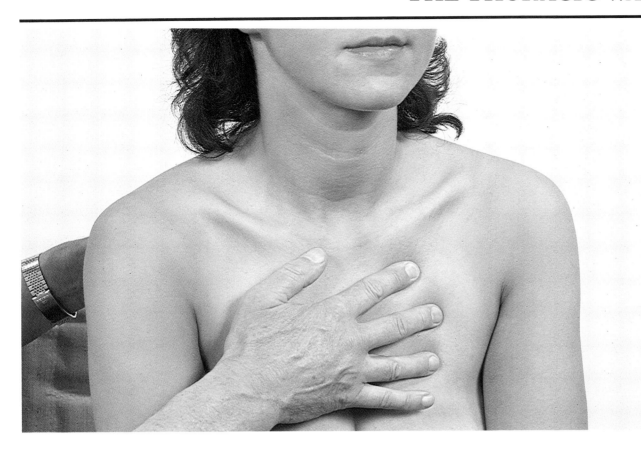

333

two, also articulate with the lower part of the body of the vertebra above and the intervening intervertebral disc. Anteriorly the ribs articulate by synovial joints only though their costal cartilages with the sternum, the upper seven doing so directly. In the cases of the 8, 9 and 10th ribs, the costal cartilages turn upwards to articulate with the one above, thus forming the inverted V of the costal margin anteriorly, which, being cartilaginous, has considerable flexibility. The 10th costal cartilage forms the lowest part of the costal margin laterally. The 11th and the still shorter 12th, the so-called floating ribs, are free anteriorly and do not join the costal margin.

Counting the ribs anteriorly is quite easy in a slim male but may be far less so in a female, due to the overlying breast.

As the first rib lies beneath the clavicle, the second is the uppermost one normally palpable. If the examiner's fingers are laid along the ribs they can be placed in the intercostal grooves, starting from 1–2, with the ribs between them, and then counting down (**333**).

From below, the lower border of the 5th rib is level with the xiphisternal joint, while the linea semilunaris of the abdomen (lateral border of the rectus abdominis muscle) points to the tip of the 9th costal cartilage (see page 242).

As the ribs and sternum are raised in inspiration, their positions relative to the vertebrae must be considered in the resting state, rising by as much as a full vertebra on full inspiration. Positions also vary with flexion and extension of the thoracic spine and some extension takes place here in full inspiration. Furthermore, the shape of the chest plays some part also; broad chested individuals tend to have more horizontally running ribs than slim people. As an average, however, the upper border of the manubrium is level with the body of T3 (a little above its spine) and the lower border (sternal angle) level with T4–5 (upper part of T4 spine). Lower levels are:

Xiphisternal joint – Body of T11 (T10 spine).
Tip of 9th costal cartilage – lower border of L1.
Costal margin (10th costal cartilage) – L3.

THE BREAST

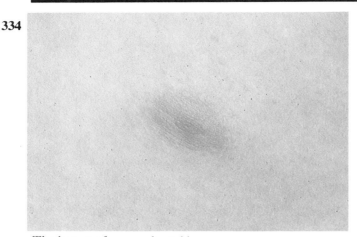

334

The breast of a prepubertal boy under reasonably warm conditions.

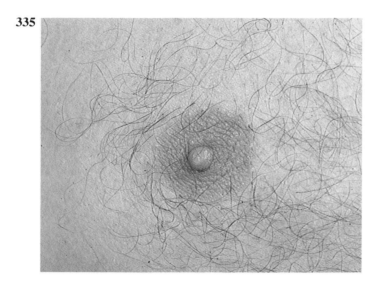

335

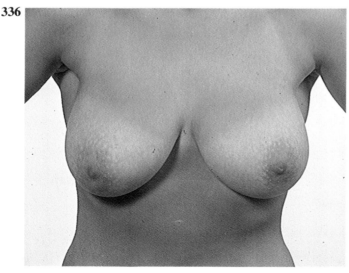

336

The breast is often a very prominent and obvious feature of the adult female but in the male or prepubertal members of both sexes it is seen only as a very small nipple and the surrounding areola. The position of the nipple varies even in the male. It is usually about a centimetre or so outside the midclavicular line (i.e. a line drawn vertically downwards from the middle of the clavicle) and lying over the fourth intercostal space. In earlier descriptions a vertically running nipple line was often used as a surface marking but in view of the variability of the position of the nipple, even in the male, the midclavicular line has now replaced it.

Before puberty the nipple is very small and surrounded, in pale skinned individuals, by a pink areola (**334**), though this is more pigmented with a darker skin colour. Under warm conditions the nipple is soft and projects little above the surrounding areola, but cold leads to contraction of the smooth muscle to produce a small projecting cone.

In the male the nipple and areola show little change with puberty (**335**). The areola may become a little more pigmented and the nipple slightly more obvious, particularly in cold conditions.

The breast region may also be involved in the characteristic male hair pattern. Although the change with puberty is slight in the male, occasionally a boy will show some swelling and hypersensitivity for a short time around puberty (gynaecomastia) in the region of the nipple, not unlike the very first signs of change as seen in the female. This reverts to normal in a few weeks, or at the most, months.

In the female the situation is quite different, for around puberty there is a gradual swelling, initially in the region of the nipple, which extends to produce a breast of such size and form as is characteristic of the person concerned. The area of the areola increases in size as also does the nipple (**336**).

The nipple and areola become obvious features at the apex of the mammary swelling. The female breast swelling, although very variable in form and size is essentially a rounded mound, extending vertically from the second to the sixth ribs; medially from the lateral edge of the sternum, laterally to the midaxillary line. In this position some two thirds of it overlies pectoralis major muscle whilst the infralateral

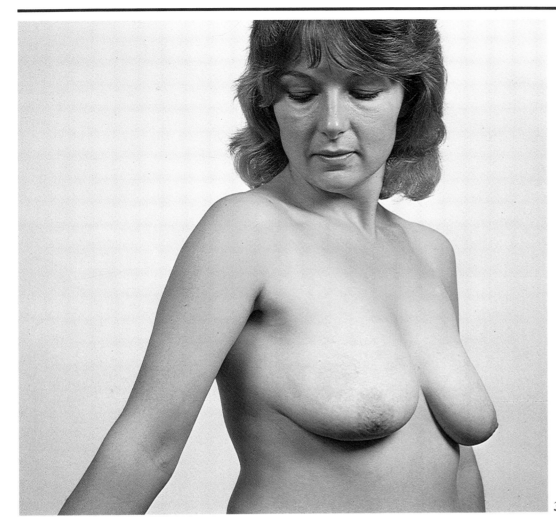

337

aspect covers serratus anterior. Although the rounded character of the breast is most obvious, one important feature is a projection extending along the pectoral muscle towards the axilla, the axillary tail. This follows the course of the major lymph drainage of the breast via the pectoral nodes to the axilla (**337**). Medially the skin remains closely related to the underlying sternum even in an obese person, so emphasising the swelling of the breasts and producing a cleavage between the two.

Embryologically the breast is a development and specialisation of some 15 or so skin glands which open at the apex of the nipple and are contained in the subcutaneous mammary fat. These are rudimentary structures in the male and prepubertal female which increase in size in the female at puberty and extend radially into the underlying breast fat but remain relatively small. Thus a nulliparous breast consists mainly of fat and supportive fibrous tissue except in the region of the nipple. During pregnancy the glandular tissue hypertrophies into the surrounding tissue in anticipation of lactation, so that by the end of pregnancy glandular tissue has become a major component of the breast which likewise shows increase in size.

The extension of glandular tissue radially into the breast creates a segmentally lobulated structure of lactiferous glands enclosed in fat, each separated from the others by fibrous intersections. Thus if one compartment of gland becomes infected to the extent of producing an abscess which needs surgical drainage, a radial incision is to be preferred, limiting the surgery to the affected lobule.

THE BREAST

The breasts are constructed mainly of fatty tissue and milk secretory glands. With the exception of the highly specialised muscle in the nipple region the breasts are not directly controlled by muscle. However, fibrous tissue within the breast is linked with the fascia over the pectoral muscles and through this also to the skin. Movements of the arms thus affect the breast, not only from the pulling of the skin but also in relation to the pectoral muscular movement.

The two cyclographs were taken from the front (**338**) and the side (**339**) as the arms were raised from the side to above the head. Note how the breast is raised with the arm.

In (**339**) it will be seen that the thoracic spine becomes somewhat straightened in raising the arm and this plays some part in the elevation of the breast but the major movement is due to the fibrous linkage with the underlying muscle fascia.

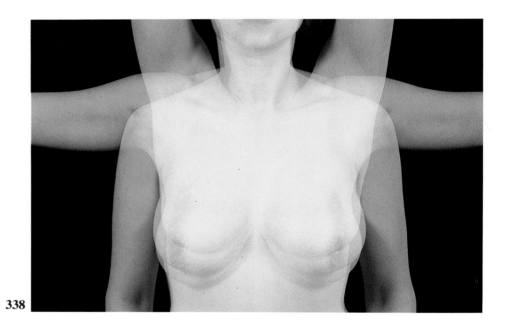

338

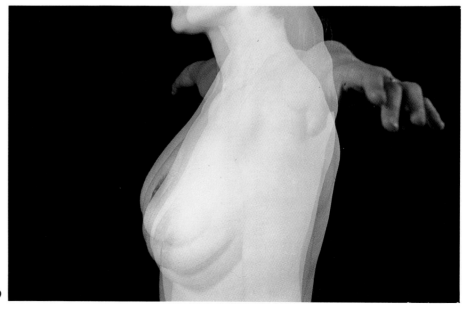

339

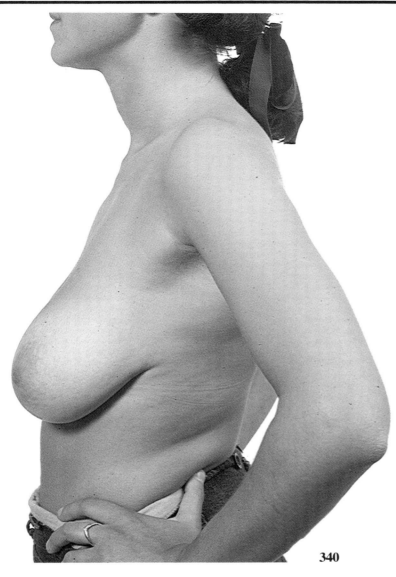

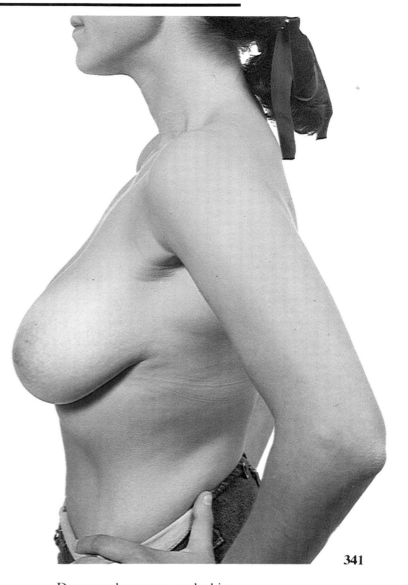

340

The arms are resting lightly on the hips and pectoralis major is relaxed.

341

Downward pressure on the hips puts pectoralis major into activity producing a marked change in the breast, lifting it so increasing its prominence and flattening the curve of the skin on its upper surface.

As the breast is essentially a structure based on subcutaneous fat, its support is largely dependent upon the fibrous intersections which link the skin with the deep fascia over the underlying muscle, particularly pectoralis major. The fibrous connections are particularly strong in the upper part of the gland where support is most needed. Here they are called the suspensory ligaments (of Astley Cooper). They usually give good firm support in a young and particularly nulliparous person but may become stretched if the breasts are unduly heavy or after multiple pregnancies and lactations.

Although there is no direct muscle control in support of the breast, the attachments of the suspensory ligaments to the pectoral fascia leads to some influence on the breast on contraction of this muscle (**340–341**).

THE BREAST

The value of the suspensory ligaments in maintaining breast form in the upright posture is made evident when the same person as shown in **340–341** lies on her back and bends forwards where in each case the suspensory ligaments are less effective in control (**342–343**).

The role of the fibrous intersections in the breast tissue may often become valuable in the early diagnosis of breast cancer, a condition responsible for the deaths of many women. Early growth may involve the fibrous tissue so that a dimple may appear in the skin even before a swelling can be palpated. The dimple may become more obvious or only appear when the underlying muscle is put into activity. This fact has been utilised in a series of procedures advocated for self examination in women by use of a mirror.

342

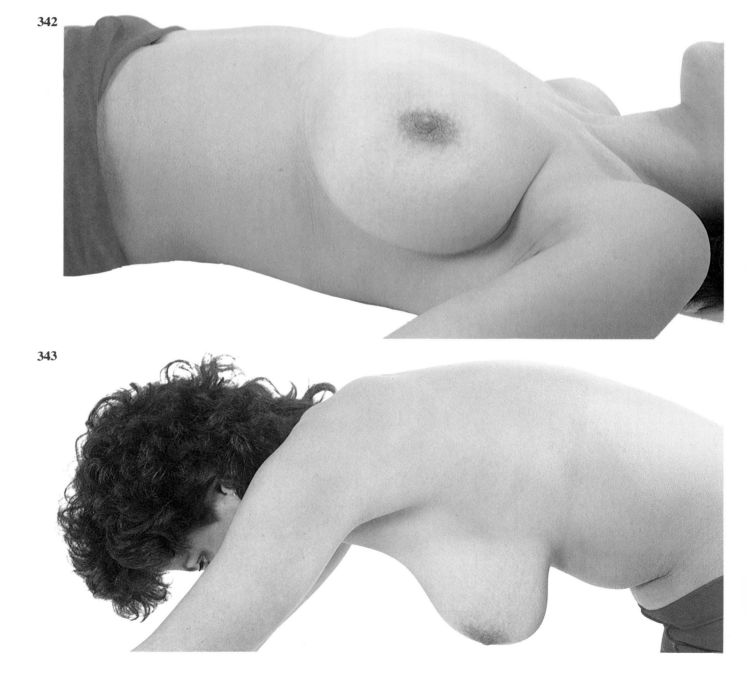

343

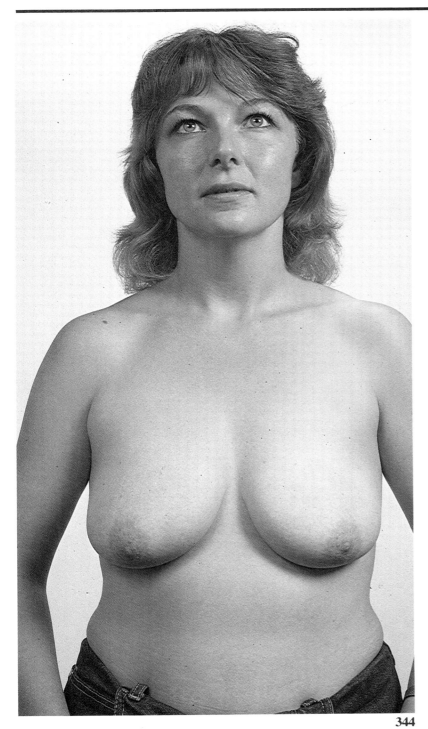

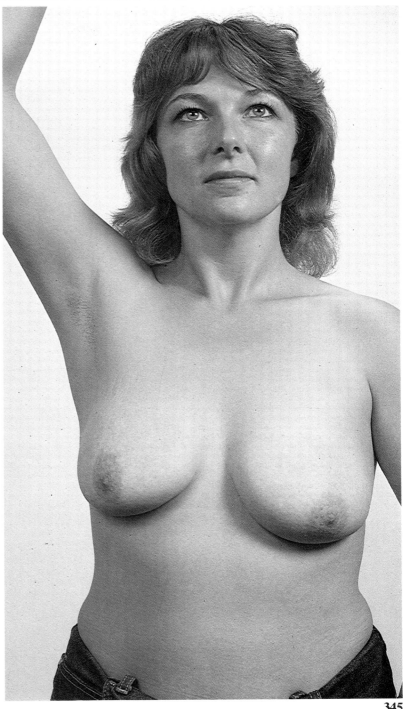

344

345

The effect can be produced as in **341** by pushing downwards with the arms to put pectoralis major into contraction. If the arms are raised above the head, pectoralis and its fascia is put on stretch and the breast raised through the suspensory ligaments as shown in (**345**).

If the arm is taken to the side somewhat a lateral pull is applied which also influences the axillary tail and the medial part of the gland.

THE BREAST

Pregnancy and lactation lead to hypertrophy and although support of the breast may return more or less to normal afterwards, sometimes stretch marks may be left in the skin (**346**), a feature which may also be seen in the abdomen after pregnancy or in the skin of a fat person who slims drastically.

The nipple and areola remain pink in a pale skinned and fair haired person but become more pigmented after the first pregnancy. However a person with white skin but darker hair may show pigmentation even if nulliparous (**342**). With darker skins the pigmentation becomes much greater (**347**).

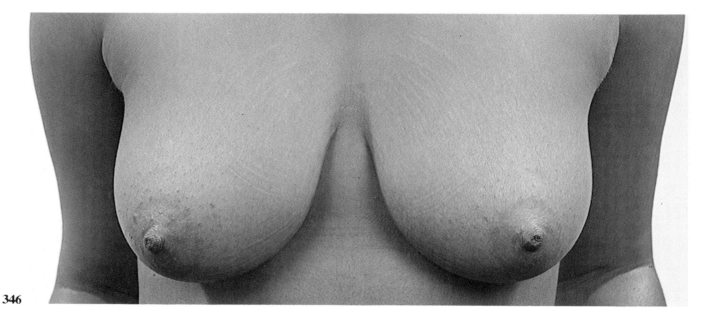

346

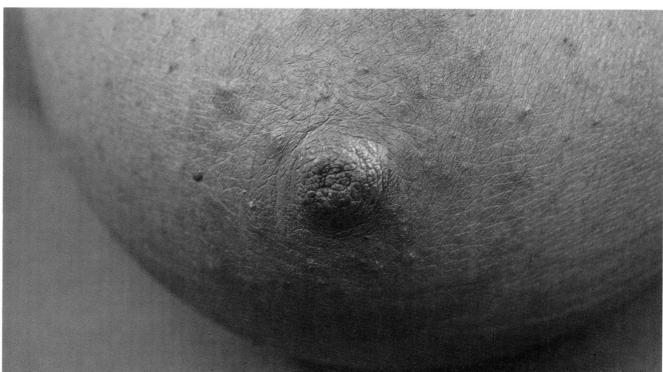

347

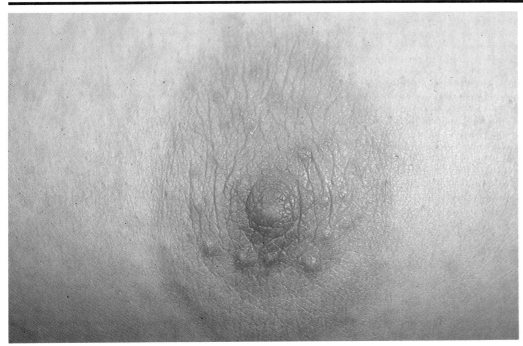

348

The effect of cold on the nipple is readily seen in 349 compared with the warm state in 348

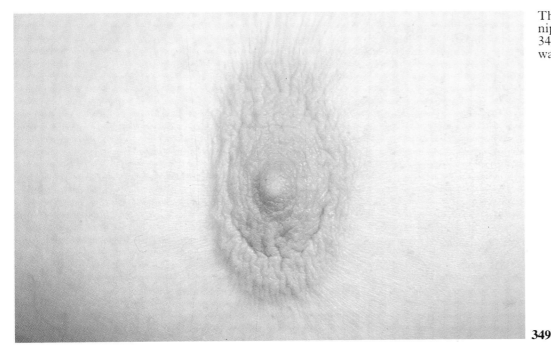

349

The region of the nipple is supplied with involuntary muscle which contracts on stimulation, constricting the areola and erecting the nipple (**349**), a feature which becomes more marked during lactation when the nipple also becomes somewhat hypertrophied for suckling.

Small swellings are apparent in the areola (**348**) caused by the areolar glands. These are specialised sebaceous glands which enlarge during pregnancy to produce an oily secretion to assist in lubricating the skin of the nipple during lactation thus maintaining it in a supple healthy state.

BLOOD SUPPLY AND LYMPH DRAINAGE OF THE BREAST

The breast receives its main blood supply from three sources; perforating branches from the internal thoracic artery medially (**350**, 1), from lateral thoracic branches from the axillary artery, laterally (2) and from the acromiothoracic artery (3), with venous drainage following the same routes. The vessels form a rich sub-areolar plexus while the medial and lateral supplies converge and commonly anastomose mainly in the regions below the nipple. Here the veins may be seen through the skin, particularly when enlarged during pregnancy and lactation. Thus circumferential incisions in the lower part of the breast, following resting stress lines (see page 11) are the most likely to avoid major blood vessels.

The lymphatics are of particular importance as a route of spread of cancer of the breast, unfortunately a very common condition. It is often said that drainage tends to follow segmental routes but such a description can be misleading. By far the most important route is along the pectoralis major muscle and fascia, via pectoral lymph nodes (**351**, 1) thence to central and apical axillary nodes (2) from whence main drainage is into the venous system of that side of the body. Spread does occur upwards to infra and supraclavicular lymph nodes (3), medially to nodes along the internal thoracic vessels (4) and downwards into the upper abdomen and even the inguinal nodes (5). Spread to the other breast and thence axilla is described but it is worthy of note that the less usual routes may open up when the usual routes are blocked by secondary involvement.

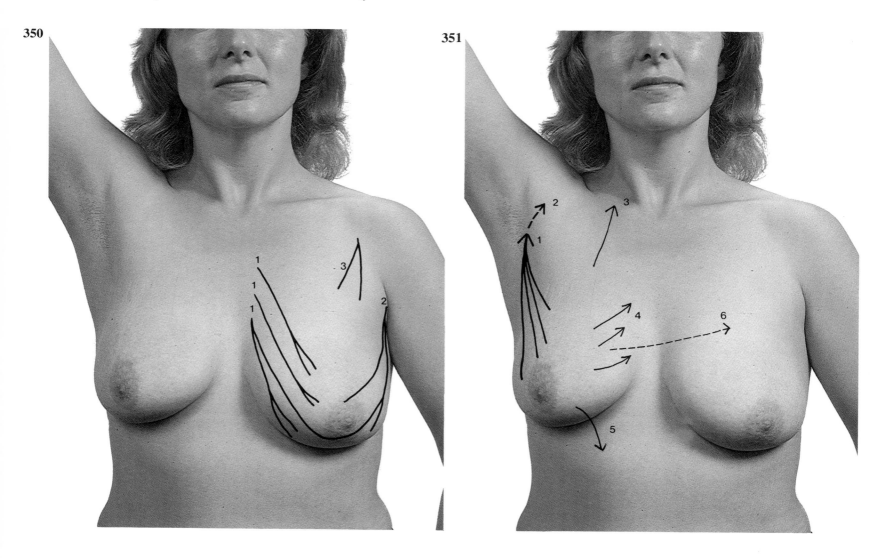

The sternal angle (of Louis), the junction of manubrium and sternum proper, is at the same level as the lower part of T4 vertebra. It is a very important level in the thorax, where a considerable number of things happen (**352**).

The aorta arches backwards behind the lower half of the manubrium and thus above the sternal angle. The left brachiocephalic vein lies above the upper half of the manubrium as it crosses to join the right vein to form the superior vena cava on its right border. This is joined by the vena azygos at the level of the sternal angle having arched forwards over the root of the right lung.

The trachea runs down to divide at the sternal angle to form the two main bronchi which run to the hila of the lungs. The upper parts of the hila are at the level of the angle and here also the pulmonary artery runs under the arch of the aorta to divide into its two branches, one to each lung. In the fetus the left pulmonary artery is joined to the aorta by the ductus arteriosus but after birth this constricts, ceases to carry blood and forms the ligamentum arteriosum around which the left recurrent laryngeal nerve runs to go up to the larynx, having left the vagus. The superficial cardiac nervous plexus lies in front of the ligamentum arteriosum with the deep one behind. These receive parasympathetic contributions from the vagus and sympathetic ones from the cervical sympathetic trunk.

The thoracic duct begins its course upwards in the thorax to the right but crosses over to the left and, although this is somewhat variable in level, it is usual to describe it as being at T4.

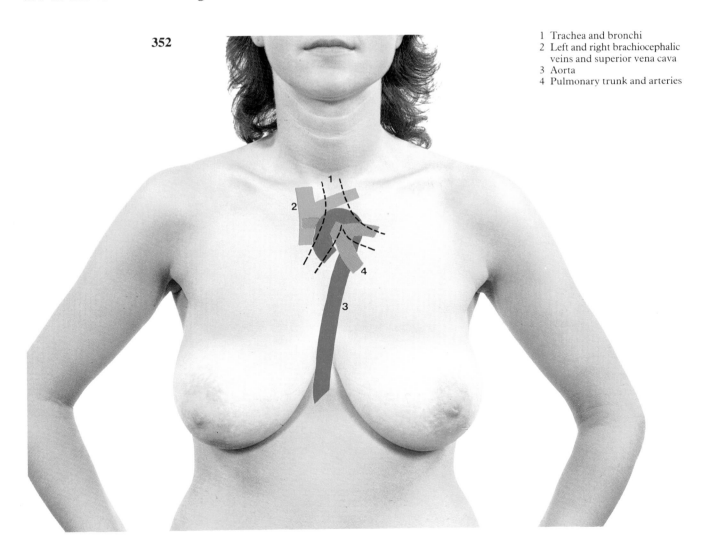

352

1 Trachea and bronchi
2 Left and right brachiocephalic veins and superior vena cava
3 Aorta
4 Pulmonary trunk and arteries

THE PLEURA AND LUNGS

The lungs form the greatest volume of the thoracic contents and, because of their rôle, this volume varies considerably with the phase and needs of respiration. The pleura, having the function of providing a relatively friction-free surface on which the lungs can move within the thoracic walls, has a parietal layer which conforms with movements of the walls and a visceral layer which moves with the lungs. The parietal layer lines the thorax to the maximal extent of inflation of the lungs. Thus in the resting stages of respiration there is a marked difference in the extent of pleural cover of the thoracic walls and the lungs within. The main differences are on the costal and diaphragmatic margins where the potential space of these recesses can be filled by lung as the depth of respiration increases. In the recesses, which are largest between costal and diaphragmatic surfaces (costo-diaphragmatic recess), the two parietal layers are in contact but will be separated by the expansion of the lung. Elsewhere the lungs generally conform to the pleural lining of the chest wall (**353**).

The apex or dome of the thoracic cavity extends above the medial third of the clavicle to an extent of some 2–3 cm in quiet respiration. It is covered by the suprapleural membrane (Sibson's fascia) which extends from the anterior

1 Oblique fissure
2 Transverse fissure
3 Back border of long
4 Back border of pleura
5 Anterior border of lung
6 Anterior border of pleura

353

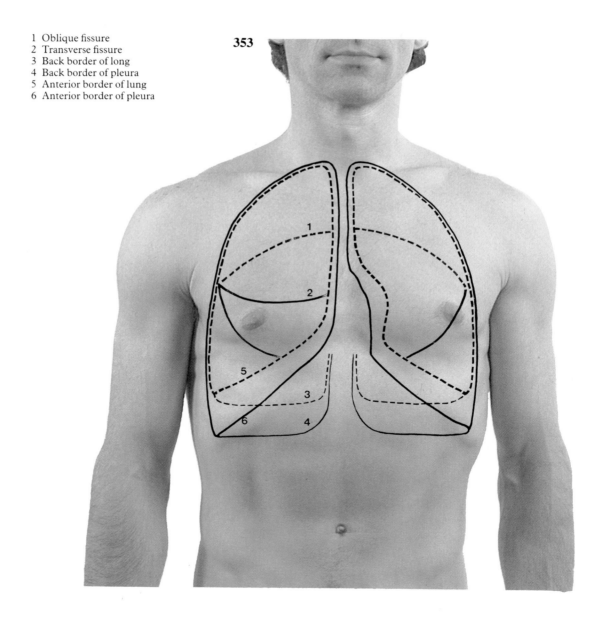

tubercle of the transverse process of the C7 vertebra to the inner margin of the first rib. In some 50% of cases this is supplemented by muscle, the scalenus minimus. In addition the dome is protected anteriorly and laterally by the scalene muscles and anteriorly it lies behind the sternomastoid muscle. As part of the projection of the lung above the clavicle is due to the slope of the first rib, in deep inspiration the chest wall will be raised and with it the clavicle, so reducing the height of the dome above it. For a similar reason the height is greater in asthenic than in broad chested individuals.

From the junction between the medial and middle thirds of the clavicle, both pleura and lung follow the chest wall closely except at the sternal margin (and at the lung fissures). The sternal reflection of the pleura crosses the sterno-clavicular joint to approach the midline at the sternal angle from whence the pleurae of the two sides approach closely down the sternum. On the right side the pleural limit moves laterally at the junction of the seventh costal cartilage and sternum and then follows around the chest wall behind the 8th rib at the midclavicular line, the 10th rib at the midaxillary line and the 12th rib below the medial border of the scapula (and lateral margin of erector spinae). More medial to this it runs below the 12th rib towards the transverse process of L1 vertebra, to form a subcostal pleural triangle. Here the pleural cavity is said to be vulnerable particularly in surgical exposure of the kidney. However it is protected here by the quadratus lumborum and erector spinae muscles. The great danger is when the 12th rib is very short, the incision can run up inadvertently to the 11th rib.

On the left side the course behind the sternum is essentially the same as the right down to the fourth costal cartilage where a cardiac notch carries the pleura out to the left of the sternum down to the seventh costal cartilage, and then the lower margin is the same as on the right side. Posteriorly both lungs and pleura have a medial margin some 2–3 cm lateral to the midline, i.e. along the vertebral bodies except on the left side where the aorta intervenes.

Anteriorly the lung follows behind the sternum, with only a slight separation from the pleural reflection on the right, down to the level of the 6th costal cartilage. From here it follows around the chest wall some 2 ribs above the pleural reflection i.e. 6, 8 & 10th ribs at the three lines. On the left side the cardiac notch carries the lung laterally much more than the pleura, going to some 2–3 cm opposite the 5th costal cartilage and then moving in a little at the 6th before following the same lower course as on the right side.

It is important to stress that the lines of lung markings relative to the costo-diaphragmatic recess and the cardiac notch as given are essentially static i.e. with breathing stopped. They will not vary much in quiet respiration, where flow of respiratory gas is small. In deep respiration, however, the lungs will expand towards the limits of the recesses. They will cover the heart anteriorly to the lateral margin of the sternum in deep inspiration and extend down laterally in the midclavicular line to some 5 cm of the costal margin; here in full respiratory excursion the movement of the lower lung margin will be of the range of some 5–7 cm.

Lung fissures. The left lung is divided into two lobes, an upper and a lower, by the oblique fissure. The lingular lobe is not separated by a fissure and is a component of the upper lobe. The right lung has an oblique and a transverse fissure dividing it into upper, middle and lower lobes. The oblique fissures of the lungs can be shown on the surface by a line drawn around the chest wall from some 2–3 cm from the midline, a little below the spine of T3 vertebra, to the 6th costal cartilage anteriorly. Alternatively, if the arm is raised above the head the fissure follows the medial border of the scapula. The transverse fissure lies anteriorly behind the 4th costal cartilage and runs horizontally laterally to meet the oblique fissure in the midaxillary line. The transverse fissure passes above the nipple in the male while the oblique passes below it, though the fissures both run below it in deep inspiration.

THE PLEURA AND LUNGS

Broncho-pulmonary segments. As the anatomy of the lung is based on the repeatedly dividing bronchi these have come to be known as the bronchial tree and like the branches of a tree, each branch is a self contained unit (**354**). Blockage of the bronchial branch removes aeration of that segment of the lung which will collapse as the air is absorbed. The branches of the pulmonary artery run parallel with the bronchi and their branches are likewise isolated to that particular segment as are the veins. Thus blockage of one of these vessels leads to death of that segment of lung. This bronchopulmonary segmental pattern of the lung is therefore of major functional and clinical importance.

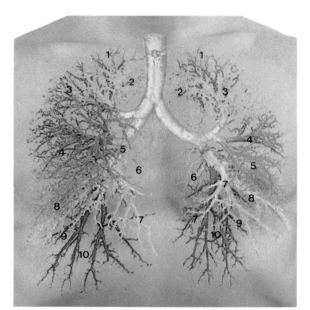

354

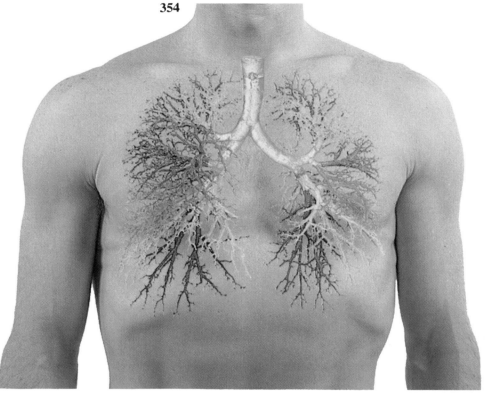

The trachea divides behind the manubriosternal joint (sternal angle). The right, larger, main lobe bronchus runs down almost vertically for 1.0–1.5 cms. before dividing into upper and lower lobe bronchi, at the right border of the sternum behind the upper border of the 3rd right sternocostal joint. The upper lobe bronchus divides into three primary divisions for the three primary bronchopulmonary segments, apical (1), posterior (2) and anterior (3). The lower lobe bronchus runs on in line with the main bronchus. Behind the third intercostal space, some 1.0–1.5 cms from the sternal border, it gives a posterior branch to the apical segment of the lower lobe (6) and an anterior, middle lobe branch which, in turn, divides into lateral (4) and medial (5) branches. The lower lobe bronchus then continues to give medial (7), anterior (8), lateral (9) and posterior (10) basal branches.

The left main lobe bronchus is about three times as long as the right, as it has to pass across and under the arch of the aorta before reaching the hilum of the lung. Here it divides into upper and lower lobe bronchi approximately behind the junction of the 3rd rib with its costal cartilage. The upper lobe bronchus gives three comparable branches to those on the right and also superior (4) and inferior (5) lingular branches. The lower lobe bronchus gives a lower apical branch (6) and the same basal branches as on the right, though the medial basal may be small due to the space taken by the heart.

The bronchial cast shows only the major branches, the more peripheral ones having been removed for clarity.

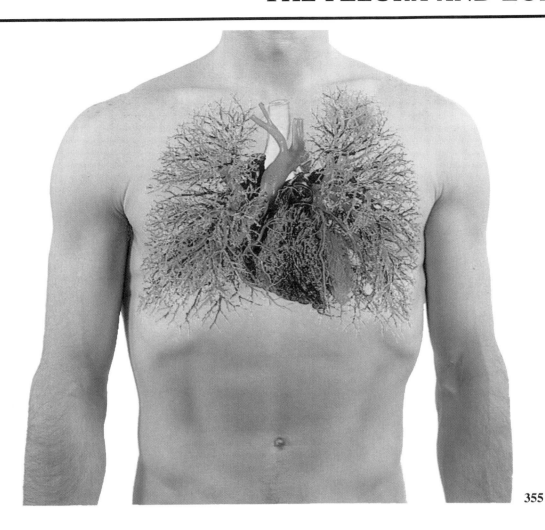

355

The close relationship between the branches of the bronchial tree (pale yellow), pulmonary arteries (blue) and veins (red) is shown in **355**, together with a cast of the heart chambers. The left ventricle of the heart is filled in red, as is the auricle of the left atrium, as well as the aorta. This artery can be seen arching over the left bronchus (behind the lower half of the manubrium sterni). The origins of the brachiocephalic, the left common carotid and subclavian arteries can also be seen. The superior vena cava and the cavities of the right atrium and ventricle are shown in blue.

The reversal of the usual arterial/venous colouring is due, in the lungs, to the pulmonary arteries carrying the systemic venous blood from the right side of the heart to the lungs for respiratory exchange, i.e. oxygenation and removal of carbon dioxide, while the veins carry the blood back to the left atrium and thence left ventricle for transmission as systemic arterial blood.

THE PLEURA AND LUNGS

On the right side the upper lobe is divided into three primary bronchopulmonary segments, apical, anterior and posterior and these are also found in essentially similar positions in the upper lobe of the left lung. The right middle lobe has medial and lateral segments, while the equivalent lingular component of the upper left lobe has superior and inferior segments. The lower lobe on each side has a lower apical segment at the back which extends upwards deep to and medial to the scapula as high as its spine. Below that are anterior, posterior, medial and lateral basal segments, placed as their names imply (**356–357**).

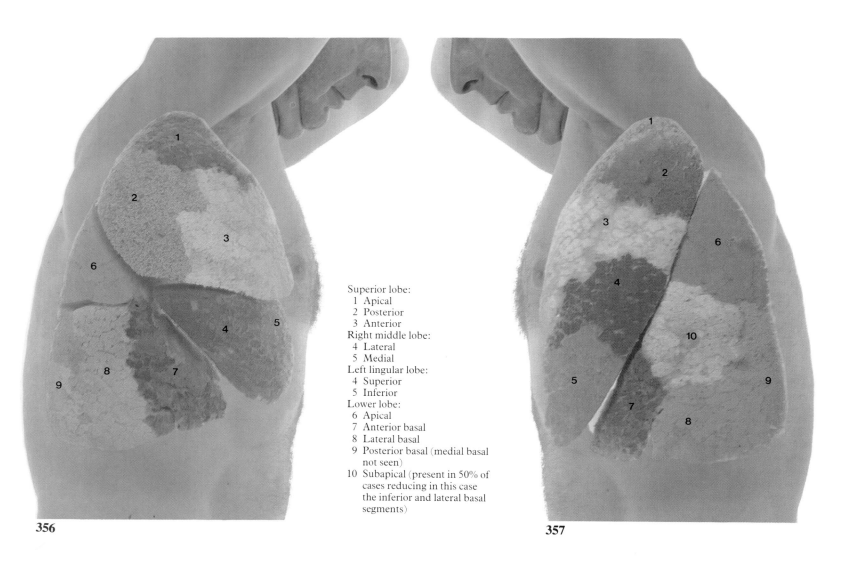

Superior lobe:
  1 Apical
  2 Posterior
  3 Anterior
Right middle lobe:
  4 Lateral
  5 Medial
Left lingular lobe:
  4 Superior
  5 Inferior
Lower lobe:
  6 Apical
  7 Anterior basal
  8 Lateral basal
  9 Posterior basal (medial basal
    not seen)
10 Subapical (present in 50% of
    cases reducing in this case
    the inferior and lateral basal
    segments)

356

357

of normal lung can be estimated by this means (**358–359**). If the middle finger (usually) of one hand is placed palmar surface against the chest wall and hit by the tip of the bent middle finger of the other hand, the movement occurring at the wrist, the air-filled lung gives a resonant sound, which becomes dull if there is solid tissue or fluid beneath. By this means it is possible to estimate if there is any consolidation in the lung or fluid in the pleural cavity or fissures. Auscultation e.g. by the use of a stethoscope, also allows the observer to hear variation from the normal sounds of air flow in the lungs during breathing.

358

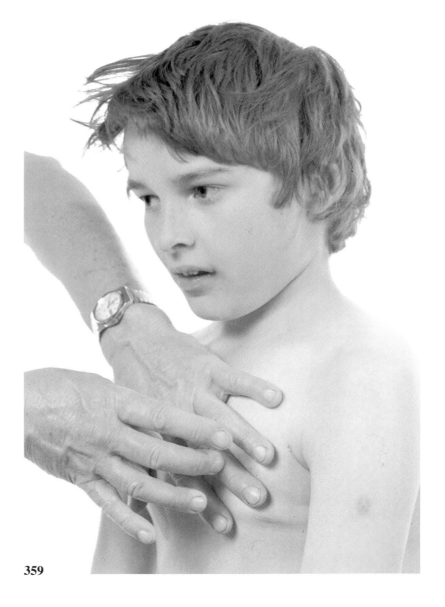

359

Examination of the lungs. As the lungs have an essentially respiratory rôle, their examination depends upon their effective inspiration and expiration of air, which in turn depends upon the movements of the chest wall. This can readily be observed as the patient breathes but variations between the two sides are less easily found. However, if the two hands are placed with the fingers to the sides of the chest and the thumbs touching in the midline in expiration, as the patient breathes in, the thumbs will normally be pulled apart to an equal amount on each side. Being air-filled the lungs give a resonant quality to the person's own voice and also to percussion of the chest, rather like a drum. Thus the extent

THE HEART

The heart fills the central part of the thorax, which is commonly called the middle mediastinum, and is covered by a loose fibrous coat, the fibrous pericardium, with a lubricating serous lining, the serous pericardium. This allows the heart to beat with minimal friction against the surrounding tissues. From its central position the apex of the heart extends towards the left (**360**). Like the lungs the heart is subject to movement, varying in shape and position, not only due to its own beating but also with respiration. With the raising of the diaphragm in expiration the heart comes to lie more transversely and thus appears shorter in height in a radiograph. In inspiration it lies more vertically and so appears narrower. The apex and the apex beat therefore vary in position with the phase of respiration. The twist in the interventricular septum induces a change in cardiac form, in addition to contraction, dependent upon the phase of the beat. Thus in systole (cardiac contraction) the heart twists with rotation towards the right. The ventricles are thus not only reduced in size because of the muscular contraction of their walls but a greater proportion of the left ventricle appears on the anterior aspect and even a little more of the left atrium may appear at the root of its auricle. In addition the way the heart lies in the chest depends somewhat on its shape and the normal height of the diaphragm in that person. In a broad chested individual and those with a naturally higher diaphragm, the heart lies more transversely whereas the narrower chested person has a more vertically lying heart. Distension of the stomach can also affect the position of the heart which tends to be pushed over to the right; thus overeating can materially embarrass an already stressed and particularly dilated heart. All these influences affect the normal position of the heart and thus the apex and apex beat which is usually described as being just inside the midclavicular line in the 5th intercostal space. The apex beat is that part of the heart which can normally be felt against the chest wall but as this is normally so close to the true apex the two tend to be treated together.

From the front the right border of the heart is made up entirely of the right atrium (**360**, 1). The superior vena cava (2) runs down the right side of the manubrium and sternum to the level of the 3rd costal cartilage where it enters the

1 Right atrium
2 Superior vena cava
3 Inferior vena cava
4 Arch of the aorta
5 Pulmonary artery
6 Left auricle
7 Left ventricle
8 Right ventricle

360

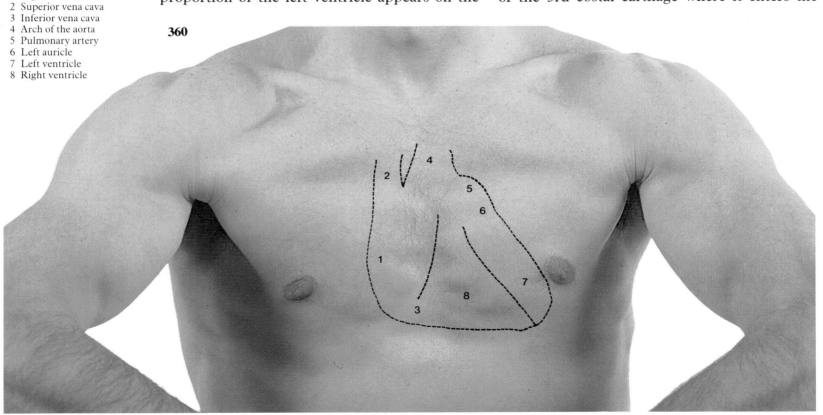

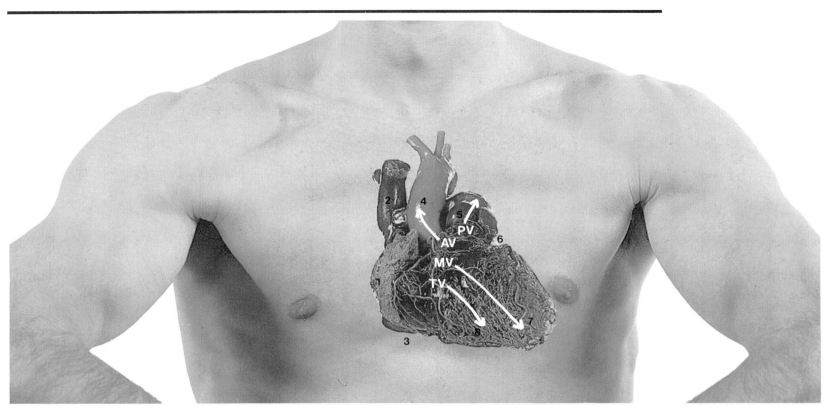

361

atrium. This then follows down with a curve a little outside the right border of the sternum to the 6th costal cartilage or the xiphisternal joint. The inferior vena cava enters from below (3). On the left side the arch of the aorta (4) lies behind the lower half of the manubrium sterni and just below this the pulmonary artery (5) and its left branch form a bulge evident on an anteroposterior radiograph. These two form the aortic and pulmonary knuckles of the radiograph. Below this and extending some 2.5 cm to the left of the sternum and behind the 2nd intercostal space and the 3rd costal cartilage, a small portion of left auricle appears (6). The rest of the left border of the heart is made up of the left ventricle (7).

The lower border of the heart has the inferior vena cava opening into the right atrium to the right but most of this aspect is made up of the two ventricles, being some two-thirds right ventricle (8) and then the apical third the left ventricle, though this last increases somewhat in systole due to the twist of the heart.

As the left ventricle runs somewhat behind the right, it forms much of the posterior aspect towards the apex but above this the left atrium forms the major upper part of the heart. This lies immediately in front of the oesophagus and so any left atrial dilatation will tend to compress the oesophagus. It may produce difficulty in swallowing, a common sympton of left sided problems in the heart.

The valves of the heart all lie on the same plane, surrounded by a fibrous ring on which the contractile muscles of both atria and ventricles are mounted. However, as the heart lies obliquely in the chest the plane of the valves is also oblique. As an easy guide, if a line is drawn from the medial end of the third left costal cartilage downwards and to the right towards the right border of the sternum, level with the 4th intercostal space, the four valves lie on that line in the order pulmonary (PV), aortic (AV), mitral (MV) and tricuspid (TV). The mitral valve linking the left atrium and ventricle lies a little behind the tricuspid (the right atrio-ventricular valve) and the aortic lies a little behind the pulmonary valve.

A cast of the cavities of the heart and the origins of the great vessels, with the heart in diastole. The coronary arteries can be seen in red, coursing over the surface of the cast of the heart.

PV = Pulmonary valve
AV = Aortic valve
MV = Mitral valve
TV = Tricuspid valve
The arrows indicate the direction of the blood flow and extend to the sites for auscultation of the valves.

THE HEART

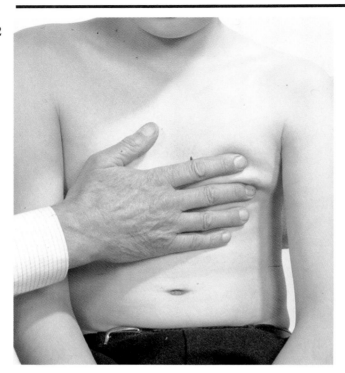

362

Clinical examination of the heart. Observation of the chest in a slim person may show evidence of pulsation at the apex beat usually in the 5th intercostal space. This is particularly likely to be seen if the heart is beating forcefully as after hard exercise or if the person is bending forwards a little to bring the heart closer to the chest wall. Palpation of the apex beat is usually quite easy in a slim male particularly if the fingers are separated and laid along the intercostal spaces.

In a female with anything but small breasts or in a more obese male, the situation is less easy. In a female it is necessary to raise the breast and place the hand beneath it and along the spaces and allowing the breast to fall over the examining hand (363–364). If there is difficulty in palpation it may be helped if the person bends forwards somewhat.

The heart is usually higher and further to the left in a child. Here the beat could be felt through the 5th rib.

363

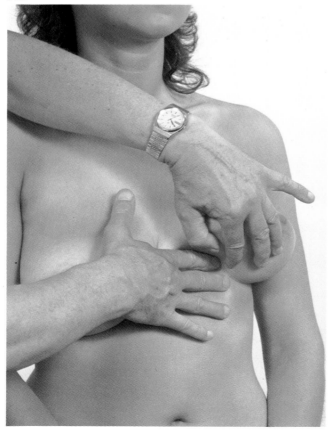

364

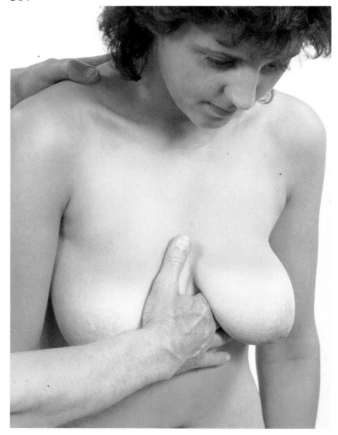

THE HEART

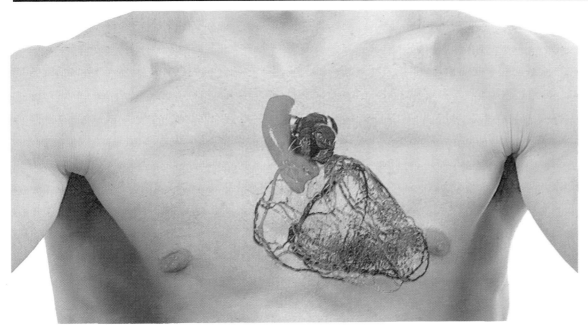

A cast showing the regions of the aorta (red) and the pulmonary artery (blue) with their respective valves closed. The details of the pocket-like cusps of the three valves of each artery can be seen. The two coronary arteries (red) run from the sinuses above the left and right anterior aortic valves. The right artery shows clearly as it runs around the heart in the atrioventricular groove. The left artery runs behind the pulmonary artery posteriorly in the atrioventricular groove, having given the large and very important anterior interventricular artery. The cardiac veins are shown in blue, terminating in the main in the coronary sinus which enters the back of the right atrium though the anterior cardiac veins enter separately.

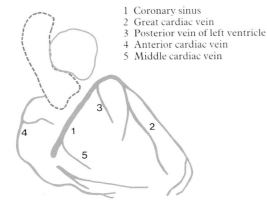

1 Coronary sinus
2 Great cardiac vein
3 Posterior vein of left ventricle
4 Anterior cardiac vein
5 Middle cardiac vein

A Aorta
P Pulmonary artery
1 Right coronary artery
2 Left coronary artery
3 Right marginal artery
4 Posterior interventricular artery
5 Anterior interventricular artery
6 Left marginal artery
7 Circumflex branch of left coronary artery
8 Atrial branch of left coronary artery

A rough estimate of the size of the heart may be obtained by percussion. By using the same technique as in the lungs. The finger is laid on the chest surface parallel to but outside the heart. Percussion will produce normal lung resonance and the finger is gradually moved until the sound changes to the dullness to be expected over a solid body. By repeating percussion around the heart a reasonably good map of its size can be drawn. Though obviously not so accurate as can be achieved by such diagnostic tests as radiography, ultrasonics etc. it is remarkably good for routine clinical purposes. However it should be remembered that it is less effective in a barrel shaped chest where overlying lung tissues may blur the edges.

Auscultation of the sounds generated by blood flow and valve closure etc. can give valuable information and is most commonly carried out by means of a simple stethoscope. It is important to realise that the sound is propagated via the blood after it has passed the valves. There is little point therefore in listening over the valves at the sites shown in **361**. For the mitral and tricuspid sounds, these must be looked for below and to the left of the valves, the mitral most effectively over the apex beat area. The aortic and pulmonary sounds can be heard over the origins of these vessels above the valves (**365**).

OTHER THORACIC STRUCTURES

The *thymus gland* lies immediately behind the manubrium and sternum and in an adult extends as a lobulated structure from the upper border of the manubrium down to the 4th costal cartilages (**366**). As it develops from the 3rd branchial pouch and moves down into the thorax its position is somewhat variable, although not so much as the inferior parathyroid which, developing from the same pouch, can be anywhere in position from the back of the thyroid to the thorax along with the thymus.

Before birth the thymus fills a large part of the thorax at the expense of the unexpanded lungs but with the expansion of the lungs at birth the position changes and, as the rest of the body grows, the thymus becomes relatively smaller. However it does not reduce in weight into adult life and become degenerate, as was previously thought, unless the person suffers a period of ill-health. This latter explains why the gland is commonly degenerate at postmortem.

The *Aorta*. As indicated in **367** the artery leaves the heart behind the sternum roughly level with the third costal cartilage and runs upwards behind the sternum towards the right border before arching backwards behind the lower half of the manubrium sterni. As it does so it moves slightly to the left, so meeting the left side of the lower part of the body of T4 vertebra. It then descends against the bodies of the thoracic vertebrae, producing a flattening which gradually moves to the front as the artery leaves the thorax through the diaphragm in front of T12 (i.e. some 7–8 cm below the xiphisternal joint). As the heart moves with both systole and the movement of the diaphragm, these affect the position of the ascending part and arch of the aorta but not its descending portion.

The *Oesophagus*. The oesophagus enters the thorax in the mid-line behind the trachea (**367**). The position of the trachea can be seen as a band of greater translucency in a radiograph in the centre of the vertebral bodies until it divides at the level of the sternal angle. The oesophagus, although pushed slightly to the right by the aorta at about T4, carries on downwards in front of the aorta moving to the left to leave the chest opposite T10, some 2–3 cm to the left and 4–5 cm below the xiphisternal joint.

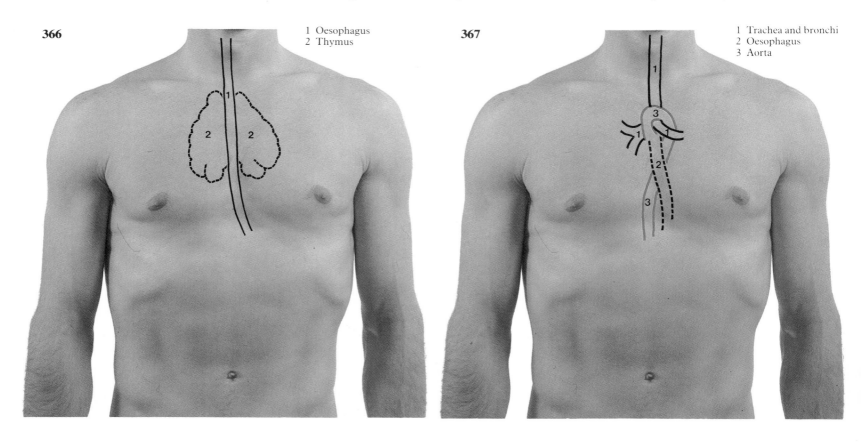

366

1 Oesophagus
2 Thymus

367

1 Trachea and bronchi
2 Oesophagus
3 Aorta

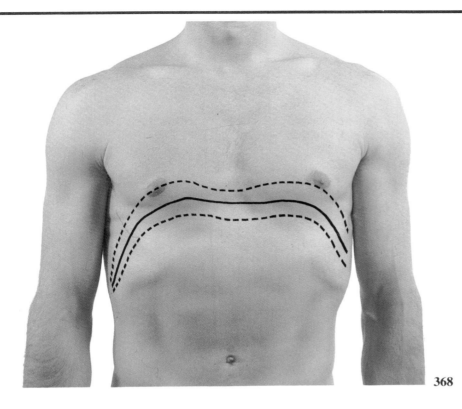

368

The diaphragm is a musculotendinous dome forming a roof to the abdomen and arching upwards into the thorax (**368**). Although described as a dome, it is lower in the middle where it is tendinous than on the two sides, and higher on the right where it overlies the liver than on the left, which is above the stomach. Anteriorly it is attached by short muscle fibres to the xiphisternum, then by longer fibres around the inside of the lower six costal cartilages and the related ribs close to the costal margin, where it interdigitates with the transversus abdominis muscle. Posteriorly it has strong muscle bundles, the crura, running almost directly upwards from the bodies of the upper 3 lumbar vertebrae (3 on the right and 2 on the left) as well as fibres from the arcuate ligaments (fascial thickenings over the quadratus lumborum and psoas muscles and, medially, the aorta). The main pull is posteriorly from the crura and to the sides where the muscle fibres run into a central tendon through which the inferior vena cava passes, so that when the muscle contracts the caval passage is pulled open.

The level of the diaphragm in the body depends upon not only the state of respiration but also the build of the person. In a broad chested individual it tends to lie relatively higher than in a narrow chested person. In a neutral respiratory position the right side of the dome can be said to lie at the level of the 5th costal cartilage (T10-11 or the 4th rib in the midclavicular line) and the left at the 6th costal cartilage (T11–12 & 5th rib) with the central portion level with the xiphisternal joint. It may, however, be a full vertebra higher with the left side raised more, dependent upon the contents of the stomach. The diaphragm also tends to be higher in a person lying supine, and one or other side may be raised when lying on that side. When sitting or in a half lying and sitting position, when the abdominal wall is at its most relaxed, the diaphragm sinks to its lowest relaxed level, thus explaining why people with respiratory problems (dyspnoea) prefer to sleep in a half-sitting position, and find difficulty in breathing when the diaphragm becomes raised when lying down. However it is important in the half-sitting position to support the back and prevent spinal flexion as this allows the abdominal contents to push the diaphragm upwards and limits respiratory range.

DIAPHRAGM

The main muscle power is to the back, and that muscle runs more vertically, while the anterior muscle is short and runs only slightly upwards, therefore the major movement of the diaphragm is to the back and to a lesser extent to the sides. It will already have been noted that the dome of the diaphragm rises to a higher level on the left than the lower border of the heart which is nearest to the anterior chest wall. Thus the greatest movement of the diaphragm is to the bases of the lungs, affecting the heart relatively slightly.

During quiet respiration the diaphragm moves vertically little more than a centimetre. In deep or forced respiration its vertical range varies greatly between individuals but can be anything from 3–10 cm. Some individuals, particularly females, appear to make little use of the diaphragm for respiration, a phenomenon which appears in young women shortly after puberty but obviously is likely to be aggravated by pregnancy. Conversely athletically active people and particularly trained singers and wind musical instrumentalists make great use of the diaphragm. In such people inspiration may lead to some 3–4 cm drop in the dome and a considerably greater range on full expiration from the neutral position. And the important feature in such people is that with training, the expiratory control, in balance with the upper abdominal muscles, is extremely precise.

Powerful contraction of the diaphragm is used with the abdominal wall muscles to increase intra-abdominal pressure, with relaxation of components of the pelvic diaphragm, in defaecation, urination and parturition. With concurrent contraction of the pelvic diaphragm this pressure is used to compact the abdominal contents to give trunk strength in lifting (see page 225). Before lifting it is usual to take a deep breath to contract the diaphragm followed by the abdominal wall and then to stop breathing. Intrathoracic pressure is commonly built up during this phase of activity, which explains the backpressure on the veins of the head and neck.

The nerve supply of the diaphragm comes from the cervical nerves due to the embryological origin of the muscles in the neck, being pushed down by the developing lungs. The phrenic nerve is mainly C4 with quite a large contribution from C5 and a small amount from C3. Sometimes the C5 contribution runs down separately. The nerve starts in the neck and runs down over scalenus anterior where it can be either stimulated electrically to induce breathing, or anaesthetised to still the diaphragm (as in persistent hiccup due to spasmodic bursts of activity in the muscle) or in diaphragmatic pain (see page 74). Loss of nerve supply leads to stilling and raising of the dome of the diaphragm. Before the availability of drugs for the effective treatment of pulmonary tuberculosis it was common practice to destroy the phrenic nerve on the affected side to stop movement of the diaphragm on that side in order to rest the affected lung so assisting healing of the lesion.

1 Oesophagus
2 Right vagus with recurrent laryngeal
3 Left vagus with recurrent laryngeal
4 Right phrenic nerve
5 Left phrenic nerve

369

The lungs are highly elastic structures which collapse like deflated rubber balloons if taken from the controlling influence of the thoracic wall. In fact the lungs do collapse in the chest to a very small size if the potential space of the pleural cavity is opened, as by an open chest wound, or if air escapes into the cavity from the lung itself. The natural response of the isolated lung is to collapse, i.e. expiration, unless held out by the chest wall and this is usually described as the elastic recoil of the lung. The recoil which is supported by the elastic relaxation of inspiratory muscles and with the effect of gravity on the chest wall is the main expiratory force in quiet respiration. The dynamic activity is in inspiration, to pull out the elastic lungs and so suck air in. In deeper and forced respiration extra muscular activity comes into play, not only in inspiration but expiration also.

It is usual to divide respiratory activity into thoracic and abdominodiaphragmatic but this is only an analytical convenience as both should work in concert. In addition other muscles can be brought in to give extra power when needed; the so-called accessory muscles of respiration.

Muscles involved. Much of the basic thoracic movement comes from the muscles of the thoracic wall itself. The intercostals, lying between the individual ribs, are in two strata, external and internal. The external fibres run downwards and laterally, forwards or medially, dependent upon the direction of the rib. These shorten as the ribs are raised and thus can be accepted as inspiratory muscles, while the internal intercostals, running at right angles to the above, are expiratory. However both muscles act to maintain the integrity of the intercostal spaces against the pressure variations upon them, particularly in deep respiration. On the inner chest wall are three muscle systems which, lying in the same morphological plane as the transversus abdominis muscles, are therefore collectively known as the transversus thoracis group. They consist of muscles at the front, the sternocostalis, running from the lower sternum to the higher costal cartilages and ribs; the intercostales intimae, whose muscle fibres run over the inside of the lateral chest wall in the same direction as the internal intercostals, while the subcostalis muscles are at the back. All these are expiratory muscles. The levatores costarum also at the back act as inspiratory counters to the subcostalis muscles.

Muscles outside the chest wall acting from above are the scalenus group which support the first rib in quiet respiration, but, although producing relatively little actual movement in deep inspiration on this short rib, have a profound effect when this is transferred to the much longer lower ribs. Serratus posterior superior runs from the cervical spines to the upper ribs at the back and acts as an inspiratory muscle, while the serratus posterior inferior, running from the lumbar spines to the lower ribs is the expiratory counter.

The erector spinae muscles play an important rôle in respiration, much more than is often appreciated. A stiff thoracic spine limits respiratory movement. A stiff straight spine tends to maintain the chest in an inflated position, while a stiff curved spine, so commonly seen in ankylosing spondylitis, grossly limits inspiratory range. But in addition to freedom of spinal movement, a minor amount of which produces much when transmitted through the long ribs, the longissimus group and, to a greater extent the iliocostalis, play a major part in controlling the rib cage, being attached quite a distance out (iliocostalis) along the ribs. Those attached from above elevate the ribs while those from below depress. Quadratus lumborum also controls and depresses the 12th rib.

The diaphragm is the most important individual muscle and has been said to be responsible for some 60–70% of respiratory movement. However these figures are upper limits and by no means a universal phenomenon. Loss of the phrenic nerves does not normally produce respiratory distresses as might be expected were such high figures the norm.

CONTROL OF RESPIRATION

Diaphragmatic movement requires reciprocal activity of the upper abdominal muscles. As, with the exception of any contained gas, the abdominal contents are incompressible, being essentially fluid, contraction of the diaphragm must be compensated for by a comparable stretching and expansion of the upper abdominal wall, unless totally wasteful increases in pressure are to be the norm. This usually only occurs where there is deficiency in functional control but of course must be expected in respiratory distress (dyspnoea). Controlled reciprocal contraction of the upper abdominal muscles works in coordination with diaphragmatic relaxation to allow the lungs to contract by their own elasticity or, in more urgent or fuller respiratory effort, give added dynamic impulse. Although all the upper abdominal muscles play their part in the respiratory rôle only the transversus abdominis is capable of the necessary contractile range to produce full expiratory effort, in view of its attachment to the inside of the lower chest wall and the involvement of its muscle fibres through into the posterior wall of the rectus sheath (372), though the oblique muscles assist by pulling down the chest wall.

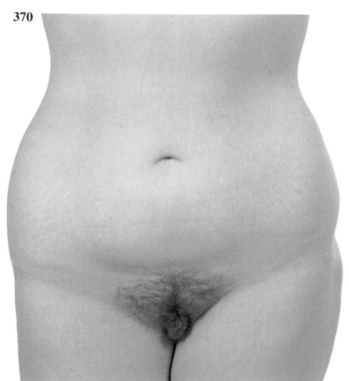

370

The lower chest and abdominal walls are seen in the quiet phase of respiration.

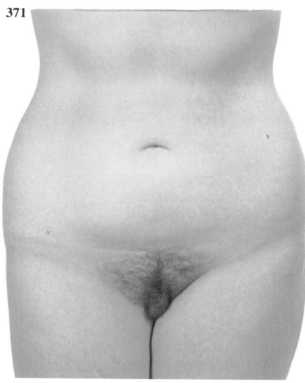

371

On expiration without undue effort the supra-umbilical portion of the abdominal wall can be seen to have been contracted, the rib margins becoming more obvious, as also is the lateral margin of the rectus abdominis muscle (linea semilunaris) due to the contraction particularly of the transversus abdominis muscle. Note that there is no change in the lower abdominal wall.

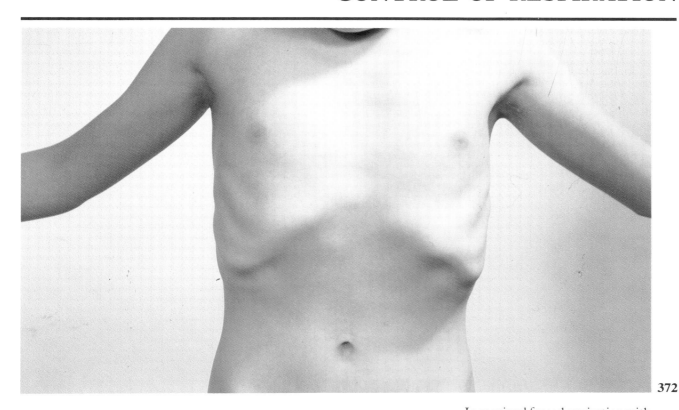

372

In maximal forced expiration with contraction of the abdominal wall the constricting effect of the transversus abdominis muscles can be seen, acting from within the rib cage. In order to achieve this degree of abdominal contraction the other abdominal muscles must relax so that they can be pulled in with the wall. However their lower fibres remain active in support of the subumbilical region.

Accessory muscles of respiration are those which come into play to give support in times of respiratory stress. Several muscles are available for this purpose.

The sternomastoid can pull up the sternum and clavicle if the head is fixed and can be assisted to some extent by the small strap muscles in the neck. The sternocostal fibres of pectoralis major together with pectoralis minor can also be powerful elevators of the ribs if the arms are fixed i.e. the functions of the muscles are reversed from their more usual rôles. After severe exercise an athlete will often fix the hands on the hips for this purpose. The 'heart table' running across a hospital bed was also designed for a similar purpose of holding the arms during respiratory distress and allows the pectoral muscles to work on the chest.

The component of the latissimus dorsi running into the ribs also allows it to act as an accessory expiratory muscle, amplifying the increased activity of the abdominal muscles.

Serratus anterior is often described as being an accessory muscle of respiration but, although it acts in the spasmodic action of coughing, there is little evidence that it has any other part to play in respiration.

ANTERIOR ABDOMINAL WALL

The anterior abdominal wall is made up of a dynamic 'corset' of three sheets of muscle each running in different directions, on each side. These are incorporated by their fibrous aponeuroses into controlling sheaths around the longitudinally running pair of rectus muscles, anteriorly, thus giving a close functional inter-relationship between all muscle components of the wall.

The *rectus abdominis* runs from a broad superior muscular attachment to the superficial aspect of the 5–7 costal cartilages and runs down to a narrower lower attachment to the pubic crest with a medial tendinous component linking with its fellow of the opposite side on the front of the symphysis pubis. It (usually) has three tendinous intersections affecting the major anterior part of the muscles; one below the xiphisternum, one intermediate between this and the umbilicus and a third at that level. Although these are often described as being evidence of an embryological segmental origin, in fact they can be trained to act separately one from the other. As the fibrous intersections are attached to the anterior wall of the rectus sheath, this arrangement allows for the remarkably fine control of which the supra-umbilical part of the anterior abdominal wall is capable (**373**).

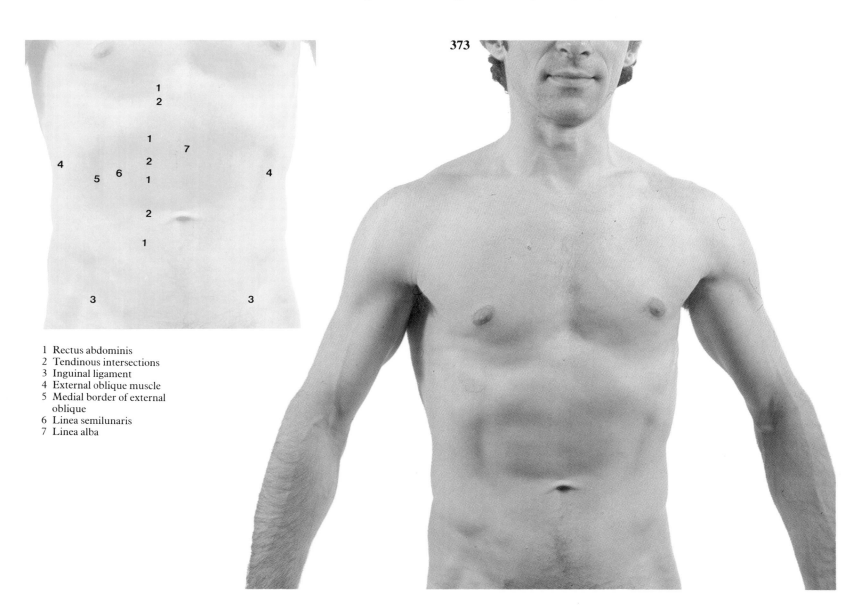

373

1 Rectus abdominis
2 Tendinous intersections
3 Inguinal ligament
4 External oblique muscle
5 Medial border of external oblique
6 Linea semilunaris
7 Linea alba

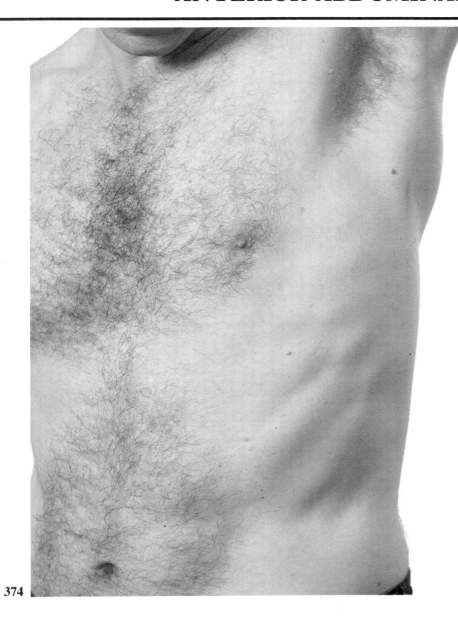

374

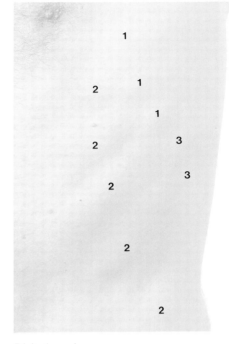

Digitations of:
1 Serratus anterior
2 External oblique
3 Latissimus dorsi

The muscle is supplied by lower six intercostal and the subcostal nerves.

The *externus obliquus abdominis* muscle is the largest and outermost of the three controlling the major part of the abdominal wall. It is attached by fleshy slips to the outer aspects of the lower 8 ribs. The upper four slips interdigitate with the lower four of the serratus anterior muscle and below that with the latissimus dorsi (**374**). The lowest slips run down almost vertically to the outer lip of the anterior part of the iliac crest, so giving the muscle a free posterior border. The higher slips join to run downwards and forwards to end by forming a tendinous aponeurosis roughly in a curved line running from the tip of the 9th costal cartilage to the anterior superior iliac spine (see 373), with no fleshy fibres passing a line drawn from the umbilicus to the anterior superior iliac spine. The aponeurotic fibres continue downwards and medially forming a major part of the anterior wall of the rectus sheath, to meet their fellow of the opposite side at the linea alba, which extends from the xiphoid to the pubis. The lowest fibres of the aponeurosis form the inguinal ligament (see page 228).

The *internus obliquus abdominis* lies deep to the external oblique and its fibres generally run at right angles to it, i.e. upwards and medially. The lowest attachment is to the outer two-thirds of the inguinal ligament, the anterior part of the iliac crest and then above from the thoracolumbar fascia. The upper fibres run upwards and anteriorly into the margins of the lower ribs; below that they form an aponeurosis which divides into two laminae, the superficial joining that of the external oblique to make up the anterior wall of the rectus sheath while the deeper runs to the posterior wall of the rectus sheath down to the level of the arcuate line, about midway between the umbilicus and the pubis. The division of the aponeurosis into laminae forms the linea semilunaris which is also, in effect, the lateral margin of the rectus muscle and runs from the tip of the 9th costal cartilage to the pubic tubercle (**375**). Although the fibres from the iliac crest and above run upwards and forwards (medially), the lower ones below the umbilicus run transversely, while the lowest, related to the inguinal canal, run downwards and medially to form the conjoined tendon with the transversus abdominis.

The *transversus abdominis* forms the deepest layer and this is the true constrictor muscle of the abdomen, with transversely running fibres. The lowest fibres come from the lateral half or so of the inguinal ligament, then the iliac crest, the thoracolumbar fascia and the inner aspect of the cartilage of the lower six ribs, interdigitating with the diaphragm. The lowest fibres run down to be involved in controlling the inguinal canal but the rest run transversely to form an anterior aponeurosis which joins the deep part of that of the internal oblique to make up the posterior wall of the rectus sheath. The upper fibres remain muscular into the sheath and behind the rectus almost to the linea alba.

The functions of the abdominal muscles are far more complex than the obvious one of support for the abdominal wall and hence the abdominal contents. A degree of compression from the enclosing muscles' tone and activity not only plays an important part in support of the abdominal contents but also builds a higher pressure zone which influences venous return to the low pressure thorax and the right side of the heart. An increase in abdominal pressure is obviously valuable for such propulsive efforts as defaecation and urination as well as in vomiting and parturition.

The abdominal muscles generate a major part of the vital control over the vulnerable lumbar spine. The two rectus muscles act as the flexor antagonists of the erector spinae system but these muscles work on the levers of the ribs and the pelvis and not directly upon the lumbar vertebrae as do the erector spinae components. The lumbar vertebrae have no ventral control other than the psoas muscles, which tend to accentuate the lumbar lordosis by pulling the vertebrae forwards, even on their resting tonus, and especially so when acting as hip flexors, were the lumbar spine and pelvis not securely controlled. Hence the rectus muscles can give the necessary pelvic control but the lumbar spine depends upon the equally important compressive force of the other abdominal wall muscles upon the essentially incompressible abdominal contents to give a firm trunk and thus intrinsic control of the lumbar spine. Weak abdominal muscles mean a weak and vulnerable lumbar spine. For heavy lifting, powerful contraction of the abdominal walls, including the diaphragm and that of the pelvis compressing the abdominal contents gives the necessary dynamic strength for the lift without danger to the lower lumbar spine. Ideally this should remain vertical leaving the legs to do most of the active lifting.

375

1 Linea alba
2 Linea semilunaris
3 Medial limit of external oblique
4 Tip of 9th costal cartilage

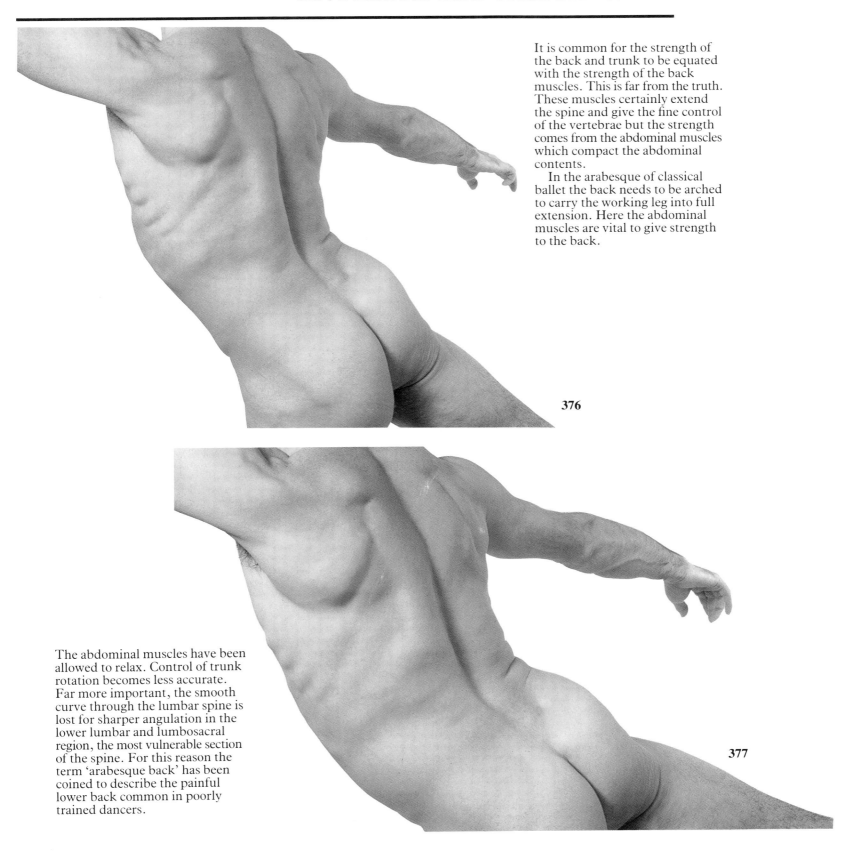

It is common for the strength of the back and trunk to be equated with the strength of the back muscles. This is far from the truth. These muscles certainly extend the spine and give the fine control of the vertebrae but the strength comes from the abdominal muscles which compact the abdominal contents.

In the arabesque of classical ballet the back needs to be arched to carry the working leg into full extension. Here the abdominal muscles are vital to give strength to the back.

376

The abdominal muscles have been allowed to relax. Control of trunk rotation becomes less accurate. Far more important, the smooth curve through the lumbar spine is lost for sharper angulation in the lower lumbar and lumbosacral region, the most vulnerable section of the spine. For this reason the term 'arabesque back' has been coined to describe the painful lower back common in poorly trained dancers.

377

ANTERIOR ABDOMINAL WALL

The important and finely controlled functions of the upper abdominal muscles have been considered in relation to respiration and in particular such activities as singing and other forms of voice control, playing wind musical instruments, etc. The infra-umbilical musculature is much cruder in function and is essentially supportive as indicated by the fact that all three layers of muscle run essentially transversely as a lower 'sling', controlling the lower abdominal wall.

The upper obliquely running parts of the external and internal oblique muscles are the prime power rotators of the lower thoracic spine (**378**). The external oblique of one side, attached to the ribs, works with the internal oblique of the other side, acting on the iliac crest, through their natural intervening aponeuroses and the rectus sheath. The posterior, almost vertically running fibres of the external oblique also act with the quadratus lumborum as lateral flexors of the lumbar spine (**379**).

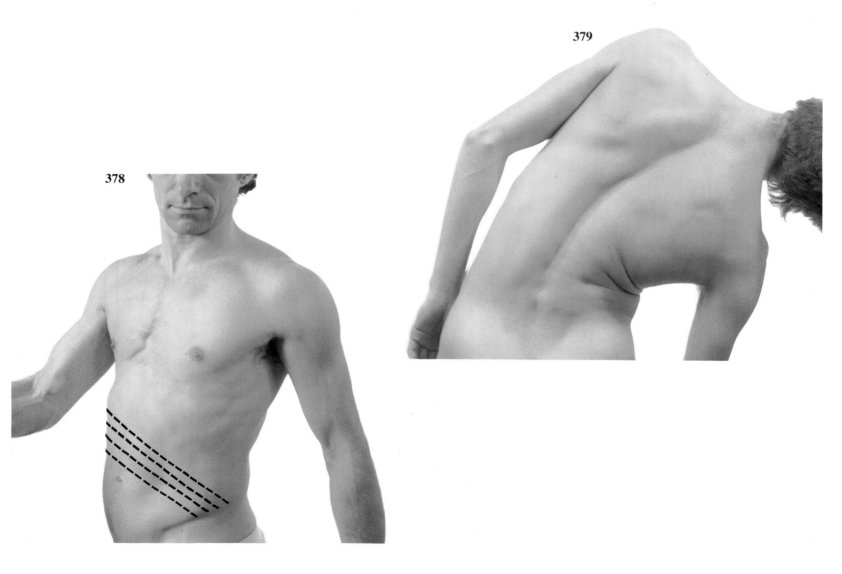

378

379

The *fasciae of the anterior wall*. In the usual fascial pattern of the body the skin is separated from the muscles by subcutaneous fat or superficial fascia and then a deep fibrous sheet, the deep fascia. In the abdominal wall a major area anteriorly already has a fibrous aponeurotic sheet from the external oblique muscle which also acts as a deep investing fascia of the rectus abdominis muscle. Thus in the region of the aponeurosis the fascia is limited to the superficial layer though over the muscle itself in the flanks a normal relatively thin deep fascia is present.

Above the umbilicus the superficial fascia is essentially fatty but below that level there is a gradually increasing amount of fibroelastic tissue in the deeper layers. The superficial fascia is thus divided here into superficial fatty and deeper membranous layers though there is generally no real separation one from the other. Medially in the male the membranous material is increased to form the suspensory ligament of the penis and more diffusely as the mons pubis in the female.

One important feature is that the membranous layer runs into the perineum to become attached to the posterior border of the perineal membrane and the boney margins behind the external genitalia. Thus any fluid collecting in the superficial perineum, as in a rupture of the urethra in a male, not only fills this perineal pocket back to the space between the genitalia and the anus but is free to track up into the anterior wall of the abdomen. At the inguinal fold the skin is bound down to the deep fascia of the leg (below the inguinal ligaments) and this prevents any fluid tracking down from the abdominal wall to the legs (**380**).

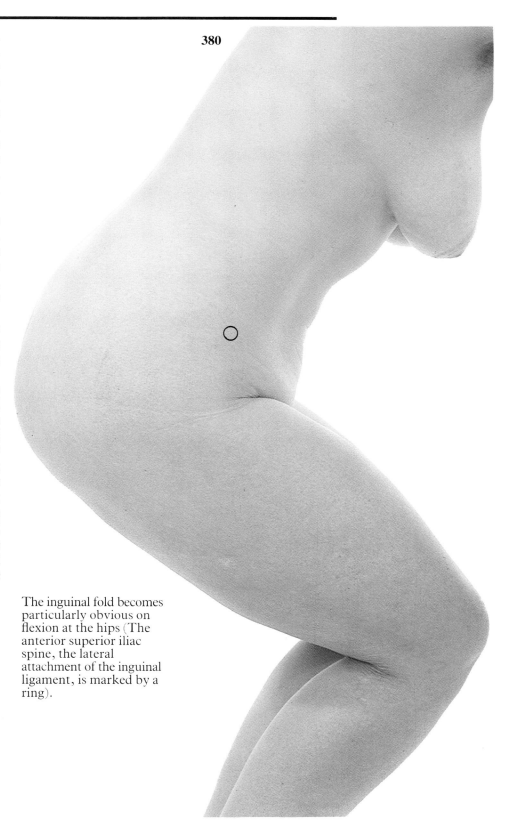

380

The inguinal fold becomes particularly obvious on flexion at the hips (The anterior superior iliac spine, the lateral attachment of the inguinal ligament, is marked by a ring).

THE INGUINAL REGION

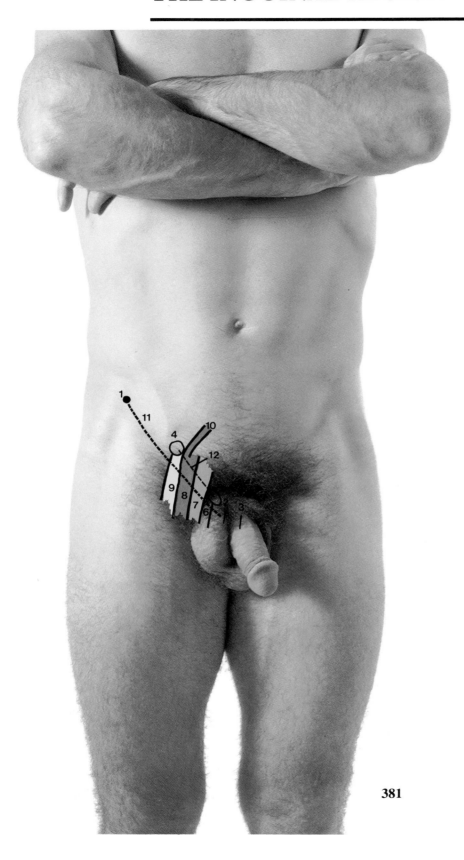

This is an important region clinically, particularly in the male, as it includes the passage serving and linking the testis with the body. As such it is a potential site for hernia as well as a variety of other related problems. During embryological and fetal life, the testes develop within the abdomen and a column of mesenchyme, the gubernaculum testis, maintains an undifferentiated channel through each side of the developing abdominal wall and a core for the scrotum. Shortly before birth this mesenchyme is invaded by the processus vaginalis from the abdomen and through which the testis will descend from the abdomen to the scrotum, after which the processus normally closes. The inguinal canal so formed in the abdominal wall remains after testicular descent, as an oblique canal running through the muscles of the lower abdominal wall, immediately above and parallel to the inguinal ligament, carrying the ductus deferens and the vessels and nerves of the testis.

The inguinal ligament represents the lower border of the aponeurosis of the external oblique muscle of the abdomen. But it is also a fascial confluence between the external oblique above and the deep fascia of the leg below. Joining from above and behind and thus producing a fascial gutter are the fascia iliaca, laterally, and the transversalis fascia (the lining fascia of the abdomen). Behind the inguinal ligament another channel links the abdomen and the leg, the femoral sheath containing three passages; medially the femoral canal, essentially a fat supported lymphatic channel, then the femoral vein and the femoral artery, while the femoral nerve runs lateral to the sheath. Like the inguinal canal the femoral canal is also a possible site for hernia and hence it is important to be able to differentiate the one from the other. Inguinal hernia comes from above the inguinal ligament and a femoral hernia below.

It is essential not to confuse the inguinal fold with the inguinal ligament. The former is a flexion crease linking skin to the deep fascia and runs more transversely and below the ligament; some 2 cm medially and 3–4 laterally (**381**).

381

1 Anterior superior iliac spine	9 Femoral nerve
2 Position of pubic tubercle	10 Inferior epigastric artery
3 Pubic symphysis	11 Inguinal ligament
4 Internal inguinal ring	12 Inguinal canal
5 External inguinal ring	
6 Femoral canal Within	
7 Femoral vein femoral	
8 Femoral artery sheath	

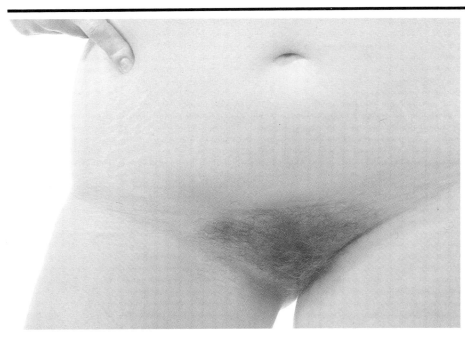

382

The finger is pressing into the abdominal wall immediately above the spine which is palpable below the finger. Note the inguinal fold well below this level.

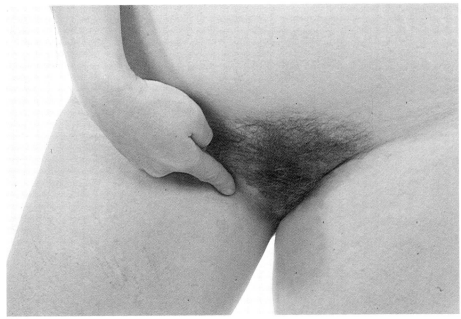

383

Her finger now points to the tendon of adductor longus running up to the pubic tubercle.

Whereas inguinal hernia is more common in males, femoral hernia is more common in females, where the often greater amounts of subcutaneous fat may make the identification of the bony attachments of the inguinal ligament more difficult. Furthermore, while a femoral hernia appears below the inguinal ligament it may produce swelling above the inguinal fold.

The inguinal ligament runs from the anterior superior iliac spine (**382**) which is usually palpable, to the pubic tubercle, which may not be. However the tendon of adductor longus runs up to it and this usually stands out if the leg is abducted (**383**). (In a very fat person resisted adduction from this position will help but this is rarely necessary.)

THE INGUINAL REGION

The inguinal canal runs from the internal inguinal ring, an opening in the transversalis fascia, to the external inguinal ring, an opening in the external oblique aponeurosis. The internal ring is about 2 cm above the mid-point of the inguinal ligament (**384**). Immediately medial to the internal ring the inferior epigastric artery, a branch of the external iliac artery just before it changes its name to femoral, runs up into the abdominal wall. The inguinal canal runs round and in front of this artery. The arteries are usually said to lie at the mid-inguinal point, i.e. midway between the anterior iliac spine and the symphysis pubis (hence just medial to the mid-point of the inguinal ligament, **385**). The external inguinal ring lies some 2–3 cm above and lateral to the pubic tubercle.

In the male the peritoneal processus vaginalis, through which the testis has passed in descent, may not close but remain patent throughout life, either in its whole length or some part. Such a patent channel may allow a herniation from the abdomen through the inguinal canal, i.e. running obliquely through the anterior abdominal wall and hence called an oblique inguinal hernia.

384

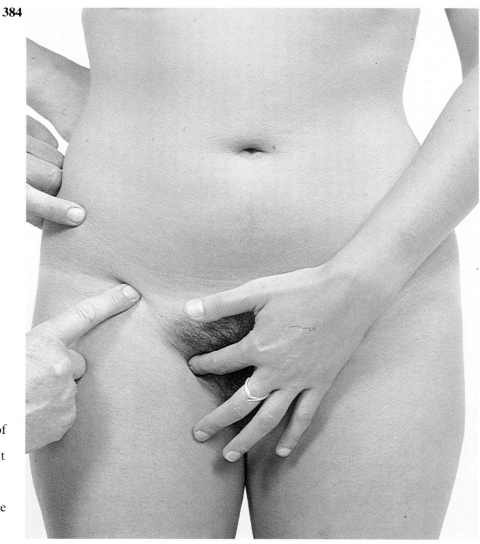

The subject's index finger now identifies the lower attachment of the inguinal ligament while the examiner points to the mid-point of the inguinal ligament immediately above which is the internal inguinal ring. The subject's left thumb indicates the position of the external inguinal ring.

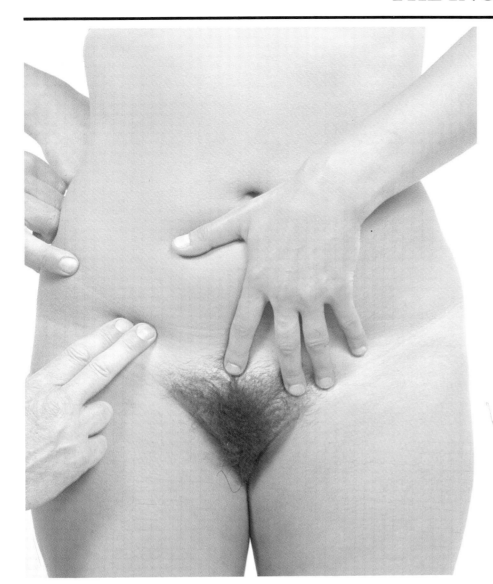

385

The examiner's middle finger now indicates the mid-inguinal point (midway between the anterior superior iliac spine and the symphysis pubis, indicated) and thus overlies the femoral artery and points to the inferior epigastic artery just medial to the internal inguinal ring.

The internal inguinal ring is protected anteriorly by the muscle fibres of the internal oblique muscle from the inguinal ligament and often some of the transversus. These fibres then join together to arch medially and backwards over the inguinal canal to run down as the conjoined tendon behind the external inguinal ring. As the inguinal region is a weak zone in the abdominal wall, herniation can occur directly through deficiencies in the wall. This is the more likely type of hernia in the older age groups.

Although the male is far more vulnerable to inguinal hernia than the female, she also develops a gubernaculum in the embryonic stages and a small processus vaginalis can develop before the normal female pattern of development takes over. If the processus develops to any size, the so-called canal of Nuck, indirect herniation can occur in the female.

THE EXTERNAL GENITALIA

In the female the major part of the external genital region of the perineum shows the two antero-posteriorly running labia majora (singular-labium majus). They run backwards from the pubic arch anteriorly to end at the posterior commissure about 2–3 cm in front of the anus. They are fibro-fatty cushions which carry a posterior extension of the pubic hair (**386–387**). Between them are the labia minora, much narrower folds, which may be almost totally enclosed between the labia majora or project a very variable distance below them. Anteriorly they enclose the tiny homologue of the penis, the clitoris, with the urethra opening immediately behind it. The entrance or vestibule of the vagina lies behind this, extending to the commissure. Although the vagina is a potentially wide canal it is, under normal circumstances, effectively sealed as is to be expected when it is realised that from the vagina an opening exists through the uterus and then the two uterine tubes to the abdominal cavity wherein the ovaries lie. The labia, with a degree of mucoid secretion, give good closure externally unless the legs are abducted quite widely. Within the vagina the anterior and posterior walls meet, so that in cross section the tube comes to resemble a letter H. The walls also have prominent transversely running folds which interlock and, with the mucoid secretions give a most effective seal though readily dilatable as required.

The term vulva or pudendum is often given to the complete external female genitalia which fill the anterior part of the perineum. Behind the vagina and in front of the anus is an important central tendon, the perineal body, which acts as a central axis for the pelvic diaphragm, a muscular system which not only provides important support for the potentially vulnerable female genital passage but also for the muscular sphincteric system of the anus. Damage to this muscular system as may occur in childbirth may leave the female vulnerable to prolapse of the uterus and other problems. Thus care must be taken of this perineal region, not only during the period of childbirth but also to build up the muscular efficiency of the system in the postpartum period.

386

387

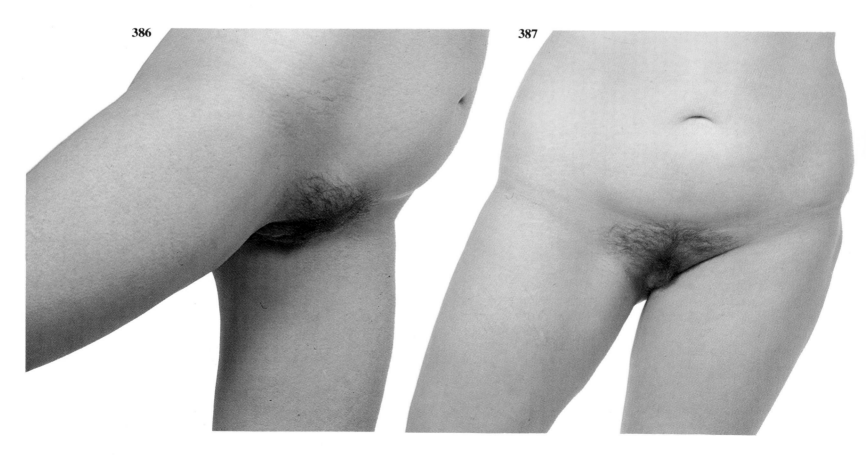

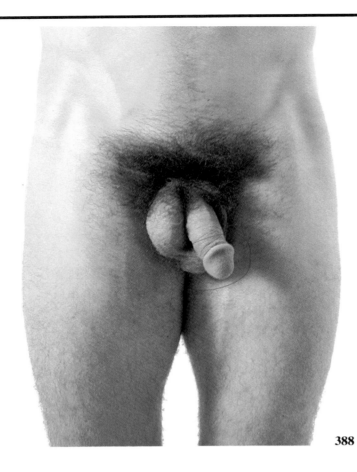

388

In the male the penis is the most obvious anterior feature, hanging down from the pubis but with its root curved backwards along the perineal membrane, which gives a firm base, particularly important when the organ is erected. It is covered by loose skin which is carried down as a protective but retractile sheath over the glans, the sensitive tip of the organ (**389**). Probably for hygienic reasons which have been incorporated into several religious customs and social practices, the terminal sheath or foreskin is often removed (circumcision) to leave the glans permanently exposed (**388**). If the foreskin is retained in some individuals it may fit too tightly around the distal part of the glans so that if retracted it may not be readily returnable and produce severe constriction around the base of the glans (paraphymosis).

The scrotum lies behind the penis. Embryologically this is a fused homologue of the labia majora and the line of fusion is marked by an antero-posteriorly running ridge on the surface.

The scrotum contains the two testes and epididymes. These, having descended into the scrotum to the necessary cooler environment needed for spermatogenesis, rely on the mechanics of the scrotum for temperature maintainance. Failure to descend, as commonly occurs, prevents spermatogenesis in that testis even if it is otherwise normal and capable of producing testosterone, the male sex hormone. Usually the left testis descends first and comes to lie lower in the scrotum than the right. Each testis hangs on a spermatic cord which includes the ductus deferens, responsible for transferring the sperms and their containing fluid. It also includes the testicular artery which is surrounded by the pampiniform venous plexus, an arrangement which allows heat transfer from the arterial blood to the now cooler venous, so reducing the temperature of blood reaching the testis. Travelling also in the cord are the artery to the ductus deferens and the lymphatics and testicular nerves. The testis is also supported

THE EXTERNAL GENITALIA

dynamically by the cremaster muscles, lateral and (usually) medial. The former comes from the inguinal ligament and the medial from the pubis, running down and interdigitating around the cord to be inserted into the root of the testicular mesentery, and are supplied by the genito-femoral nerve (L1 & 2). The cremaster muscles are much smaller and less dynamic than in many mammals who retain an open processus vaginalis and in whom the cremaster muscle pulls the testis back into the abdominal cavity under stress, or in danger. In prepubertal boys it can still be highly active but as the processus vaginalis is closed the testis can only be pulled up close to the external inguinal ring where it usually comes to lie to its lateral edge where the fascia is loosest, in the so-called superficial inguinal pouch. This often gives the impression of an undescended testis unless great care is taken in examining the boy. With the general increase in size of the genitalia at puberty the cremaster muscles become much longer and far less reactive but nevertheless still respond weakly to the cremasteric reflex.

The scrotal wall also contains muscle, the dartos, but this is involuntary and responds to temperature in a similar way to the muscle of the nipple. Its function is to maintain the testis at an even, cooler temperature some 3° below that of the body. Thus it relaxes under warm conditions taking the testes farther from body heat and contracting in colder conditions (**389–390**).

Examination of the testes should be gentle (as should all clinical examination). Pressure on the testis can be extremely painful especially if they become swollen for any reason. They are surrounded by a firm fibrous tunica albuginea which means that if the testis swells the pressure inside the fibrous coat increases, causing considerable pain. The juvenile testes are quite small and hence if retracted can easily be lost to the examiner in the subcutaneous tissues. In the adult they are some 4–5 cm in height and 3 cm in diameter with the comma-shaped collection of tubules, the epididymis, around the posterior aspect and leading off to the ductus deferens. In the neck of the scrotum above the level of the testis the cord can be felt as a soft roundish but indistinct structure but the ductus deferens is easy to feel as a firm round cord due to its very thick muscular wall.

Both urine and seminal fluid are transmitted through the penis to the opening at the tip. However on occasions the penis does not become canalised in development, the urethra opening on its under surface, much as in the female relative to the clitoris, a condition known as hypospadias.

389

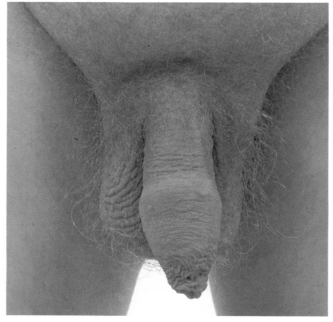

390

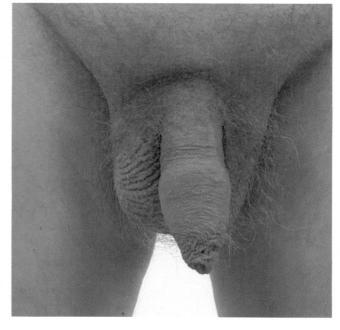

The uncircumcised penis and scrotum in moderate temperature conditions (**389**) and showing some degree of contraction of the scrotal wall on cooling (**390**). Note that even the size of the penis is much influenced by temperature as is to be expected in a highly vascular organ.

The general innervation comes from the segmental spinal nerves. Posteriorly the posterior primary rami innervate the erector spinae muscles and send cutaneous supply to the central skin of the back, roughly as far out as the outer edge of the extensor muscles but with some overlap with the anterior primary rami, which may reach as far as the posterior axillary line. Here the nerves supply areas of skin (with inter-segmental overlap) appropriate to the vertebral level of the nerve i.e. cervical, thoracic, lumbar and sacral.

Anteriorly the position differs. All of the anterior primary rami in the brachial plexus area (C5–T1) go to the arm and those in the lumbo-sacral plexus to the leg. Thus C4 cutaneous innervation runs down over the shoulder and clavicular regions to be succeeded by T2 in and around its segmental band (with a similar jump from upper lumbar to lower sacral in the perineal region). Therefore in the thorax the segmental nerves run around the chest wall in the intercostal spaces, supplying thoracic wall musculature and giving cutaneous branches (**391**). A major lateral branch is homologous with those branches to the brachial plexus and comes through in the mid-axillary line to give a posterior division and a larger anterior division. The posterior division supplies the lateral aspect of the back while the anterior runs on to supply the antero-lateral aspect of the trunk. The lower six thoracic and first lumbar run on down to give a similar supply to the abdominal wall, though T12 & L1 give little supply to the flank but run down to the gluteal region over the hip.

391

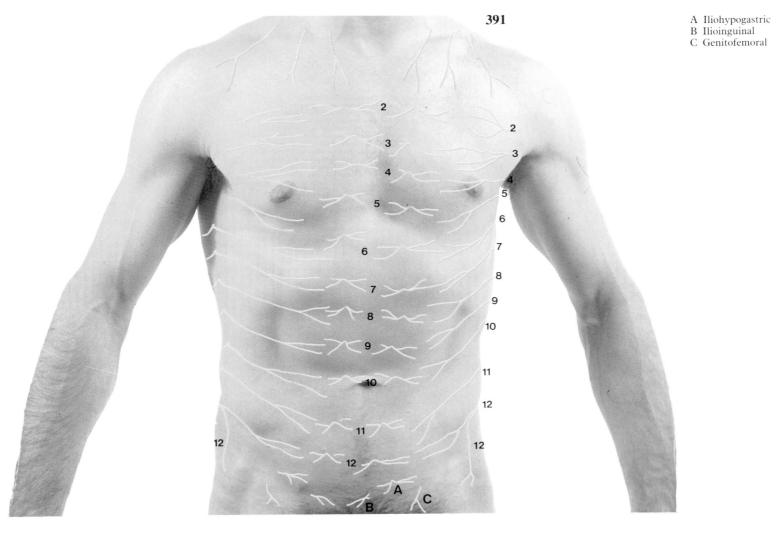

A Iliohypogastric
B Ilioinguinal
C Genitofemoral

NERVES OF THE THORACIC AND ABDOMINAL WALLS

The main nerves then continue round to the front of the trunk, giving terminal sensory branches to the skin. The lower six thoracic and first lumbar run into the lateral aspect of the rectus sheath deep to the muscle and supply and pierce it before supplying the skin. L1 divides early into iliohypogastric and ilioinguinal. The former supplies skin around the pubis and the latter runs through the inguinal canal, supplying skin of the medial part of the groin and the anterior parts of the penis (clitoris) and scrotum (labia). This root also supplies the lowest part of the internal oblique and transversus abdominis muscles and thus it is often considered that its loss predisposes to inguinal hernia due to reduced motor control over that component of the muscles covering the inguinal canal. T10 gives the segmental supply to the umbilicus (**392**).

Although anatomical diagrams tend to give a clear cut segmental picture it must be remembered that, as elsewhere in the body, there is considerable overlap. Thus a segmental nerve will usually supply its own segment, with considerable amounts to those immediately above and below and some to the ones above and below those. Thus loss of an individual segmental nerve, as after an abdominal operation, usually passes unnoticed – but not always.

The root of the penis or clitoris and the anterior parts of the scrotum or labia majora receive their sensory innervation from the ilioinguinal (L1) and the genitofemoral nerves (L1 & 2) but immediately behind that the innervation drops to S 2, 3 & 4 from pudendal nerves. These latter supply the major part of the skin of the penis or clitoris and the external genital and anal regions. This arrangement of innervation of the perineal region is particularly important as, for instance, a low spinal anaesthetic block gives excellent control for much of the perineal region but care must be taken not to move too far anteriorly where the region supplied by L1 & 2 will not be anaesthetised.

From time to time local anaesthetic block of the intercostal nerves is valuable. The main nerve runs along the lower margin of the rib (with the vein deep to the margin of the rib and the artery between it and the nerve). Thus the needle can be inserted close to the lower border of the rib wherever needed, taking care that the tip has not punctured the lung (this will be confirmed if the plunger is withdrawn a little; air indicates that the needle is in the lung and should be withdrawn a short distance). It is also useful to know that if the injection is made posteriorly near the angle of the rib, anaesthetic will travel up and down in the paravertebral gutter for a segment or two giving a wider area of anaesthetisation from a single injection, either for the chest wall or, in the lower nerves for abdominal surgery (though muscular relaxation may be poor). Such an injection may also be valuable for pain in the segmental area such as from fractured ribs etc.

Each nerve gives the major supply to the skin along its segmental axis but in fact supplies a much broader band of skin with considerable overlap of its segmental neighbours.

392

236

Referred pain. It is important to be aware that most deep structures, particularly in the thorax and abdomen, have poor sensory localisation, unlike the skin and the mucous membranes of the mouth and for a short distance up the anus and the vaginal canal. Here the special modalities (pain, touch, pressure, temperature etc.) are readily identifiable. Deep sensation lacks these qualities, though pain from locomotor structures in a limb may be well localised. From the viscera even that localisation is missing and may be referred to a superficial region away from the original site (**393**). Thus pain from heart or lungs (unless parietal pleura is involved) tends to be diffusely concentrated behind the sternum. Pain from the diaphragm and the related pericardium may however be referred to the C4 (& 5) skin areas shared with the diaphragm. Pain thus appears in the shoulder region (C4) or running down the arm (C5). Pain in these regions on the left side may thus be of cardiac origin particularly if it is also associated with sternal pain. However, pain of angina pectoris (i.e. true heart pain) may also appear on the left side of the sternum and spread down the medial side of the arm (T1–5).

In the abdomen, pain from the viscera tends to be localised to the mid-line. Stomach and upper abdominal structures are referred centrally to the epigastrium though an indication of left or right may come from the stomach or liver and gall-bladder. Hypersensitivity or pain from these structures may also affect the area below the scapulae to left or right. The intestines refer generally to the umbilical region with the transverse and descending colons centrally but below. If, however, inflammation etc. affects the parietal peritoneum (or the pleura in the chest) then localisation is good to that area of the surface, as the surface nerves become involved. Thus the characteristic pain of appendicitis is initially to the umbilical region as a dull ache but later inflammation may affect the overlying peritoneum in the right iliac fossa, where the pain becomes sharper and localised (though in a retrocaecal appendix the localisation may be less obvious).

Pain from the kidneys may be referred to the loins as a dull ache but where it affects the pelvis of the kidney or ureter it becomes more localised to the inguinal regions. The pelvic organs including the bladder generally give suprapubic pain.

Although the pain does not originate in the referred area, nevertheless the latter often exhibits hypersensitivity and may even become redder. The pain may also be obliterated by local anaesthetisation of the referred area.

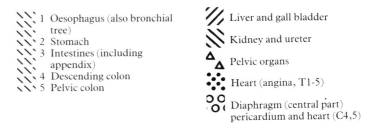

1 Oesophagus (also bronchial tree)
2 Stomach
3 Intestines (including appendix)
4 Descending colon
5 Pelvic colon

Liver and gall bladder
Kidney and ureter
Pelvic organs
Heart (angina, T1-5)
Diaphragm (central part) pericardium and heart (C4,5)

393

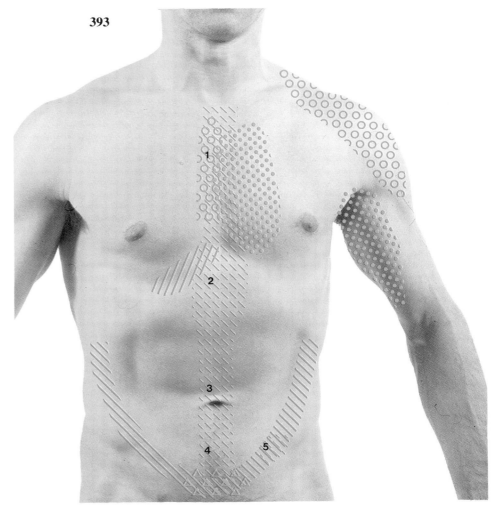

BLOOD VESSELS OF THE THORACIC AND ABDOMINAL WALLS

The body wall receives a rich blood supply with excellent anastomoses, which can often play a major part in providing an alternative route if the axial vessels of the arm or leg are lost proximally.

Dorsal arterial supply comes from arteries running about the lower borders of the ribs in the intercostal spaces, from the aorta and below that in the lumbar region. These arteries, the intercostal and lumbar arteries, follow essentially the same course as the segmental nerves and give similar areas of supply. However, they are supplemented anteriorly by longitudinally running intersegmental arteries with which they anastomose and which come from the origins of the main limb arteries. In the thorax, thoracic branches of the axillary and subclavian arteries give a major lateral and anterior supply anastomosing with the intercostal arteries (**394**). From the axillary artery a small superior thoracic artery supplies the upper anterior chest wall, anastomosing medially with internal thoracic and intercostal arteries. The thoraco-acromial (acromiothoracic) artery supplies the lateral anterior part of the chest wall, while the lateral thoracic runs down approximately in the anterior axillary line. More posteriorly, large vessels form an anastomosis around the scapula, the circumflex scapular, subscapular and suprascapular arteries, this latter from the subclavian via the thyrocervical trunk. Anteriorly the internal thoracic (mammary) artery, is a major branch of the subclavian artery, and runs down from an origin about 2 cm above the medial end of the clavicle, inside the chest wall, 1–1.5 cm from the lateral border of the sternum. Here it anastomoses directly with the intercostal arteries, which thus have anterior as well as posterior vessels of supply, giving an excellent anastomosis between the descending aorta and the subclavian arteries. As well as supplying the diaphragm and intrathoracic branches, the internal thoracic sends segmental perforating branches through the chest wall. In the female the upper branches (2, 3 & 4) are large to supply the mammary gland on its medial aspect while the thoracoacromial artery gives lateral supply. These branches increase considerably in size during lactation. The main trunk then continues downwards, passing the diaphragm, in the gap between its xiphoid and costal attachments, to

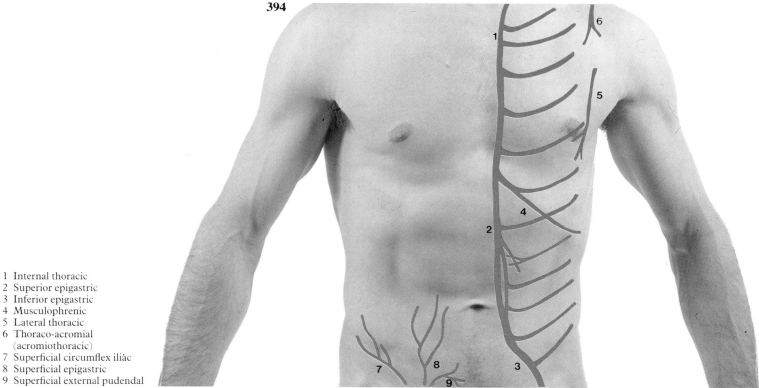

394

1 Internal thoracic
2 Superior epigastric
3 Inferior epigastric
4 Musculophrenic
5 Lateral thoracic
6 Thoraco-acromial
   (acromiothoracic)
7 Superficial circumflex iliàc
8 Superficial epigastric
9 Superficial external pudendal

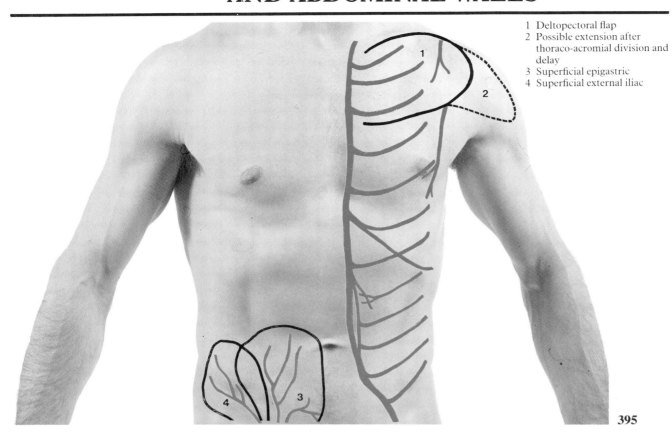

1 Deltopectoral flap
2 Possible extension after thoraco-acromial division and delay
3 Superficial epigastric
4 Superficial external iliac

395

enter the abdomen. Here it becomes the superior epigastric artery. This runs down in the rectus sheath behind the muscle and continuing the intercostal anastomoses before entering the rectus abdominis muscle which it supplies and here anastomoses with the inferior epigastric artery.

Inferiorly the external iliac artery gives off the inferior epigastric artery which passes upwards medial to the deep inguinal ring and then deep to the rectus abdominis muscle, to anastomose with the lower intercostal arteries and the superior epigastric artery. The deep circumflex artery also runs from the external iliac to the lower lateral abdominal wall and anastomoses with arteries of the gluteal region. Slightly more distally the femoral artery gives superficial epigastric and circumflex iliac arteries (as well as pudendal). These originate about 1 cm below the inguinal ligament and run up to supply the lower abdominal wall.

The veins follow essentially the same routes but in the thorax drain posteriorly into the azygos system.

Axial vascular flaps. The rich anastomoses in both the upper and lower trunks offer excellent opportunities for axial vascular skin flaps to be prepared when needed for repair (to which can be added myocutaneous flaps based on the vascular pedicle of the muscle e.g. pectoralis and latissimus dorsi, as well as fasciocutaneous flaps). An excellent long cutaneous flap can be raised on the upper perforating arteries from the internal thoracic and running out towards the deltoid region – the deltopectoral flap (**395**). (If the thoracoacromial artery is first divided and the raising of the flap delayed to allow anastomoses to increase in the flap it can be extended even farther laterally). It can give good soft and thin skin cover for either the face or neck.

The superficial epigastric and circumflex iliac vessels also give good axes for the transfer of lower abdominal skin, e.g. for repair of a hand or elsewhere as a free flap. The skin is good and thin but the superficial epigastric area includes the pubic hair bearing area which is not present in the case of the superficial circumflex iliac flap.

SURFACE FEATURES OF THE ANTERIOR ABDOMINAL WALL

Other than the hair bearing area, the umbilicus is the most obvious feature of the anterior abdominal wall (**396**). It is however an extremely variable structure in form and even in position. Being essentially a scar of the umbilical cord the pattern of degeneration of the structure determines its form. As a scar it is often subject to herniation particularly in young children. Initially it carried the umbilical vein and the two umbilical arteries, while the midgut and the urachus, the terminal part of the developing bladder, also extended into the early umbilical cord. The obliterated umbilical vein, the ligamentum teres, linking the umbilicus with the liver, can be a route for venous dilation in portal hypertension, dilating periumbilical veins to resemble the snake-laden head of the mythical Greek Medusa – and is hence named the caput Medusae. The small intestine may retain a Meckel's diverticulum which may be attached to the umbilicus, possibly leading to important clinical problems, while the bladder always retains a link, the median umbilical ligament. This latter link may be reflected on stimulation of the umbilicus, when the normal T 10 sensory innervation may be supplemented by a diffuse supraumbilical sensation characteristic of the bladder.

396

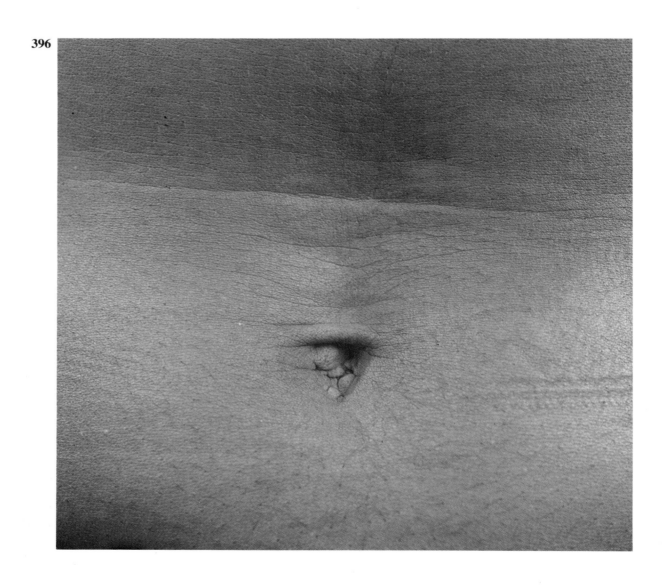

SURFACE FEATURES OF THE ANTERIOR ABDOMINAL WALL

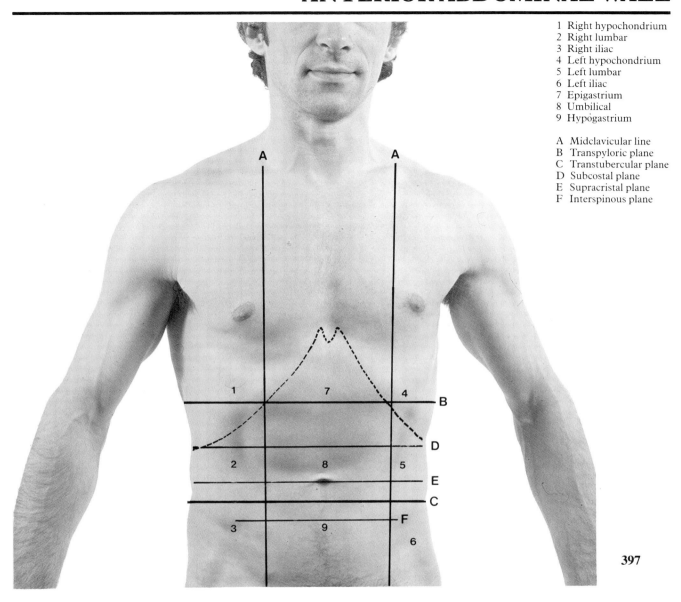

1 Right hypochondrium
2 Right lumbar
3 Right iliac
4 Left hypochondrium
5 Left lumbar
6 Left iliac
7 Epigastrium
8 Umbilical
9 Hypogastrium

A Midclavicular line
B Transpyloric plane
C Transtubercular plane
D Subcostal plane
E Supracristal plane
F Interspinous plane

397

Although somewhat variable, the umbilicus is usually at the level of L3 vertebral spine but may even be as low as L5, particularly in a stocky individual with a protuberant abdomen. The only bony landmarks are at the upper and lower limits; above, the xiphisternum and the costal margins and below, the pubis and laterally the ilia. The anterior superior iliac spines are usually obvious (**397**). Behind this the iliac crest curves upwards and backwards with a lateral flare which is usually more obvious in the broader pelvis of a female. Some 5 cm behind the anterior spine a prominence, the tubercle, may be palpable in a slim person. A similar distance farther back the ilium reaches its highest point, the true crest. The only other features of the anterior abdominal wall at all obvious in a slim muscular person are the mid-line linea alba and, to the lateral border of the rectus abdominis muscle, the linea semilunaris. These lines are made more obvious if the rectus muscle is contracted, whilst the anterior limits of the external oblique muscle may also be seen.

SURFACE FEATURES OF THE ANTERIOR ABDOMINAL WALL

As a result of the relatively featureless expanse of the abdomen in many people, a number of planes are described to help delineation. Of these perhaps the transpyloric plane is the most important. As originally described, it is midway between the suprasternal notch (upper border of the manubrium sterni) and the upper border of the pubis (**398**). Clinically this is of little value in view of the wide exposure of the patient needed and hence an approximate alternative is midway between the xiphisternal joint and the albeit variable umbilicus (**399**). Perhaps more effective is the patient's hands breadth below the xiphisternal joint (**400**). The plane is also at the level at which the linear semilunaris meets the costal border at the tip of the 9th costal cartilage.

Posteriorly it is at the level of the lower border of L1 vertebra and its spine.

Although called the transpyloric plane this is only strictly true, as described, in a cadaver, for when the living person is standing the pylorus may be from 3–10 cm below this level. However it may be more acceptable when the patient is supine and, in this position, is helpful in identifying the position of several other structures. The gall-bladder is usually described as being behind the tip of the right 9th costal cartilage. The renal vessels run across to the hila of the kidneys from the aorta or superior vena cava at this level though the kidneys, like the stomach, drop in upright posture. The superior mesenteric artery is given off from the aorta at this level

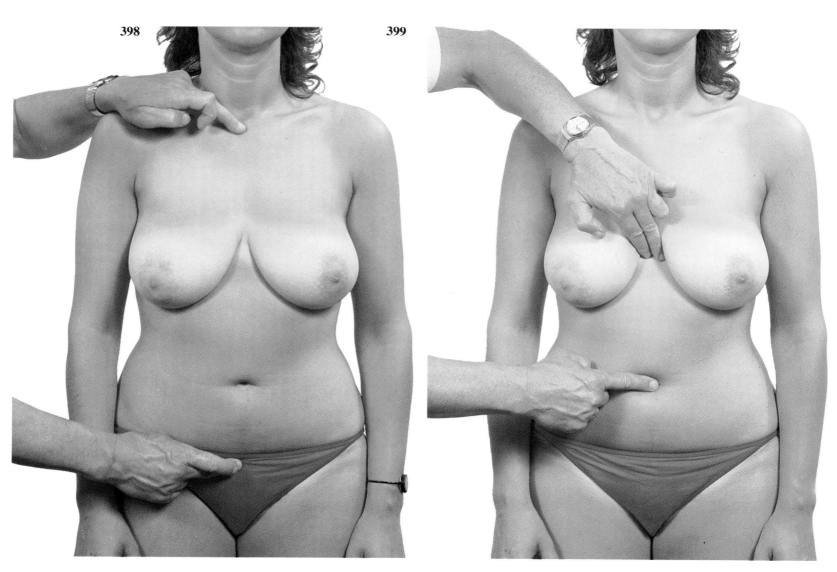

398   399

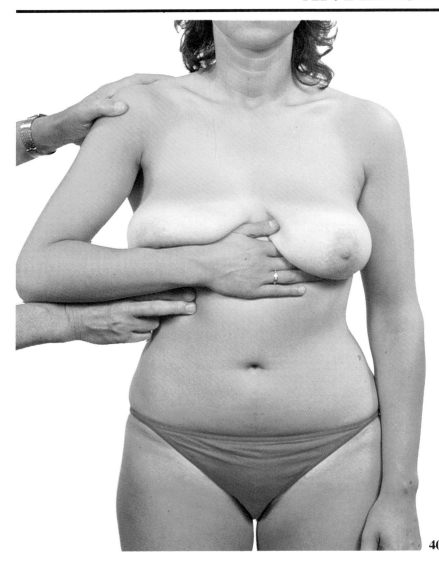

400

which also is the level of formation of the portal vein. Here also some 3–5 cm to the right of the mid-line is the aditus to the lesser sac of peritoneum and, in front of that, the hepatic vessels and the common bile duct run in the free edge of the lesser omentum.

Other useful levels are:

Xiphisternum	Body of T11 (spine of T10)
Iliac crests (Supracristal plane)	L4 spinous process
Iliac tubercles (Intertubercular plane)	L5 spinous process
Anterior and posterior superior iliac spines	S2
Upper border of symphysis pubis (and centre of the acetabulum)	Tip of coccyx (in a female, sacrum in a male)

A subcostal plane is often described (i.e. 10th costal cartilage) but this varies, not only with build but also with posture and state of respiration. It is however usually at L3 when the subject is relaxed and lying supine.

By using the transverse lines of the transpyloric and intertubercular planes with vertical ones drawn down from the middle of the clavicles to the mid-inguinal point, the abdominal and lower thoracic walls can be divided into regions which often facilitate clinical descriptions (**397**).

THE VISCERA

The first and most important feature to be aware of is that the position and shape of certain of the viscera vary enormously with posture, state of respiration, the physiological state of the organ in question and the functional control of the abdominal wall. These factors must be considered before considering evidence of pathology.

The position of viscera relative to posture depends not only on gravity but also to a major extent upon the tonus of the anterior abdominal wall. The stomach at its cardiac end moves essentially with the position of the diaphragm in respiration but at the pylorus, while being at the transpyloric plane when supine, may descend some 2 vertebrae (3–10 cm) in the upright posture. The kidneys are usually described as having an acceptable descent of up to 6 cm but even greater levels of descent have been recorded in perfectly normal medical students.

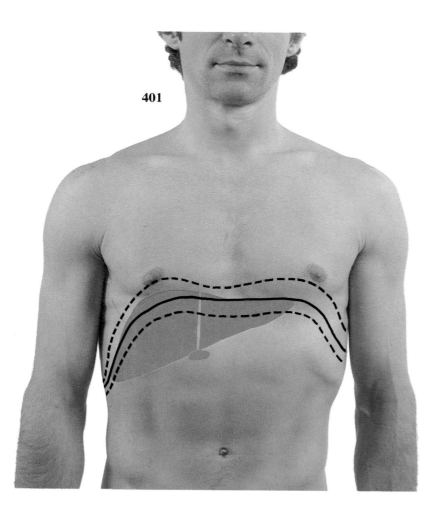

401

Upright posture also affects the transverse colon but even retroperitoneal structures such as the pancreas and duodenum are affected to some extent. The range of descent may be limited by vascular attachments e.g. the liver. It moves with respiration and the diaphragm but is firmly related to the inferior vena cava which in turn is similarly linked to the central tendon of the diaphragm. The spleen, which moves with respiration and becomes more vertical in position in upright posture, is nevertheless limited in its range by its vascular attachments. So also are the kidneys, for although they descend to a considerable distance, further drop is limited by the vessels and if movement is too free their vascular supply can be materially affected.

The positions of the liver, gall bladder, spleen and kidneys are markedly affected by the descent of the diaphragm in inspiration and use is made of this movement in their clinical examination by palpation.

The morphological form of an individual materially affects the shape and position, particularly of the stomach, while the contents of the hollow visera also add to the variations. To this must be added the intrinsic movements due to peristalsis, while the abdominal fat in the mesenteries tends to push the viscera forwards and, in the case of the stomach, elevate its greater curvature.

The Liver lies largely to the right being in the right hypogastrium and extending across the epigastrium. Although described anatomically as having right and left lobes with intervening caudate and quadrate lobes, this description is of relatively little value functionally. More properly the caudate and quadrate lobes should be included in the functional left lobe thus dividing the liver through the gall bladder at the front (tip of the 9th costal cartilage) to the inferior vena cava at the back (**401**). The organ can thus be divided by a line drawn upwards from the tip of the 9th costal cartilage. The functional left lobe thus lies to the left of this line.

The liver lies immediately below the diaphragm and thus of necessity moves with this structure in respiration. Furthermore, due to the maximal diaphragmatic movement being related to the crura, the anterior margin of the liver moves to the right in inspiration. The upper surface of the liver corresponds to the surface markings of the diaphragm (see p 217).

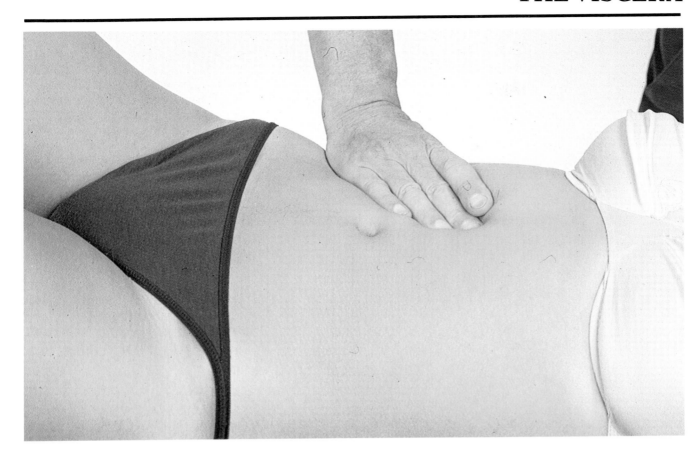

402

On the right it follows the right dome and so in quiet respiration it reaches the level of the 5th costal cartilage (or in the midclavicular line the 4th intercostal space.) The line then runs across the xiphisternal joint to the level of the 6th costal cartilage on the left. The lower margin follows the costal margin on the right and then crosses the epigastrium from the tip of the right 9th costal cartilage to the 8th costal cartilage on the left and continuing on upwards inside the costal margin to end level with the xiphisternal joint some 8–10 cm from the mid-line. In deep expiration the liver rises while in inspiration its anterior margin projects beyond the costal margin on the right but not usually to an extent which is palpable.

Direct clinical examination of the liver is limited by its being covered by the rib cage. As the liver is solid, percussion gives an area of dullness compared with the resonant lung above and the other abdominal contents below. However the upper margin is masked by the overlying lung. Although the liver lies in the epigastrium, even here it is not normally palpable. Pathological enlargement may project the anterior margin below the rib cage, especially on inspiration. If the fingers are laid parallel with the costal margin over the relaxed abdomen and the patient asked to breathe deeply the lower sharp margin may be felt moving across the fingers. (**402**).

Liver biopsy is a common clinical examination. If the patient is asked to breathe out, the biopsy needle can be passed through the lower intercostal space in the mid-clavicular line into the liver without puncturing the lung.

The Gall-bladder is normally described as being behind the tip of the 9th costal cartilage i.e. where the lateral margin of rectus abdominis joins the costal margin. As in the case of the liver it is normally impalpable and even in pathology this is usually the case. However, if the fingers are pressed as in (**402**) below the costal margin and the patient asked to breath in, pain may be induced in a diseased gall-bladder, commonly producing a 'catch' in the breath.

THE VISCERA

The Stomach lies in the hypochondrial, epigastric and umbilical regions. It is subject to numerous variations in shape and position (**403**). The oesophagus penetrates the diaphragm some 3 cm to the left of the midline at the level of T10 or behind the upper part of the 6th costal cartilage. It becomes the stomach a little lower, behind the 7th cartilage. The line of the right side of the oesophagus continues downwards, curving to the right as the lesser curvature of the stomach to the pylorus which lies some 1–2 cm to the right of the midline, at or about the transpyloric plane if the person is supine and the stomach empty. The left border bulges upwards to the left to form the usually gas filled fundus, which rises as high as the 5th rib, in the mid-clavicular line. From here the greater curvature follows a very variable course to the pylorus, depended upon the position, build and muscular state of the individual, contents of the stomach, contents of the other viscera and the muscular activity of the

stomach wall itself, among other factors. The pylorus may drop some 3–10 cm in upright posture and the lower margin of the greater curvature i.e. the pyloric antrum, may descend even more, particularly when full, in a slim built asthenic individual, to well below the umbilicus and into the false pelvis. In a broadly built person the stomach tends to lie more transversely and have the so-called 'steerhorn' shape, whereas the slim asthenic person is likely to have a J shaped structure.

Because of the soft nature of the organ, even when full, it is normally difficult to feel. Occasionally the pylorus is hypertrophic in a young infant when it may be felt as a hard lump, particularly on inspiration. The stomach commonly exhibits a high pitched resonance to percussion though this is largely lost after feeding. However it is often difficult to differentiate the stomach resonance from that of the underlying transverse colon.

Position of a transverse type of stomach when lying supine (solid line) and when standing (dotted line).

403

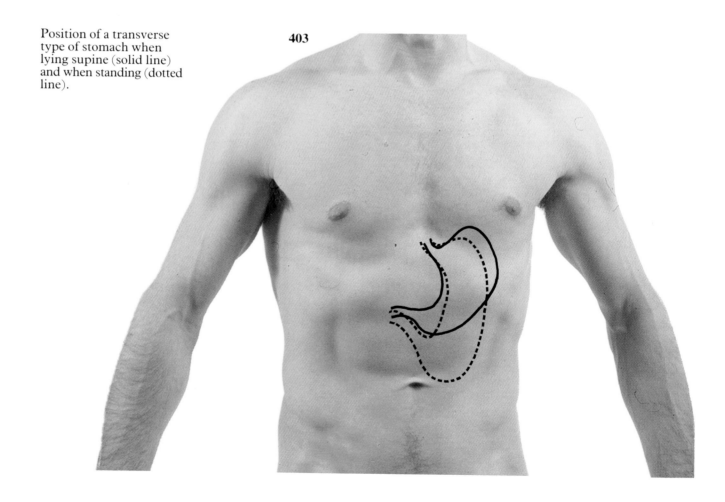

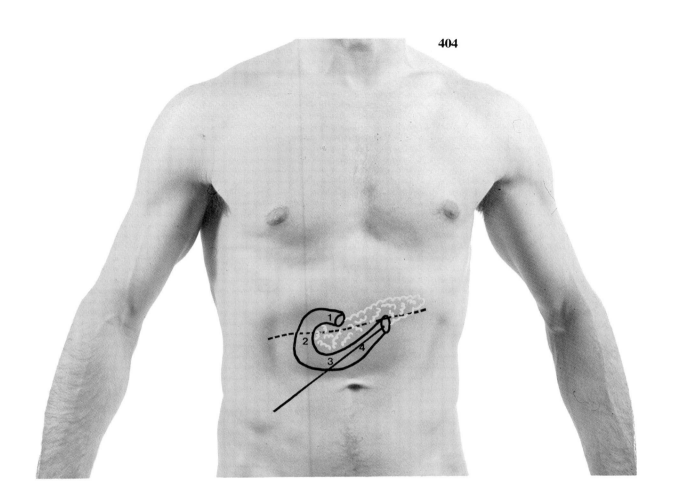

404

The duodenum begins some 2–3 cms to the right of the mid-line at, or below, the transpyloric plane and arches around the head and part of the body of the pancreas. The root of the mesentery of the small intestine is shown as a solid line running from the duodeno-jejunal junction towards the anterior superior iliac spine. The root of the transverse mesocolon is shown as a dotted line. The pancreas is shown in yellow with its tail pointing to the hilum of the spleen. The four parts of the duodenum are numbered.

The Intestines

The duodenum continues from the stomach and curves around the head of the pancreas (**404**). Its first 2–3 cm are carried on a mesentery and therefore exhibit the same motility as the pylorus but the second half of the transversely running first part becomes retroperitoneal and more fixed, roughly in the transpyloric plane or a little above. Some 5 cm to the right of the midline the second part runs vertically downwards for some 7–8 cm before turning again at right angles, now to the left. This is some 5 cm to the right of the midline and about level with the costal margin (L3). The third part of the duodenum then crosses the midline more or less horizontally and about 1–2 cm or so to the left it turns slightly upwards to the duodeno-jejunal junction, about 3 cm to the left of the midline in the transpyloric plane. The position of the junction is held fairly stable by the suspensory ligament of the duodenum (Treitz).

The remainder of the small intestine, the *jejunum* and the *ileum* form a long twisting tube which packs much of the abdomen and pelvis. However it is maintained on a mesentery, the root of which runs obliquely downwards and to the right from the duodeno-jejunal junction to the caecum, i.e. towards the anterior superior iliac spine.

247

THE VISCERA

The caecum lies in the roughly triangular area bounded by the intertubercular line and the lateral half of the inguinal ligament (**405**).

The appendix is a narrow diverticulum of the caecum some 2 cm postero-medial to the ileo-caecal junction. The position of the appendix is so variable that the position of its origin is the only reasonable surface marking i.e. at McBurney's point, at the junction of the middle and lower thirds of the line joining the umbilicus with the anterior superior iliac spine (**406**).

1 Anterior superior iliac spine
2 Tubercle of ilium
3 Crest of ilium
4 Line of inguinal ligament
5 Caecum
6 Root of appendix
   (McBurney's point)
7 Ileum
8 Ascending colon

405

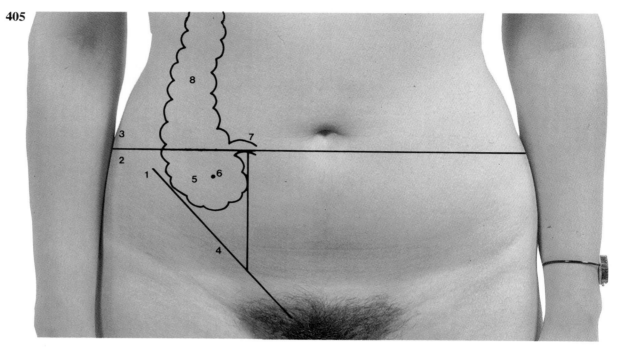

406

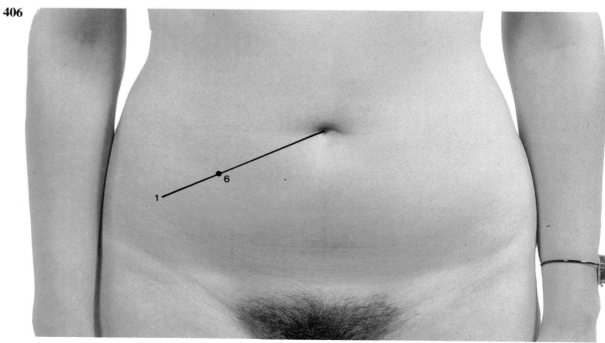

407

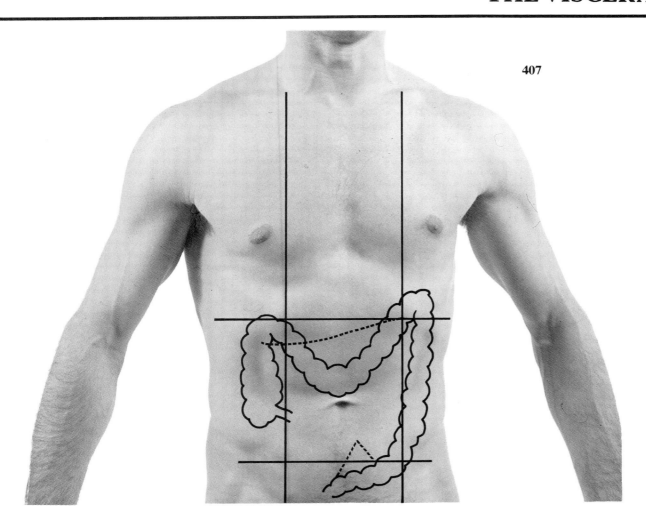

Surface projection of the colon, though the loop of the transverse colon varies. The lines at the transverse and pelvic mesocolon are indicated. The positions of the mid-clavicular lines and the transpyloric and interspinous planes are also marked.

The ascending colon lies in the right flank and is usually impalpable (**407**). It ascends roughly to the level of the 9th intercostal space under cover of the liver i.e. just below the transpyloric plane. Here it turns at the right (hepatic) flexure into the *transverse colon*. This crosses the abdomen on the transverse mesocolon, looping downwards below the greater curvature of the stomach and usually below the umbilicus before running up to the left (splenic) flexure. This lies some 10 cm to the left of the midline and behind the 8th costal cartilage i.e. it loops above the transpyloric plane. Thus the root of the transverse mesocolon can be indicated by a line linking the right 10th costal cartilage to the left 8th. From this region the *descending colon* runs down in the flank inside the ilium. It can often be felt due to its contained faeces if the abdominal wall is relaxed. N.B. If the patient is tense when the abdomen is being examined its wall can often be relaxed by bending up the legs at the hips and knees.

The pelvic colon runs on a mesentery which forms an oblique inverted V running up from the level of the inguinal ligament to the sacral promontory and then down in the midline to about 2–3 cm below the anterior superior iliac spines, when the midline *rectum* begins, i.e. at S3.

The pancreas lies with its head to the right of the midline within the curve of the duodenum. Its neck overlies the aorta and superior mesenteric arteries and thus is in the midline of the body. Its body and tail move upwards and to the left. The tail is said to reach the hilum of the spleen but rarely does completely so in practice; roughly in the mid-clavicular line a little above the transpyloric plane (see **404**).

THE VISCERA

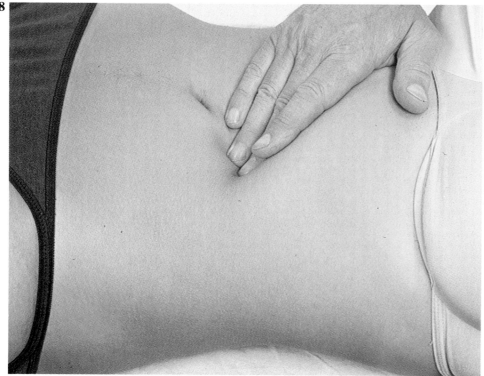

The spleen is of somewhat variable shape lying above the left kidney and behind the stomach and between it and the diaphragm posteriorly. It lies between the 9th and 11th ribs along the axis of the 10th from the lateral border of erector spinae to the midaxillary line. It is in effect on the posterolateral chest wall but separated from it by the diaphragm and pleura. It is thus vulnerable to injury from the back. In deep inspiration the lungs run down between the costodiaphragmatic recess and give it some protection. In quiet respiration the spleen can be delineated by percussion. It cannot be projected against the fingers on inspiration unless considerably enlarged (**408**).

The kidneys are two bean-shaped structures lying on the posterior abdominal wall (**409**). They are surrounded by fat on either side of the vertebrae so that their hila project anteriorly as well as medially. Each adult kidney has a height of some 11 cm and the two hila are some 4–5 cm from the midline. When lying supine the hila of the kidneys should be around the transpyloric plane. The right kidney is lower than the left due, no doubt, to the liver, so that the transpyloric plane cuts the upper part of the right hilum and the lower part of the left. From the back the lower poles of the kidneys should be about 3–4 cm above the iliac crests and the upper parts deep to the lower two ribs. In upright posture the kidneys may drop up to 6 cm and even greater descent may be found on occasions without obvious pathology.

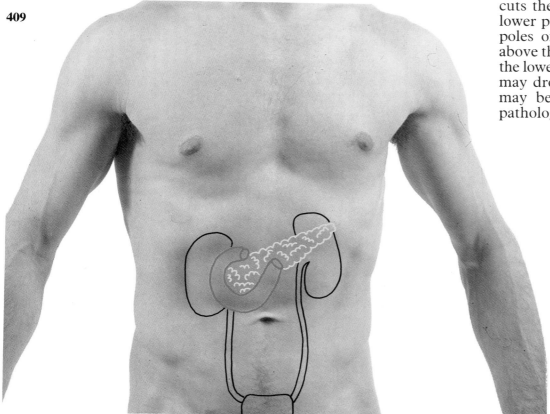

In upright posture the kidneys drop so that the hila are below the level of the transpyloric plane where they lie when supine. The ureters run down almost vertically before curving in behind the bladder.

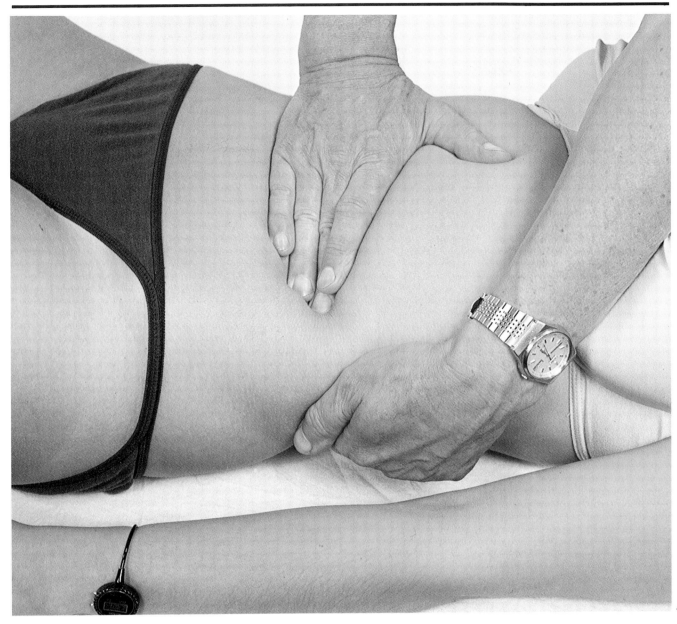

410

In a slim individual lying supine, the lower pole of the normal kidney may be felt descending on inspiration if one hand is pushed forwards from the loin and the other presses into the flank. Enlarged kidneys may be felt more easily (**410**).

The suprarenal glands lie above the kidneys and thus their lower aspects may be estimated as being some 5 cm above the transpyloric plane and on each side of the vertebrae.

The ureters leave the kidneys at the hilum and run down to the back of the bladder. In the supine position they can be delineated as running downwards from the transpyloric plane at some 5 cm from the midline. Initially they run almost vertically but then curve more medially to enter the bladder behind and a little medial to the pubic tubercles. In their course down they cross the sacroiliac joints and the common iliac arteries at their bifurcation which is at the intertubercular line about 4 cm from the midline.

THE VISCERA

The bladder lies largely behind and a little above the pubis when empty. It then has an essentially flat upper surface covered by a coil of intestine and the body of the uterus in a female. As it fills it becomes more dome shaped and a normally full bladder extends upwards to about mid-way between the pubis and umbilicus. In retention of urine, however, it may reach the umbilicus or even higher. In a baby it lies entirely within the abdomen and has a more tubular shape only reaching adult form and position in late childhood.

The bladder is not normally palpable but where it extends above the pubis its upper border can usually be delineated by percussion. In the male *the prostate* lies below the bladder in a retropubic position, and can be examined rectally. *The uterus* in an adult female lies behind and above the bladder. When the bladder is empty the uterus projects only a short distance above the pubis. As the bladder fills the normal anteverted uterus is pushed more vertically so that it projects well above the pubis as do the uterine tubes (**411**). During pregnancy it enlarges enormously and extends upwards towards the costal margins pushing the other viscera ahead. During the second half of pregnancy the uterus is easy to feel but not otherwise. It is, however, possible, to examine it per vaginam, pressing it forwards against a second hand above the publis. After child-bearing the uterus remains a little enlarged, and never returns fully to its original size.

The ovaries lie roughly level with the anterior superior iliac spine above the mid-inguinal point, though these are also pulled up by the uterus in pregnancy.

1 Bladder empty
2 Bladder moderately distended
3 Uterus with empty bladder
4 Uterine tube
5 Ovary

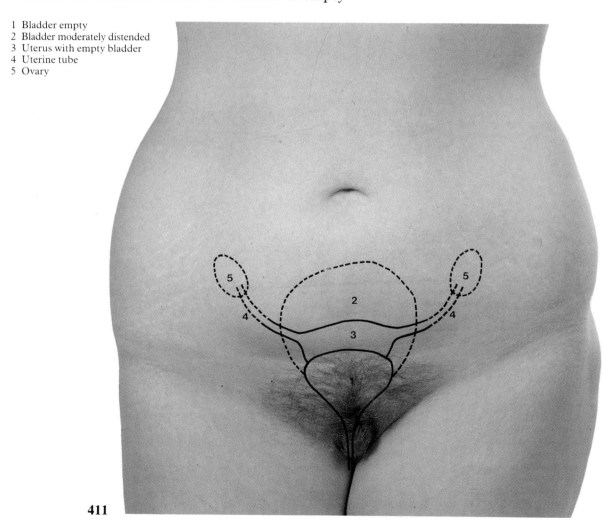

411

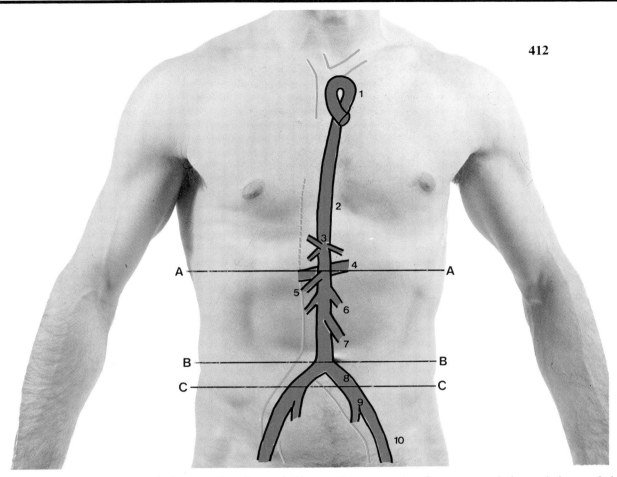

412

The levels of the brachiocephalic veins and the superior vena cava are shown as are the common iliac veins with the inferior vena cava.

A Transpyloric plane (L1/2)
B Intercristal plane
C Intertubercular plane (L5)
1 Arch of aorta
2 Descending aorta
3 Coeliac axis (T12)
4 Renal arteries
5 Superior mesenteric
6 Gonadal
7 Inferior mesenteric
8 Common iliac
9 Internal iliac
10 External iliac

The aorta enters the abdomen in the midline under the median arcuate ligament in front of T12 vertebral body, i.e. some 3–4 cm above the transpyloric plane (**412**). It runs down in the midline to end slightly to the left by dividing in front of L4 vertebra (intercristal plane) into the common iliac arteries. Within the abdomen it is about 10 cm long. The coeliac axis leaves immediately after the aorta has entered the abdomen, dividing almost immediately into hepatic, splenic and left gastric branches. The superior mesenteric artery is given off anteriorly at or a little above the transpyloric plane at which level the renal arteries also leave laterally. Slightly below, the gonadic vessels leave followed by the inferior epigastric at approximately L3, about the subcostal plane.

The common iliac arteries diverge from the aorta in front of L4 vertebral body, and each divides into internal and external branches at the sacro-iliac joints, in the intertubercular plane some 4 cm from the midline. From here the external iliac arteries flow around the pelvis, each leaving under the middle of the inguinal ligament to become a femoral artery.

The inferior vena cava is formed in front of L5 vertebral body by the junction of the common iliac veins. It thus begins at the intertubercular plane some 2–3 cm to the right of the midline and runs upwards similarly placed to pass through the central tendon a similar distance from the midline at the xiphisternal joint (T8–9).

The portal vein is formed behind the neck of the pancreas by the junction of the superior mesenteric and splenic veins. This is roughly in the midline and about 1–2 cm below the transpyloric plane from which position it runs up to the liver.

The abdominal lymphatics generally follow the aorta and therefore can be grouped with this. Those from the viscera form upon its anterior face while the body-wall lymphatics run up to its side.

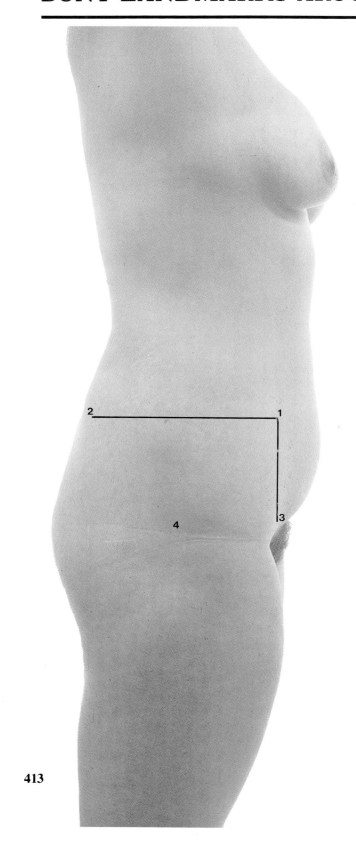

413

The anterior superior spine of the ilium is usually readily palpable, as is the greater trochanter of the femur (the so-called hip-bone). At the front, the pubis may be difficult to feel but its tubercle can be identified by running the finger up the tense adductor longus tendon, (**383** page 229). In normal stance the anterior superior iliac spine should lie in the same vertical plane as the symphysis pubis in lateral view (**413**) and at the same horizontal level as the posterior superior iliac spine and the second sacral vertebra. As indicated on page 243 the upper aspect of the pubis is at the same level as the tip of the sacrum in a male and of the coccyx in a female (the latter because of the shorter, broader sacrum). The upper aspect of the greater trochanter is also at this same level.

The greater trochanter forms a prominence on the surface, particularly in a slim male, forming the broadest part of the hips; in a female this may be a little lower because of the thicker fat which may be in this region of the thigh; the same may also be true in a muscular male due to muscle bulk. In normal posture – i.e. standing with the toes pointing directly forwards – the neck of the femur runs somewhat backwards, so that the greater trochanter lies a little behind the hip joint. Thus, in a radiograph, the greatest length of the neck of the femur is shown by turning the leg medially. With the leg laterally rotated the neck of the femur appears very short. As the lesser trochanter lies somewhat to the rear of the medial side of the femoral shaft, only a small projection is shown in the normal position, being largely overlapped by the shaft of the femur. But in lateral rotation this becomes fully prominent on the radiograph. The upper border of the greater trochanter should be level with, though behind, the centre of the hip joint. By pressing upwards into the buttock the ischial tuberosity should be palpable when the gluteal muscles are relaxed.

1 Anterior superior iliac spine
2 Posterior superior iliac spine
3 Upper aspect of pubis
4 Upper aspect of greater
   trochanter

BONY LANDMARKS AROUND THE HIP

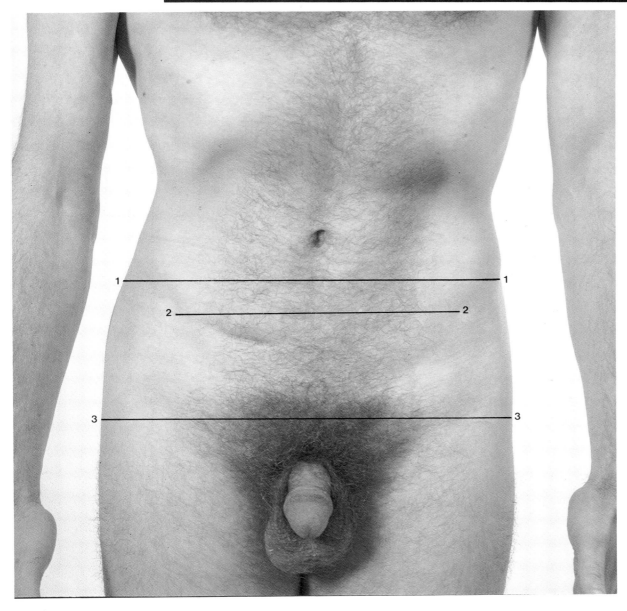

1 Iliac crests
2 Anterior superior iliac spines
3 Greater trochanters

From this stance it appears at first sight that one leg is longer than the other, but the anterior superior spines are level. The problem is one of mild scoliosis.

From a clinical point of view, any variation in leg length is important as is the site of any shortening. A line drawn across the two anterior superior iliac spines should be parallel with a line drawn across the two greater trochanters and, with the person standing, should be level (**414**).

When a person is lying supine there may appear to be shortening of one leg which may be real or just apparent. If there is variation, on standing, the anterior superior spines are not at the same level and the measured distance from the anterior superior spines to the tip of the medial malleoli are unequal, then it is important to know where the shortening is. If the lines joining the anterior spines and the trochanters are parallel then the problem lies below the level of the greater trochanters. A measure should then be made of the distances from the anterior spine to the knee, using the tibial tubercle or the top of the tibial table to the medial side of the patella and from there to the tip of the medial malleolus. Differences when compared with the other side should indicate the site of shortening.

MOVEMENT AT THE HIP JOINT

The hip joint is an extremely stable ball and socket joint between the acetabulum and the rounded head of the femur. The acetabulum is deepened by the fibro-cartilaginous lip, the labrum acetabulare, and these two structures form a cup which effectively contains a full hemisphere of the femoral head. The result is that, whereas dislocation is seen quite frequently at the shoulder joint, it is unusual in a normal hip which has no damage to the acetabular lip, though it does occur where there is congenital deformity of the acetabular cup.

The range of movement is considerable but much smaller than that of the shoulder region. It is not even as great as at the shoulder joint itself, where the joint's range is amplified by movements between girdle and trunk; this is not possible at the hip. Movement between the trunk and the pelvic girdle is minimal, no more than for some shock absorption. However the movement at the hip can be made to appear greater due to movement of the lumbar spine and this must be excluded when examining hip movement. Movements at the hip are flexion, extension, abduction, adduction, medial and lateral rotation and their combination, circumduction.

Flexion appears to allow the thigh to come up to the anterior abdominal wall as long as the knee is flexed to reduce tension on the hamstring muscles. However, much of this movement is due to flexion of the lumbar spine, which must be prevented. With the subject lying on the back the hip is flexed with a bent knee while the examiner keeps a hand under the lumbar spine in the hollow of the back. This hand records when straightening of the lumbar spine begins at the end of the normal range of hip flexion – some 120° (**415**).

Abduction and adduction can likewise be examined with the subject lying supine. The straight leg is carried out to the side (abduction) and then across the other (adduction). Care should be taken to watch for movement of the anterior superior iliac spines which indicates that movement is beginning in the lumbar spine. Abduction is possible to some 45–60°, with

415

416

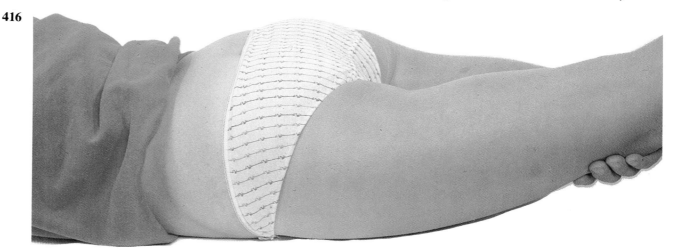

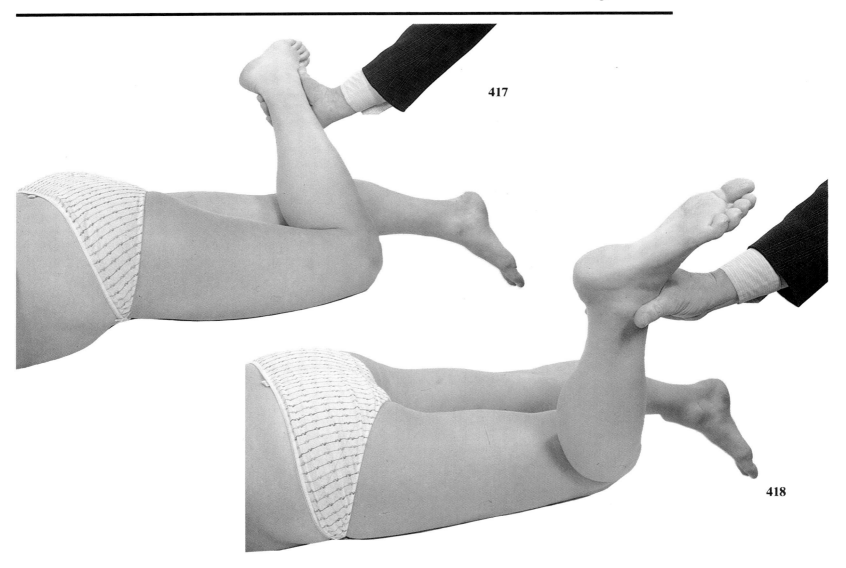

417

418

adduction also about 45°, though here movement is to some extent limited by the other leg. It is important that the leg should be maintained without rotation in this manoeuvre as lateral rotation greatly increases the range of lateral movement, a phenomenon made use of in classical ballet where 'turn-out' at the hip is used to increase the lateral range of movement of the leg.

Extension is normally limited to some 15–20° but can appear much greater, as in the arabesque of classical ballet where the leg is carried high to the back by extension in the lumbar spine (see page 225). If the subject is laid face down (prone), the leg to be examined is lifted by the examiner, the weight of the other leg, which must remain on the couch, being used to limit lumbar extension (**416**).

Medial and lateral rotation can also be examined with the subject lying prone. The knee is bent to 90°, and the thigh rotated, using the lower leg as an indicator of the angle of rotation – normally some 60–70° each way (**417–418**). Both can be somewhat greater in loose-jointed individuals. It is sometimes useful to measure the ranges of rotation with the hips flexed. This can be done either with the subject sitting when the lower leg is swung medially and laterally, or in the supine position, when the knee and hip are bent to 90° and the manoeuvre is carried out.

BONY POINTS AROUND THE KNEE

In a slim person the most obvious feature of the knee is the patella, which may make a prominent flattened knob. In a muscular male the vastus medialis may mask the upper part of its medial edge but the lower part and the whole of the lateral edge are evident, the belly of vastus lateralis being much shorter than the medial. In an obese person the bone may appear lost in superficial fat but centrally it still remains palpable in a relatively subcutaneous position overlaid by the prepatellar bursa. In even a slim female the knobbly contour is usually softened by the feminine subcutaneous fat (**419**).

The patella lies on the anterior surface of the lower end of the femur when the knee is in extension but follows around its distal end as the knee is bent (**420**). Thus with the joint bent to a right angle the patella forms the terminal feature of the thigh and, when kneeling, transmits the load of the body to the distal end of the femur.

If the quadriceps muscles are relaxed the patella can be moved medially and laterally to some extent. Lateral movement is limited by the anterior prominence of the lateral femoral condyle and this can be felt projecting close to the deep side of the lateral edge of the patella. Medially the contact between the two bones is less close as can be felt through the tissues in a slim person. The bony femoral prominence to the lateral side of the patella helps (with the medial pull of the vastus medialis) to prevent lateral dislocation of the patella which is otherwise a potential feature of the angulated knee and is in fact quite a common problem in females where the angle is greater than in males (see page 262).

The patella is a sesamoid bone in the tendon of the quadriceps muscles (though it ossifies at some four years of age whereas most sesamoid bones do not do so until nearer puberty).

Below the patella and joined to it by the ligamentum patellae is the tibial tuberosity, a prominence on the front of the upper end of the tibia. The tuberosity has a more prominent lower part into which the tendon is inserted, while the smoother upper part is separated from the tendon by the deep infrapatellar bursa.

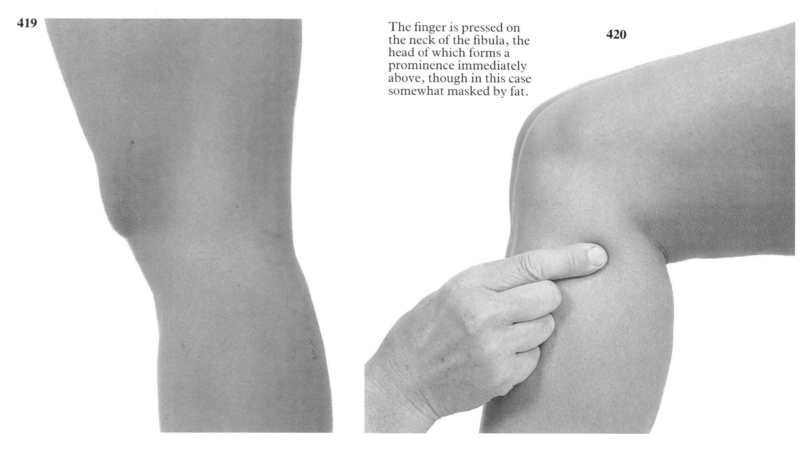

419

420

The finger is pressed on the neck of the fibula, the head of which forms a prominence immediately above, though in this case somewhat masked by fat.

BONY POINTS AROUND THE KNEE

The tibial tuberosity also has a bursa between it and skin, the superficial infrapatellar bursa. Involvement of either the prepatellar or the superficial infrapatellar bursae with swelling leads to the condition often known as housemaid's or clergyman's knee, supposedly due to too much kneeling on the prominent bony knobs.

Above the tibial tubercle and to each side of the ligamentum patellae is a hollow and in this the joint space can be felt above the sharp edge of the tibial condyles. The space behind the ligamentum patellae is filled by a soft fat pad which pushes folds of synovium into the joint space anteriorly – the alar folds. Lateral to the fat the anterior horns of the menisci can be felt, more easily as the knee is extended when the menisci tend to be projected a little.

The space of the knee joint can be followed around the sides until medially its detail is reduced by the medial collateral ligament and the overlying muscle and tendon (**421**). Laterally the iliotibial tract has a similar masking effect with the knee in extension (**422**), but in flexion the space can be felt crossed by the rounded cord of the lateral collateral ligament, running from the lateral femoral condyle to the head of the fibula. In extension this ligament is overlaid by the thick tendon of biceps femoris.

Above the joint space the medial and lateral epicondyles of the femur form medial and lateral projections of the joint region, while on the medial side the thin tendon of insertion of adductor magnus which lies to the anterior aspect of the medial hollow above the knee, leads to the adductor tubercle.

Below the joint the medial condyle of the tibia can be felt on the anterior and medial aspect, while laterally the lateral tibial condyle is supplemented by the prominent head of the fibula. Posteriorly the condyles of the femur are covered by muscle masses of gastrocnemius and the hamstrings, leaving a hollow between, the fat filled popliteal fossa.

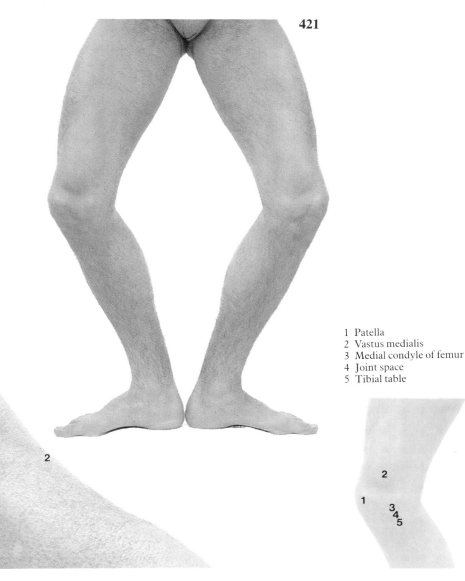

422

1 Patella
2 Tubercle of tibia
3 Tibial condyle
4 Head of fibula
5 Joint space
6 Biceps femoris
7 Iliotibial tract
8 Vastas lateralis
9 Rectus femoris

421

1 Patella
2 Vastus medialis
3 Medial condyle of femur
4 Joint space
5 Tibial table

259

MOVEMENT AT THE KNEE

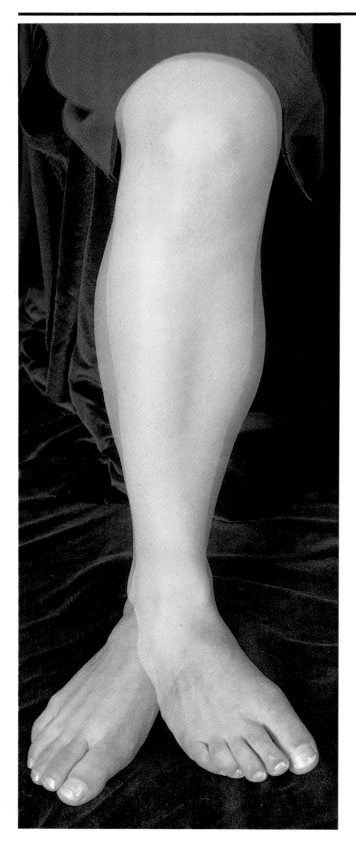

423

The knee is usually described as a hinge joint allowing flexion and extension but this simple description neglects the accessory movements which are of functional and clinical importance. Flexion is usually described as being limited by contact of the calf on the back of the thigh but as shown on page 18 this may not be achievable as an active movement with the hip extended because of the active insufficiency of the flexor muscles. Extension should be to a full 180° but is commonly more in loose limbed individuals who may well be capable of some 15–20° beyond this, producing the so-called sway-back knee.

Although usually described as a hinge joint the knee is far more complicated functionally. Lateral movement should be virtually nil but in certain individuals some may be present. This becomes important because of the load the knees have to carry; not just the weight of the body in standing on one leg but several times that when landing on one leg, even from such apparently gentle exercise as walking or jogging.

Most important in knee movement is the normally relatively small amount of rotation which occurs but which sometimes can be quite considerable. As the knee is extended there is a small amount of lateral rotation of the tibia on the femur and this is particularly so as full extension is reached, thus 'locking' the knee into a stable, close compacted state for standing. This is produced to a major extent by the twist of the cruciate ligaments which become taut in extension. The movement produces a slight turn out of the toes which, when standing to attention with the feet together may be increased slightly by a lateral rotation of the leg at the hip joint to increase lateral stability.

On the initiation of flexion, the process is reversed; the tibia is rotated medially on the femur by the more dynamic activity of popliteus muscle, a flexor rotator at the knee joint, which also by being partly inserted into the posterior horn of the lateral meniscus (semilunar cartilage) adjusts and protects this in the movement.

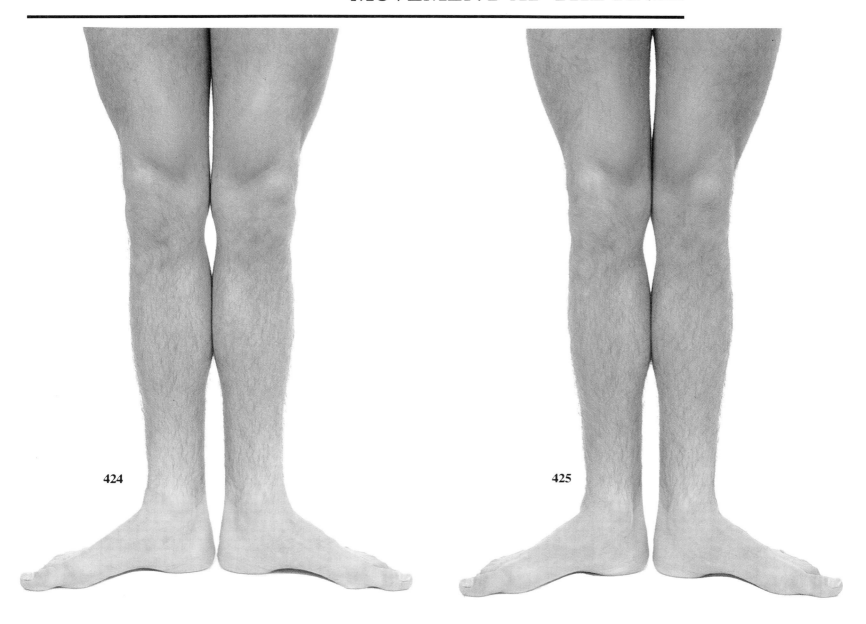

424

425

When the knee is near to extension the rotation should be essentially a feature of flexion and extension but with the knee flexed much more free range of these movements becomes possible to permit rotatory movements of the body on the standing fixed foot in dynamic activities (**423**). Unfortunately such movements often occur while twisting without proper muscle control, when the menisci (particularly the medial) may become at risk.

In classical ballet 'turn out' is an important feature, essentially at the hip joint, to free the range of lateral movement at the hip. Unfortunately for many people what matters is the position of the toes. The figure in **424** shows the movement correctly performed by lateral rotation at the hips, whereas in **425** a well trained dancer is trying to allow the movement by rotation at the knee. Note how the patella is now facing forwards. Far worse uncontrolled knee rotation can often be seen in poorly run classical dance schools where forced rotation of the knee has been permitted to produce the poor teacher's concept of "well turned out toes".

KNEE ANGULATION

To allow for parturition, the female should have a wider pelvis than the male. The two femora are thus widely separated at the hips and approach each other at the knee to allow the lower part of the legs to run vertically and parallel. There is thus a small angle from the vertical between femur and tibia, greater in the female. If there is laxity of the ligaments and muscles, particularly on the more vulnerable medial side, with overweight, this angle may become increased, producing knocked knees (genu valgum). Thus, when the knees are

426

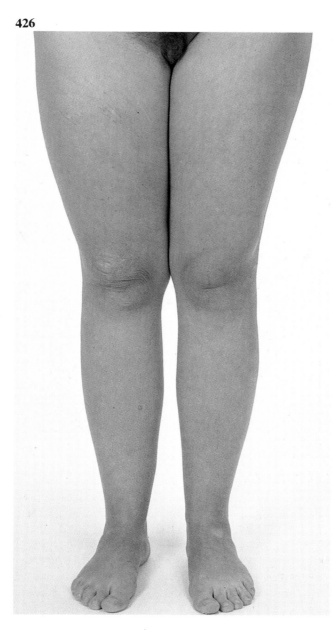

427

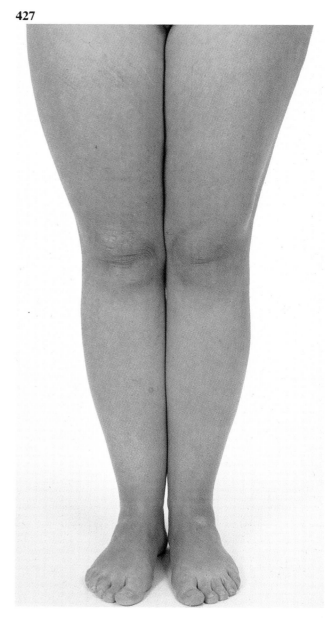

together, the feet may be some distance apart (**426**) and attempts to pull the feet together may compress the knees or even cause them to overlap (**427**). Compare the angles between the female in the colour illustration and the male inset. Overweight boys are also inclined on occasions to show a similar problem, associated with joint laxity.

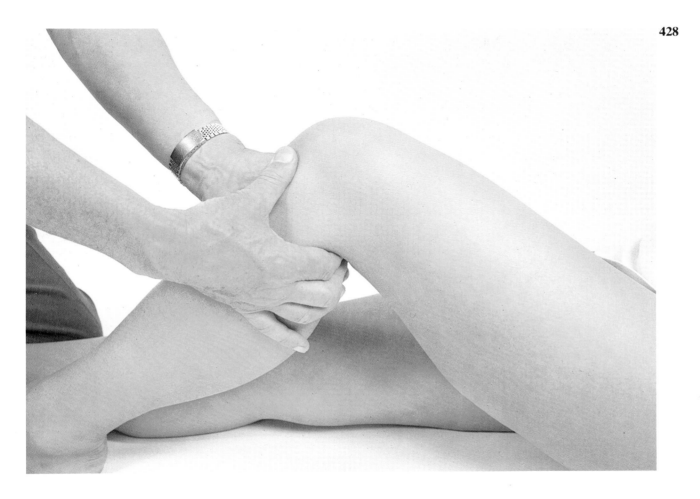

428

Owing to the angulation, laxity of the medial ligament of the knee joint is common, while this ligament is also particularly vulnerable to injury and even rupture. Examination of the collateral ligaments can be carried out by holding the leg straight, while the patient tries to relax the muscles controlling the joint, and then pressing the knee region firmly from the lateral side for the medial ligament and from the medial side for the lateral. Note that in loose jointed individuals there may be quite obvious movement and therefore it is important to compare both legs.

The cruciate ligaments create much of the internal stability of the knee joint and, in particular, prevent the femur riding forwards on the tibial table, especially when walking downhill. They are taut in extension where their twisting contributes to the locking rotation in extension. They also tighten in full flexion and are at their slackest in mid flexion. Testing of these ligaments is usually carried out in mid flexion. The foot is fixed and the upper end of the tibia is gripped and forced backwards and forwards on the femur (**428**). With normal cruciate ligaments the movement should be no more than a few millimetres.

MUSCLES ACTING OVER THE HIP JOINT

The majority of muscles acting only over the hip joint run from the pelvis and sacrum to the femur but one of the two prime flexors at the hip joint, psoas major, comes from the bodies and intervertebral discs of the upper lumbar vertebrae, running from within the abdomen and pelvis to the leg. From this position on the front of the lumbar vertebrae it could pull these forwards and thus increase the lumbar lordosis as well as flexing the hip joint unless the pelvis is firmly fixed on the trunk, a prime function of the abdominal wall muscles. Thus flexion of the leg while lying on the back is an excellent exercise not only for the leg flexors but, most importantly, the abdominal wall muscles.

The other major flexor, iliacus, comes from the inner aspect of the ilium and joins the lateral side of psoas to run down together to be inserted into the lesser trochanter of the femur. On their course they pass under the inguinal ligament and directly over the hip joint from which they are commonly separated by a bursa. These two muscles work more or less in unison and thus as iliopsoas they are powerful flexors of the leg on the trunk (**429**) but also importantly raise the trunk on the leg when getting up from the supine position.

As the insertion into the lesser trochanter lies lateral to the axis of rotation of the leg through

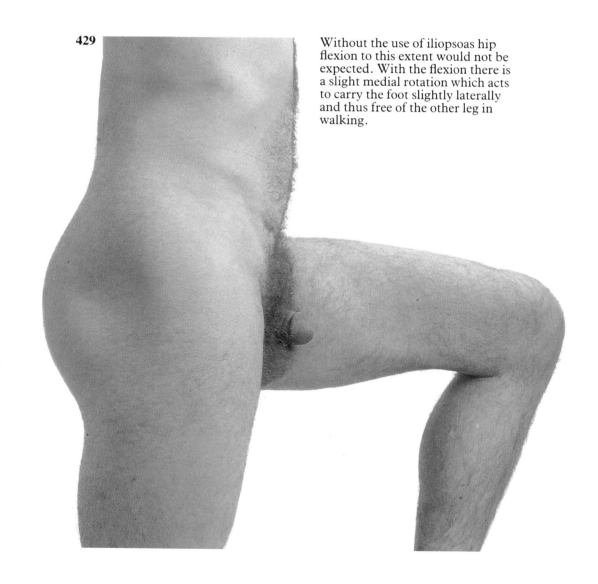

429

Without the use of iliopsoas hip flexion to this extent would not be expected. With the flexion there is a slight medial rotation which acts to carry the foot slightly laterally and thus free of the other leg in walking.

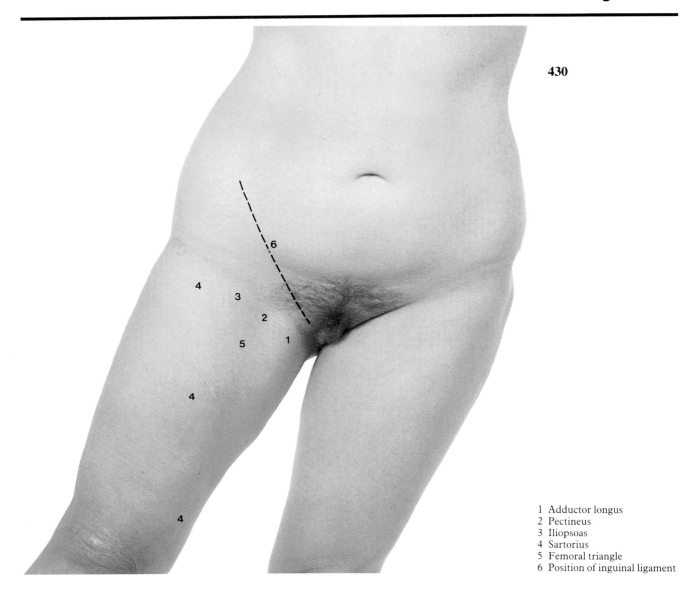

430

1 Adductor longus
2 Pectineus
3 Iliopsoas
4 Sartorius
5 Femoral triangle
6 Position of inguinal ligament

the hip joint, the iliopsoas also acts to produce some medial rotation at the hip joint. However in fracture of the neck of the femur the bone loses its axis of movement at the hip joint and, as the pull is on its medial aspect, it is now free to rotate laterally, under the pull of iliopsoas. This produces the characteristic lateral rotation typical of a fractured femoral neck, the foot coming to lie pointing laterally.

As both these muscles lie deeply they are virtually impossible to see or examine directly other than by testing hip flexor strength.

Both muscles receive their innervation from lumbar nerves, mainly L2 and L3.

Pectineus arises from the superior ramus of the pubis and runs down, medial to psoas, to be inserted into the femur below the lesser trochanter. It acts both as flexor and adductor at the hip joint together with some degree of medial rotation. It lies deeply in the medial aspect of the femoral triangle of the groin where it may be felt contracting on resisted flexion/adduction somewhat lateral to the tendon of adductor longus (**430**). It is not easy, however, to dissociate the one from the other. It is innervated by the femoral nerve (L2, L3 and L4) but may receive supply from the obturator nerve from the same roots.

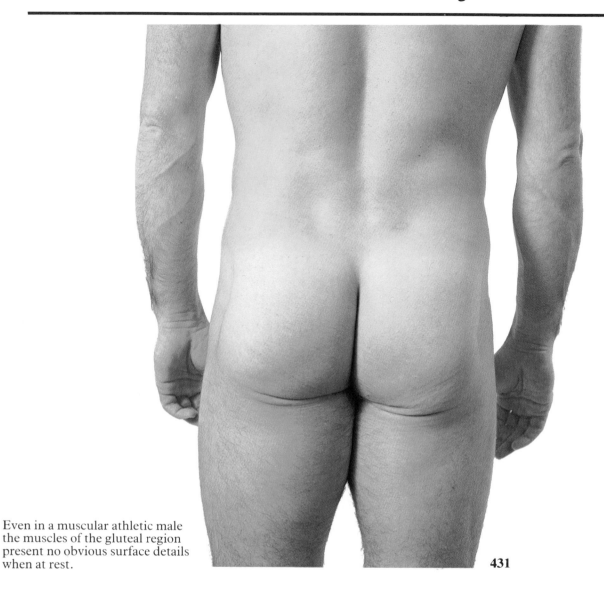

Even in a muscular athletic male the muscles of the gluteal region present no obvious surface details when at rest.

431

The three adductor muscles form a powerful mass on the medial side of the thigh and are readily palpable on forced adduction.

Adductor longus is attached to the pubis just below the pubic tubercle, by a thick rounded tendon which is readily palpable, even in an obese person, when the leg is adducted against resistance, where it acts as a useful guide to the tubercle (see page 229). It usually also stands out when put on stretch in the abducted leg (**430**). From the tendon the muscle runs backwards and laterally to be inserted in the middle of the linea aspera on the back of the femur. As such it is a flexor/adductor with some degree of medial rotation at the hip joint. Its prominence together with that of sartorius laterally produces a hollow triangle on the front of the groin below the inguinal ligament (**430**). Within this femoral triangle are the important vessels and nerves of the front of the thigh. Note that the inguinal fold, the flexor crease related to the hip, crosses rather than acts as the base of the triangle which is the higher inguinal ligament.

Adductor brevis lies immediately behind adductor longus but being shorter and deeper is not palpable from the surface. It runs from the inferior ramus of the pubis to the linea aspera above adductor longus.

MUSCLES ACTING OVER THE HIP JOINT

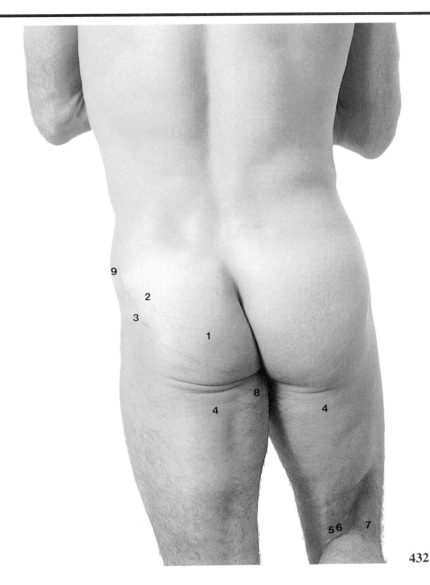

432

When one leg is raised, gluteus medius and minimus on the supporting side come into action to raise and support the pelvis, but gluteus maximus remains relaxed.

1 Gluteus maximus
2 Gluteus medius
3 Gluteus minimus
4 Hamstrings group
5 Semitendinosus (tendon)
6 Semimembranosus
7 Biceps femoris
8 Adductor magnus
9 Iliac crest

Adductor magnus is a large muscle with a wide attachment to the inferior ramus of the pubis across to the medial aspect of the ischial tuberosity. From here it is inserted into the linea aspera from below the level of the lesser trochanter distally and then along the medial supracondylar line to the adductor tubercle to which it is attached by a thin tendon. Adductor magnus forms much of the thick muscle mass on the medial side of the upper thigh behind adductor longus where it lies in a superficial position. Below, it is crossed superficially by gracilis and sartorius. However its tendon of insertion can be felt in the anterior aspect of the hollow on the medial side of the thigh above the medial epicondyle (**443**). The anterior part of adductor magnus acts as a powerful adductor while, in adduction, its lateral rotating action balances the medial rotation of pectineus and adductor longus. The ischial portion of the muscle acts with the hamstrings as an extensor at the hip joint but without their action over the knee.

All three adductor muscles are innervated by the obturator nerve supplemented in the case of the hamstring portion of adductor magnus by a branch from the sciatic nerve.

All three adductor muscles act as adductors at the hip joint, obviously carrying out this

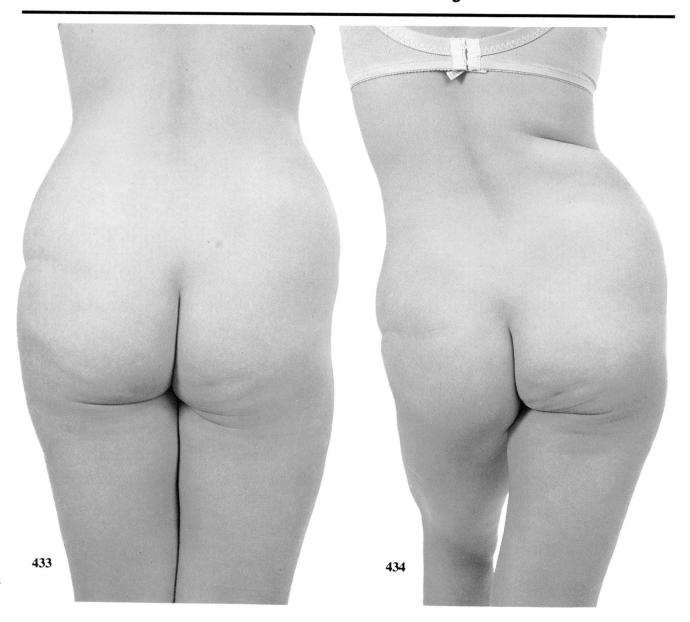

On standing with both feet on the ground all appears normal but on raising the left leg the right abductor muscles fail to support the pelvis which therefore drops.

433

434

movement as required. They also play an important part in locomotion by giving a medial balance to the hip joint. However they have a very important function which is far too often not appreciated. They act as antigravity muscles in an emergency. When a person slips these muscles come into powerful contraction to prevent the collapse of the bipod of the legs. Thus a very common sports injury is an adductor strain with pain at the pubic attachment of these muscles following a slip when the muscles have burst into activity to prevent a fall.

Gluteus medius and minimus are two large and powerful abductors at the hip joint (**431–432**). They form much of the muscular bulk of the upper lateral part of the buttock. They arise from the outer aspect of the ilium below the iliac crest and run across to the greater trochanter of the femur. Gluteus medius is the more superficial and can be felt above the large mass of gluteus maximus below the iliac crest. Gluteus minimus lies deeper and more anteriorly.

MUSCLES ACTING OVER THE HIP JOINT

If the leg is free to move they act as abductors of the thigh on the pelvis. However, their more important function is to support the trunk on the standing leg and to raise it slightly to allow the other leg to be swung clear of the ground in walking or running. The anterior fibres of the muscles, especially gluteus minimus, act as medial rotators at the hip joint and these fibres act to swing the pelvis forwards by a medial rotation on the supporting leg ready for the next step. Both muscles are supplied by the superior gluteal nerve (L4, L5 and S1). Testing for the activity of the muscles is most obviously abduction of the thigh at the hip as in **430**. However, failure of these muscles or their nerve supply will be obvious if the patient is asked to stand on that leg. The pelvis will drop on the other side (**434**). On walking the pelvis drops away from the affected leg, the so-called Trendelenburg gait. This is characteristic also of congenital dislocation of the hip, but here the cause is that, because of the dislocation, the head of the femur slips up over the ilium rather than supporting it satisfactorily at the acetabulum.

Lateral rotators. Deep in the gluteal region are a series of muscles, all of which act as lateral rotators at the hip joint. Lying deep, none is directly observable from the surface except by its action. They are obturators externus and internus, the gemelli, pyriformis and quadratus femoris.

Obturator externus arises from the bones around the obturator foramen and the obturator membrane, outside the pelvis and winds around below the neck of the femur and up behind, to be inserted into the pit on the medial side of the greater trochanter of the femur. (Nerve supply, obturator nerve L2, L3 and L4.)

Obturator internus arises from inside the true pelvis, from the bones around the obturator foramen and the obturator membrane. It leaves the pelvis through the lesser sciatic foramen, from the upper and lower aspects of which superior and inferior gemelli join it to run, collectively, into the tip of the greater trochanter. (Nerve supply L5, S1 and S2.)

Pyriformis also arises from within the pelvis from the middle parts of the sacrum and runs out through the greater sciatic foramen to be inserted with obturator internus into the tip of the greater trochanter. (Nerve supply branches from S1 and S2.)

Quadratus femoris arises from the outer aspect of the ischial tuberosity and runs across to the trochanteris crest behind the upper aspect of the femur. (Nerve supply L4, L5 and S1.)

All these muscles act as lateral rotators of the leg at the hip joint and are collectively responsible for the main power of this movement at the hip joint alone. They also play a major part in close postural support of the joint, all being closely related to the joint itself over which they can act as dynamic ligaments.

It cannot be stressed too strongly that the muscles at the hip as well as at all other joints not only produce the dynamic movement and postural control of the joint, but also normally limit the range of movement of the joint. For instance it is often stated that the ilio-femoral ligament prevents hyperextension at the hip joint; this may be true in an emergency but the real stop comes from iliopsoas. In the apparent hyperextension as seen on page 225, iliopsoas not only prevents hyperextension at the hip joint but psoas contributes to the lumbar extension by its anterior pull on the vertebrae. It is this excellent muscular control around the joint that plays such an important part in total hip replacement when virtually normal control of the joint system is so rapidly restored post-operatively.

MUSCLES ACTING OVER THE HIP AND KNEE JOINTS

Certain of the major muscles act over both these joints and, theoretically, have an action over both. However it is most important to be aware here, as elsewhere in the body, that this can limit efficiency of function of the muscle unless one or other joint is controlled by other muscles at a particular phase of movement.

Gluteus maximus is the most superficial of the muscles of the buttock and the one most involved in the production of the rounded contour with the overlying fat.

Gluteus maximus comes from the back of the ilium close to the posterior superior iliac spine, from the back of the sacrum and the sacro-tuberous and sacrospinous ligaments. It runs laterally and downwards across the buttock, where its lower and deeper fibres run to a roughened area on the back of the femur, the gluteal tuberosity. This component thus acts only over the hip joint. The major part however runs into the iliotibial tract. This is a thick fibrous sheet derived from the deep investing fascia of the leg and runs from the iliac crest to the anterolateral aspect of the tibia. The iliotibial tract thus acts as a flat tendon of insertion of gluteus maximus into that aspect of the tibia.

The total function of gluteus maximus extends over both hip and knee joints. Over the hip the control can be separated by that portion of the muscle inserted into the femur. It extends and laterally rotates the leg at the hip joint, while through the ilio-tibial tract it gives firm extension to the leg. The total picture of its function is shown in the extended leg of the dancer performing an arabesque on page 225. However in more universal usage it comes into action in standing up from a sitting position or in stepping up as in **436**, where its lateral rotating action comes into play to balance the medial rotation of gluteus medius and minimus which come into action when load is taken on that leg to control the pelvis.

435

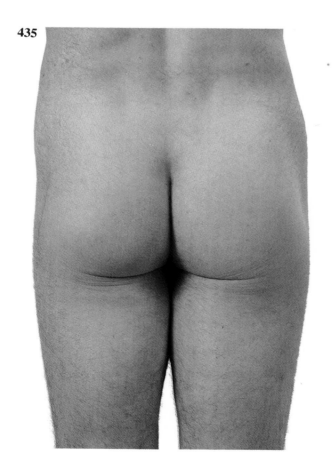

436

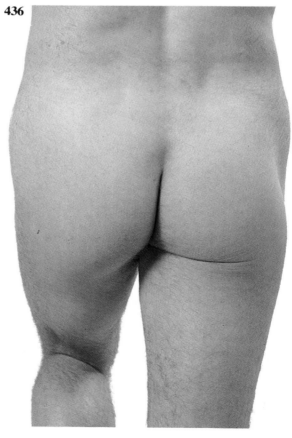

In normal standing the buttocks are soft and mobile. The gluteal muscles are relaxed even in a muscular male, as here, and are covered by a contouring overlay of fat. The two buttocks are separated by the deep natal cleft, particularly marked below the level of the sacrum and coccyx, where it extends to the anus and posterior part of the perineum. Below, the fat is tucked in by a transverse skin fold, the gluteal fold, below the lower margin of gluteus maximus but not following that edge, which runs more obliquely laterally. The more transverse nature of the fold is generated by the posterior part of the fat of the ischio-rectal fossa medial to and below the medial part of gluteus maximus.

The left leg has been placed on a step, so stretching the muscle before bringing it into action to extend the hip. It is now possible to see the direction of gluteus maximus running obliquely across from the sacral region to the back of the leg.

MUSCLES ACTING OVER THE HIP AND KNEE JOINTS

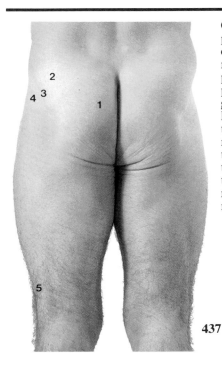

Gluteus maximus is shown in powerful activity while standing on the toes, essentially a postural role, where firm support of both pelvis and knees is vital. The pull of the muscle can be seen giving powerful extension and lateral rotation at the hips while the ilio-tibial tract is obvious running down the side of the thigh, through which extension is transmitted to the knee. Note also the bulge created by the gluteus medius and the underlying minimus.

437

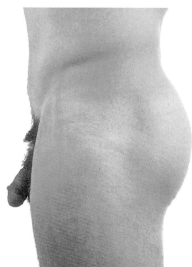

1 Gluteus maximus
2 Gluteus medius
3 Gluteus minimus
4 Tensor fasciae lata
5 Ilio-tibial tract
6 Greater trochanter

In lateral view the bulge of the gluteus maximus is evident, covered by gluteal fat, with its connection to the ilio-tibial tract extending from the iliac crest and tubercle of the ilium even with the muscle at rest. The contour of tensor fasciae latae is less obvious.

438

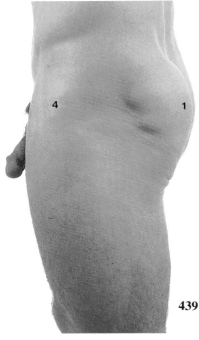

The features of both muscles become more prominent as the subject stands on his toes, giving firm anterior and posterior support to the hip joint and firm knee extension.

439

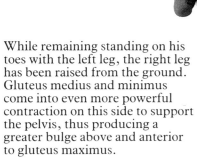

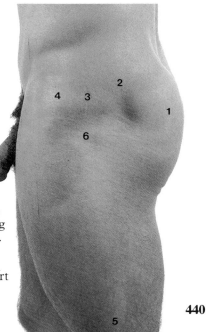

While remaining standing on his toes with the left leg, the right leg has been raised from the ground. Gluteus medius and minimus come into even more powerful contraction on this side to support the pelvis, thus producing a greater bulge above and anterior to gluteus maximus.

440

Although an extensor at the knee, this is a subsidiary activity to that of the quadriceps muscles, the prime power extensors. The extensor's role through the ilio-tibial tract only becomes effective and powerful when the knee becomes extended beyond some 50–60° of flexion, from which the power gradually increases to full extension. Probably the most important function of the pull along the ilio-tibial tract is to produce firm compacted extension of the knee.

The nerve supply comes from the inferior gluteal nerve, L5, S1 and S2.

MUSCLES ACTING OVER THE HIP AND KNEE JOINTS

Tensor Fasciae Latae can be considered to some extent as an anterior counterpart to gluteus maximus but without the same primary role over the hip joint. It arises from the lateral aspect of the ilium near to its crest and extending some distance back from the anterior iliac spine towards the tubercle. It runs downwards to be inserted into the anterior aspect of the ilio-tibial tract. It is a flexor at the hip joint and extensor at the knee. However, it can only be considered as a subsidiary dynamic flexor at the hip joint, though it does take on this role and hypertrophies to a considerable degree where the iliopsoas is lost. Its most important function is to produce an anterior postural balance to gluteus maximus in hip control while together giving extensor postural control over the knee.

It is innervated by the superior gluteal nerve, L4, L5 and S1.

The bulges created by tensor fasciae latae (1) and sartorius (2) can be seen; the latter running down from the anterior superior iliac spine with the former immediately behind.

The ilio-tibial tract (1) is pulled up by gluteus maximus and tensor fasciae latae in firm extension of the knee, coming to resemble a wide, rounded tendon which is often mistaken by the unwary for that of biceps femoris immediately behind (2).

441

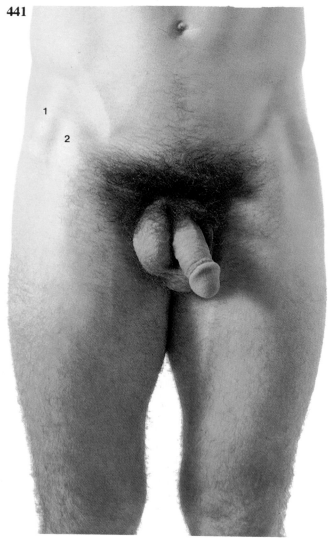

442

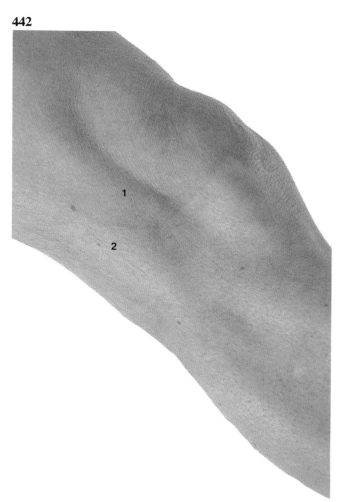

MUSCLES ACTING OVER THE HIP AND KNEE JOINTS

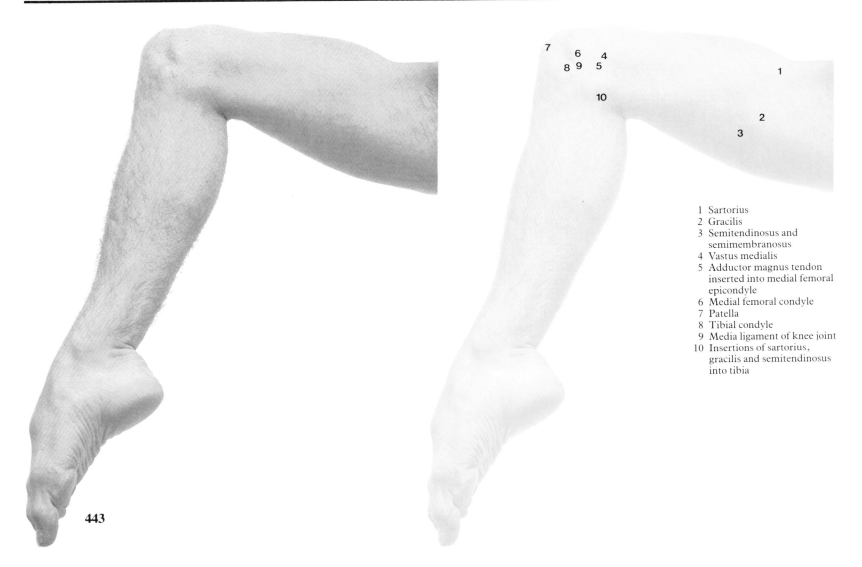

1 Sartorius
2 Gracilis
3 Semitendinosus and semimembranosus
4 Vastus medialis
5 Adductor magnus tendon inserted into medial femoral epicondyle
6 Medial femoral condyle
7 Patella
8 Tibial condyle
9 Media ligament of knee joint
10 Insertions of sartorius, gracilis and semitendinosus into tibia

443

Sartorius is a long strap-like muscle which runs from the anterior superior iliac spine region obliquely downwards and medially across the front of the thigh to be attached to the medial side of the upper part of the tibia. Its name indicates its function, sartor being the Latin name for tailor, who traditionally sat cross-legged when at work. Sartorius is therefore a flexor, abductor and lateral rotator at the hip joint and flexor, medial rotator at the knee. Even at rest the muscle influences the contour of the thigh anteriorly, where it forms the lateral margin of the femoral triangle (**430**, page 265). In contraction this feature is very much emphasised.

    Nerve supply is a branch or branches from the femoral nerve, one of which usually continues through the muscle to form the inter-mediate cutaneous nerve of the thigh.

Gracilis is also a strap-like muscle running sub-cutaneously down the medial aspect of the thigh from the body and inferior ramus of the pubis to the medial side of the tibia between sartorius (anterior) and semitendinosus. It is a weak adductor of the thigh at the hip joint and a flexor at the knee, more effective when the knee is already in some degree of flexion, when it can also act as a medial rotator. Its most important role is to give medial postural balance to both joints and especially the knee. (Nerve supply, Obturator nerve L2, L3 and L4.)

Hamstring Muscles. These are a system of muscles which act as extensors at the hip joint and flexors at the knee. They are three in number all arising from the ischial tuberosity and running down the back of the thigh, where they form the main muscle bulk. Two run down to the medial side of the knee while the third, biceps with its two heads, runs to the lateral side.

Semitendinosus has a muscular belly in its upper half which then runs into a long tendon to be inserted into the medial side of the tibia behind sartorius and gracilis.

Semimembranosus has a flattened tendon for its upper half and a thick fleshy belly below, being inserted mainly into the posteromedial aspect of the upper end of the tibia. These two muscles form essentially a single bundle, one having muscle where the other has tendon.

Biceps femoris has one head rising from the ischial tuberosity and the other from the back of the femur. The two bellies combine in the lower part of the thigh to form a tendon which is attached to the head of the fibula with the lateral collateral ligament of the knee joint.

The medial and lateral components of the hamstrings, by running medially and laterally to the leg, produce a hollow behind the knee containing fat and the vessels and nerves, the popliteal fossa (**445**).

Nerve supply comes from the sciatic nerve; semimembranosus and semitendinosus L4, L5 and S1 and the long head of biceps S1, S2 and S3 from the medial component of the nerve with the short head of biceps L5 and S1 from the lateral component (common peroneal).

The hamstrings act as powerful axial extensors at the hip joint while giving flexion at the knee (the short head of biceps giving only this movement). As they form thick medial and lateral masses to the knee they also give vital collateral support to the knee joint, while in flexion each component can give medial and lateral rotation or, perhaps more important, rotatory stability. As shown on page 18, the hamstrings cannot act effectively over the full range of both joints where they can show both active and passive insufficiency. Of the two the passive insufficiency is usually the more important as in many people the total length of the muscle is often a major limitation to full flexion at the hips with the knees extended. People with short hamstrings may not be able to touch the floor with the knees straight, whereas others may have long muscles and have remarkable freedom (**444**). Because of limitation of movement by the hamstrings it is important to measure ranges of hip flexion with the knees bent. Full flexion at the hip joint with knees extended may also pull on the sciatic nerve, particularly where this is inflamed or subject to mechanical stress as in lumbar intervertebral disc lesions.

As indicated above, the hamstrings normally act over hip and knee in different phases of movements, but in the final 'cast off' in running both are activated by the muscles.

444

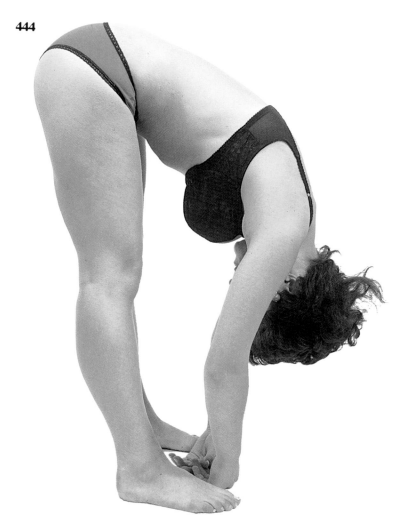

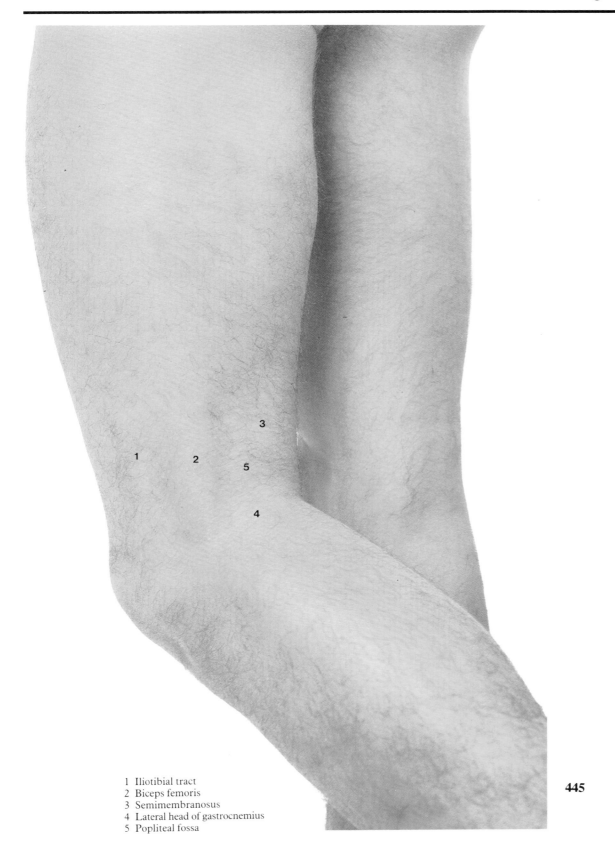

445

1 Iliotibial tract
2 Biceps femoris
3 Semimembranosus
4 Lateral head of gastrocnemius
5 Popliteal fossa

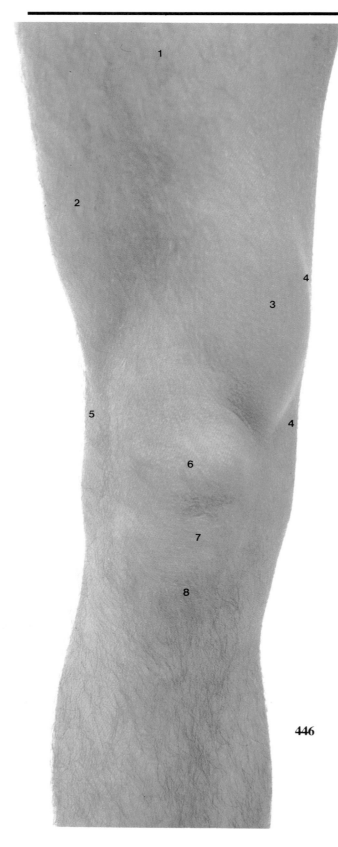

The most important muscles acting only over the knee are undoubtedly the four grouped together as the quadriceps. These muscles collectively give a most important control to both movement and stability of the joint and form the main muscle mass on the front of the thigh. Furthermore, the patella can be considered to be a sesamoid bone in the tendon, so lifting the direction of pull to give better leverage for knee extension (**446**).

Rectus femoris is the one muscle of the four to cross the hip joint, though its action over this joint is probably slight as a flexor and more of postural significance under normal circumstances. It is attached by straight and reflected heads from the anterior inferior iliac spine and the region behind it above the acetabulum. The muscle runs down in a superficial position to the patella. In a muscular person it is easily seen on contraction of the quadriceps as the most superficial and centrally running muscle mass.

Vastus intermedius is a broad mass of muscle which arises from the front and sides of the upper two thirds of the femur and covers the front and sides of the bone deep to rectus femoris.

Vastus lateralis is a broad mass of muscle which arises from the greater trochanter and down by an aponeurotic sheet along the upper half of the linea aspera, from which the muscle fibres arise to overlie the lateral aspect of vastus intermedius.

Vastus medialis arises from the trochanteric line, the spiral line, the medial lip of the linea aspera, the upper part of the medial supracondylar line of the femur and then from the tendon of adductor magnus and the medial intermuscular septum. It thus extends its origin far more down the leg than the other muscles.

The central components of the quadriceps, mainly rectus (entirely) and vastus intermedius run into the patella and through this in turn to

1 Rectus femoris
2 Vastus lateralis
3 Vastus medialis
4 Tendon of adductor magnus
5 Iliotibial tract
6 Patella
7 Patella ligament
8 Tibial tuberosity

446

MUSCLES ACTING OVER THE KNEE JOINT

the ligamentum patellae and the inferior part of the tibial tubercle. Laterally an aponeurotic sheet is formed above the level of the patella and this runs to the lateral side of the patella and links with the ilio-tibial tract and the capsule of the knee joint before reaching the tibia. On the medial side the muscle fibres of vastus medialis run almost horizontally into the medial side of the patella and also form an aponeurosis through the medial side of the joint to the tibia.

Thus the quadriceps forms an extensor mass working with maximal mechanical efficiency through the patella as a powerful extensor at the knee joint but also embracing the anterior half of the joint in a wide extensor and joint supportive structure. The vastus medialis also exerts a most important medial pull onto the patella to prevent the lateral displacement which is always a possibility because of the angulation of the knee. The double function of vastus medialis as a knee extensor and a medial controller of the patella is emphasised by the fact that these components of the muscle receive separate nerve branches. The muscle is to a major extent responsible for the stability of the knee joint and weakness of the quadriceps commonly leads to synovitis of the knee due to lack of support, even on mild exercise such as walking. For this reason it is advisable for anyone having to spend more than a few days in bed to maintain quadriceps exercises unless contraindicated. Failure to do so may often mean a return to bed to treat the resultant synovitis once activity is started on a knee without adequate quadriceps support. (Nerve supply, Femoral nerve L2, L3 and L4.)

Articularis genu is a muscle component deep to vastus intermedius which runs from the femur to hold up the deep suprapatellar bursa. This synovial fold projects some 3 fingers' breadth above the patella as an extension of the knee joint synovium, and its presence is of particular clinical importance in synovitis of the knee joint.

Popliteus is a small muscle which runs from the back of the upper part of the tibia to the lateral condyle of the femur and to the posterior horn of the lateral meniscus. As described on page 260 it acts as a medial rotator of the tibia on the femur with flexion and in so doing unlocks the compacted, extended knee. (Nerve supply, medial Popliteal nerve L4, L5 and S1.)

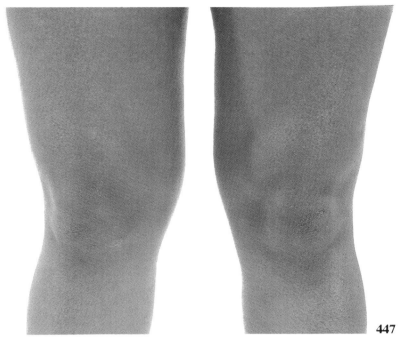

447

In a female the muscular pattern may be less obvious owing to a greater amount of subcutaneous fat.

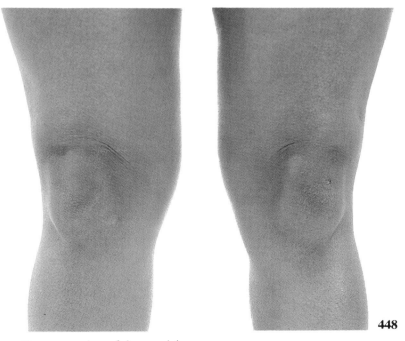

448

On contraction of the quadriceps the patella is pulled up with good medial control in spite of the angulation of the knee.

BONY FEATURES OF THE ANKLE AND FOOT

The subcutaneous and sharp anterior border of the tibia (the shin) runs down the whole length of the lower leg subcutaneously, from the tibial tubercle to the ankle. In the lowest part the extensor tendons cross anteriorly on their way to the foot but the medial malleolus forms a prominent feature, the medial of the so-called ankle bones (**449**). The medial malleolus, rather longer anteriorly than posteriorly, projects downwards from the medial side of the tibia to articulate with the medial side of the talus. Laterally the head of the fibula is readily palpable at the knee but then becomes overlaid by muscles, becoming subcutaneous again in its lowest quarter or so, which continues as the lateral malleolus (or ankle bone) (**450**). This is triangular in shape and projects further down the lateral articular surface of the talus than does the medial malleolus. (In lateral radio-

graphs the differences in length and shape of the two malleoli are important in separating the one from the other.) Posteriorly the lateral malleolus shows a prominent notch in the bone but although called the digital notch it is not palpable through the skin though this aspect of the bone is readily palpable as a sharp projection. Behind the malleoli are hollows and behind them the tendo calcaneus (Achillis) running into the prominent projection of the calcaneum at the heel.

Below the lateral malleolus and slightly anterior to its tip the peroneal tubercle can be felt. In front of the lateral malleolus the talus is palpable for a short distance before sinking to its neck. However if the foot is inverted the head of the talus forms a marked projection on the superolateral aspect of the foot some 3 to

1 Fibula to lateral malleolus
2 Peroneal tubercle
3 Talus (distal end)
4 Extensor digitorum brevis muscle
5 Calcaneum
6 Base of 5th metatarsal
7 Peroneal tendons
8 Tendo calcaneus
9 Calcaneum
10 Tibia to medial malleolus
11 Sustentaculum tali
12 Tubercle of navicula
13 Base of 1st metatarsal
14 Head of 1st metatarsal

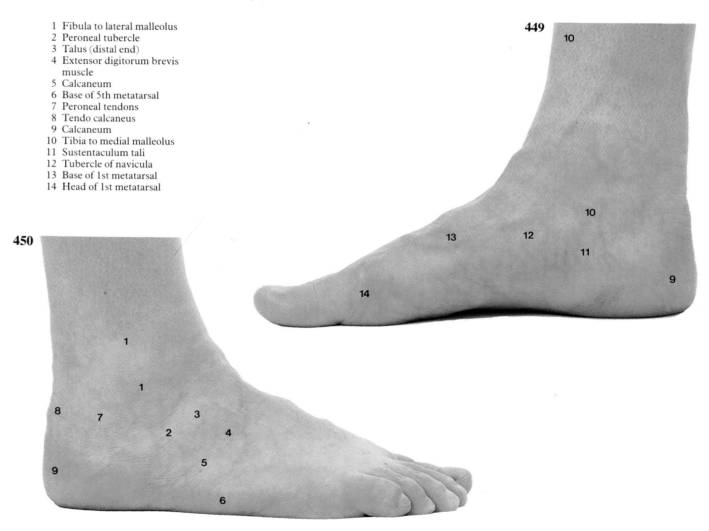

4 cm in front of the lateral malleolus but in the midposition it tends to be masked by the subjacent extensor digitorum brevis muscle mass. In a slim foot the distal end of the calcaneum may be felt laterally but then the hollow over the cuboid leads to the next prominence, the base of the fifth metatarsal.

On the medial side it may be possible to feel a little of the talus just below the medial malleolus, particularly if the foot is everted in plantar flexion, with the shelf of the sustentaculum tali below. There is a medial hollow below that, in the calcaneum, and then the prominence of the heel. More anteriorly on the medial side, the tubercle of the navicular forms a low bony prominence followed by the medial cuneiform; the base of the first metatarsal may be palpable. On the dorsum of the foot the base of the first metatarsal forms a large knob in some people which can lead to uncomfortable pressure from shoes. The shafts of the metatarsals can usually be felt through the extensor tendons while the first and fifth are prominent on the borders of the foot and leading to their heads. The head of

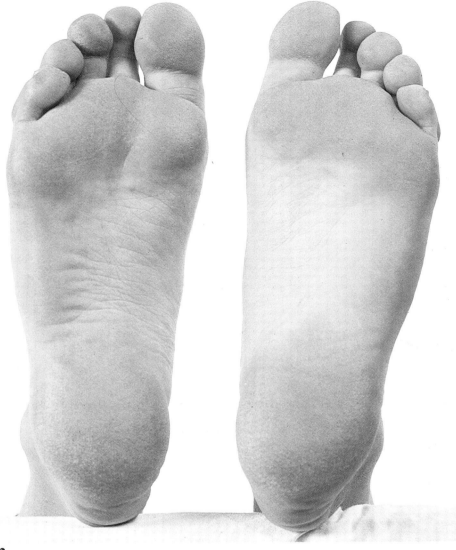

452

451

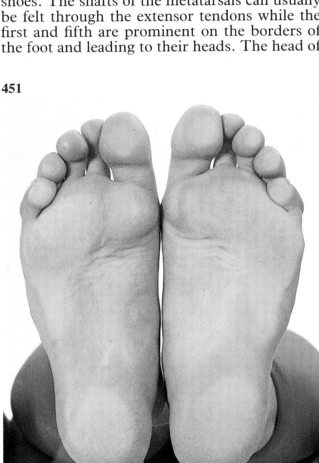

the first may project to a considerable extent when it may be overlaid by a bursa, particularly in hallux valgus.

On the sole of the foot the heads of the metatarsals are overlaid by a thick pad of fibrofatty material with sesamoid bones in the tendons of the first and sometimes other toes (**452**). This is the normal load bearing area of the foot, together with the heel and the lateral border. The area of contact between heel and metatarsal heads on the medial side will depend upon the height of the medial arch on standing. Contact between the pads of the toes and the ground will depend upon their mobility and normality of position.

MOVEMENTS OF THE ANKLE AND FOOT

The ankle joint is probably as near a uniaxial hinge as any in the body, permitting only flexion and extension (plantar and dorsiflexion), of the foot. In the normal standing position with the foot at right angles to the leg, the foot should be capable of some 30 to 40° of dorsiflexion and some 60° or more of plantarflexion (**453**). However this varies enormously with the patterns of utilisation of the feet. Many women who have worn high heeled shoes constantly without walking at normal foot level may not even be able to reach 90° angulation and may not be able to put the heel to the ground without pain in the calf muscles; the same problem may affect patients who have been nursed for a long time with the feet held in plantarflexion by bed covers. There may be shortening of both calf muscles and the dorsal capsule of the ankle joint.

In the normal standing position and in dorsiflexion the talus fits snugly between the two malleoli and the foot can be considered to be in a stable close-packed position at the ankle joint. However, the malleolar surfaces of the talus are not parallel and, being narrower posteriorly, when the foot is plantarflexed at the ankle, there is sufficient room for it to move between the malleoli. Thus when standing on the toes (or in high heeled shoes) the ankle joint loses its lateral stability and becomes free to rock unless firmly supported by the long muscles to the foot, medially tibialis anterior and posterior, and laterally the peroneal muscles.

453

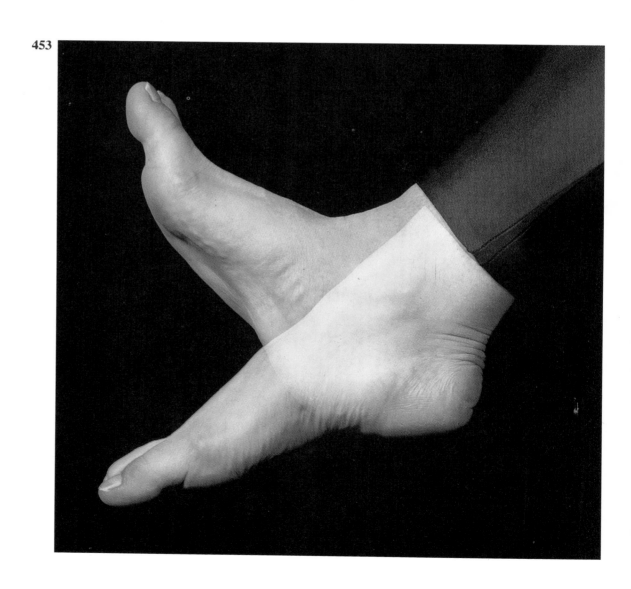

From the ankle the axis of the foot runs to the medial side towards the first three toes. The great toe and the adjoining two can be said to be the termination of the dynamic component of the foot. The lateral side with its shorter toes plays a much more static role, taking the load when standing, a load which increases considerably when standing at ease with the feet apart. This side of the foot therefore makes contact with the floor throughout its length when standing (**451**). Although a lateral longitudinal arch is present it is really little more than a low bony arch to allow the passage of the peroneus longus tendon, and runs from the calcaneum through the cuboid to the fifth metatarsal. Medially the longitudinal arch is a much more important structure, producing the medial hollow and running from the calcaneum at the heel through to the medial three metatarsal heads. The object of this arch is that it forms a cantilever spring-like mechanism when landing, as from a jump, and a dynamically sprung lever when driving off or jumping to allow a freely flowing movement through the foot. Thus the importance lies in the muscle controlled dynamic mobility of the arch system rather than the arch itself.

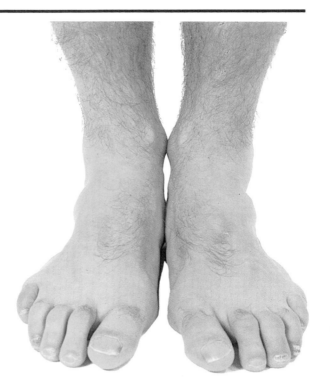

454

The feet of a highly trained dancer may appear relatively flat when at rest. When standing on toes however the medial arch develops to a remarkable extent. Note how the three medial metatarsals and toes take most of the load and would be responsible for the drive if jumping or produce a sprung system on landing. It is easy to see by the squeezing out of the blood from the toes how much load these are being subjected to. An efficient foot makes considerable use of the power of the toes.

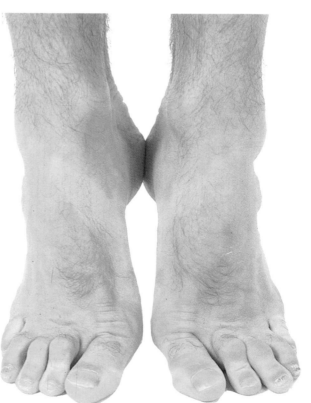

455

Although a mobile arched system is the ideal many people have a relatively flat, immobile foot which can be extremely efficient. A fixed high arch usually makes a most inefficient foot however and is commonly associated with clawing of the toes; the interossei, the prime flexors at the metatarsophalangeal joints, tend to be converted into extensors because of the degree of dorsiflexion at the joints and this is commonly a problem with people who wear high heeled shoes but do not maintain mobility of the joints, which become fixed into hyperextension.

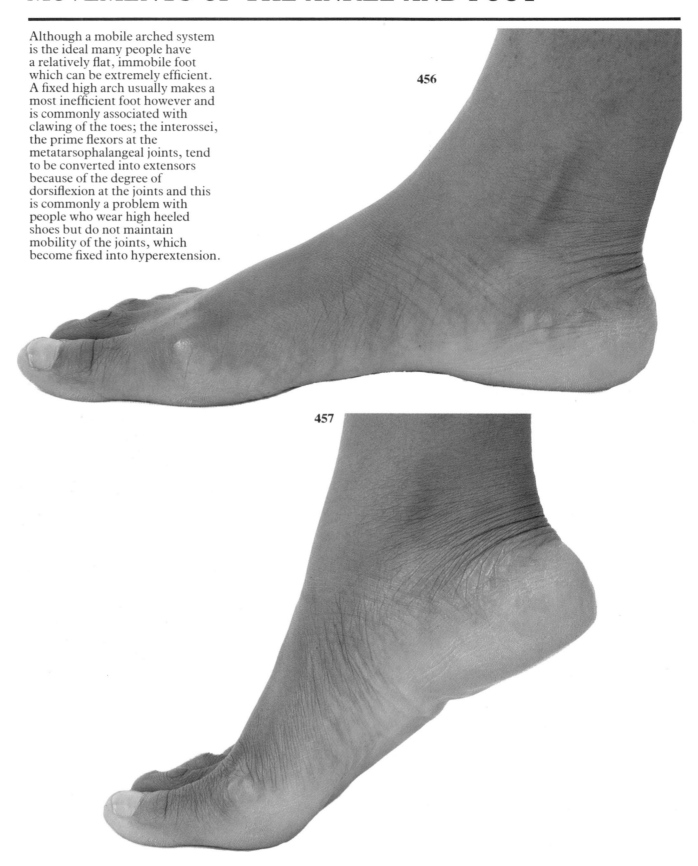

456

457

MOVEMENTS OF THE ANKLE AND FOOT

As the medial three toes form the dynamic component of the foot, these are the ones most directly involved in the rotatory movement of the foot, which is designed to allow it to adjust to variable surfaces. This component of the foot must move as a unit. The lateral aspect of the foot follows around the medial axis, then adjusts to load bearing as required. In fact when examining the bones of the feet, they readily split into medial and lateral components. The medial one consists of the talus, navicular, the three cuneiforms, the three medial metatarsals and their toes, while the lateral consists of the calcaneum, cuboid and the lateral two metatarsals and toes. The medial component forms the sprung cantilever which must also rotate on its axis from the ankle. Thus the head of the talus fits in a ball and socket joint into the navicular, which permits flexion, extension and rotation. The navicular has a similar but shallower type of joint system with the combined three cuneiforms, but thereafter rotation is blocked by the base of the second metatarsal being held between the distal parts of the medial and lateral cuneiforms. Thus movement is thereafter mainly flexion and extension of the toes though some abduction and adduction should be available at the metatarsophalangeal joints. The lateral part of the foot moves around the axis, initiated by a twisting movement between talus and calcaneum and then the cuboid follows round and increases the range of the distal end of the calcaneum. By these means the sole of the foot can face somewhat medially (inversion) or laterally (eversion), the movement being at the midtarsal joints where flexion and extension also occur, mainly on the medial side of the foot. The range of inversion is usually far greater than eversion, which may be quite limited (**458**).

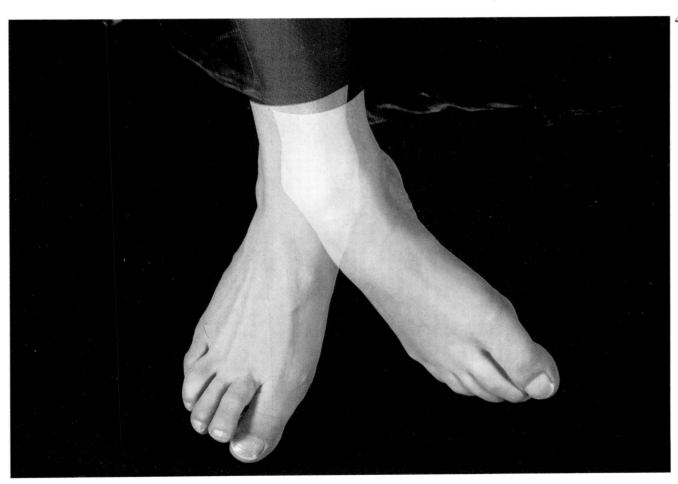

458

MUSCLES ACTING OVER THE KNEE AND ANKLE

Gastrocnemius is the muscle of particular importance in this rôle though it is combined both structurally and functionally with soleus which acts only over the ankle joint. Gastrocnemius forms the major bulge in the calf in its upper part. It arises by two heads from each of the two supracondylar regions of the femur. They run down inside the tendons of insertion of the hamstring muscles and join below the popliteal fossa, to make a single muscle mass. Thus the popliteal fossa can be described as a diamond shaped space formed from the division of the hamstrings to their respective sides of the knee above and the gastrocnemius below. Both these muscle systems act as flexors at the knee and at the same time their components offer rotation in flexion. They also have the very important function of giving vital lateral control to a joint where the bones offer remarkably little stability but which has to play so essential a rôle in the movement and support of the body; even the ligaments offer relatively little support. In fact it is remarkable how the muscles can give both a stable and efficient function in the knee even after loss of ligaments.

When the two bellies of gastrocnemius join together below the knee their combined mass comes to overlie the upper part of soleus and the two muscles then run down to form the common tendo calcaneous (Achillis). Gastro-

1 Biceps femoris tendon
2 Lateral head
2* Lateral belly of gastrocnemius
3 Medial head of gastrocnemius
3* Medial belly of gastrocnemius
4 Semimbranosus
5 Combined tendon of gastrocnemius and soleus whose muscle belly is attached to its deep aspect (6)
7 Tendo calcaneous (Achilles)
8 Calcaneum
9 Flexor digitorum longus
10 Peroneus longus and brevis

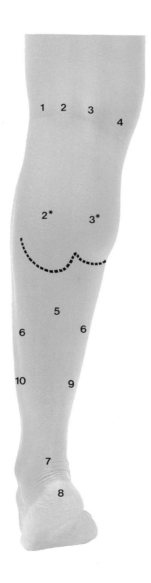

459

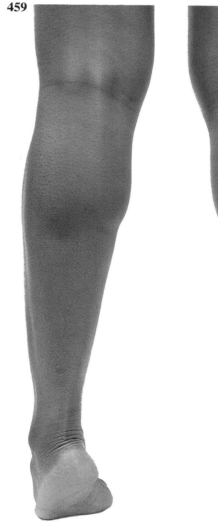

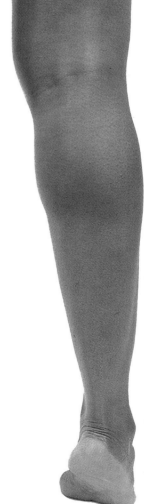

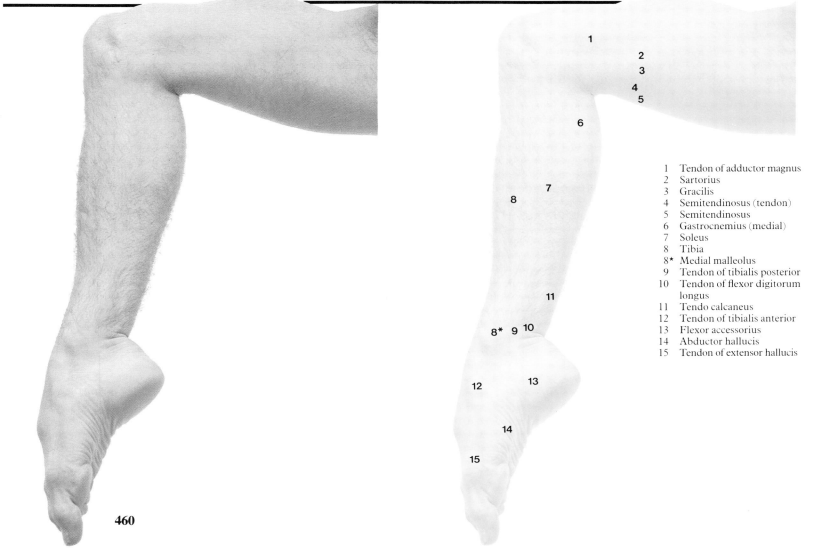

1   Tendon of adductor magnus
2   Sartorius
3   Gracilis
4   Semitendinosus (tendon)
5   Semitendinosus
6   Gastrocnemius (medial)
7   Soleus
8   Tibia
8★ Medial malleolus
9   Tendon of tibialis posterior
10 Tendon of flexor digitorum longus
11 Tendo calcaneus
12 Tendon of tibialis anterior
13 Flexor accessorius
14 Abductor hallucis
15 Tendon of extensor hallucis

460

cnemius is thus a prime flexor of the knee and, working with soleus, an extensor at the ankle joint (**459**).

Soleus takes origin from the back of the medial border of the tibia, its soleal line, and then from a fibrous arch over the popliteal vessels and the tibial nerve to the upper quarter or so of the fibula. The soleal fibres can be seen bulging to each side of the lower part of gastrocnemius when both are in action (**460**).

Although the soleus/gastrocnemius complex acts as the power plantarflexor at the ankle joint and thus plays a vital role in walking, running and jumping, it must also be stressed that it is responsible for preventing the body falling forwards in standing, and maintaining the body in balance over the feet.

Plantaris is a very small muscle and relatively unimportant, but since the long tendon can be of great value as a graft it is important to be able to find it easily. The muscle has a small belly which arises from the lateral supracondylar ridge above that of gastrocnemius. It then runs down deep to gastrocnemius to appear on the medial side of the tendo calcaneus to be inserted into the calcaneum. Here it can be found by a small incision some two fingers' breadth behind the medial malleolus and just in front of the tendo calcaneus. From this small opening the whole tendon can be harvested by using a stripper (e.g. Brand's). All three muscles are supplied by the tibial nerve S1 and S2.

MUSCLES ACTING OVER THE ANKLE AND FOOT

The long muscles acting over the ankle and foot can be divided into three groups; the extensors (tibialis anterior and extensors hallucis and digitorum longus), which cross in front of the ankle, the flexors (tibialis posterior and flexors digitorum and hallucis longus) passing behind the medial malleolus and the evertor flexors (peroneus longus and brevis) passing behind the lateral malleolus.

Tibialis anterior forms a considerable muscle belly arising from the tibia and running down immediately lateral to its sharp subcutaneous border. It runs across the ankle in front of and a little lateral to the medial malleolus where its tendon raises a thick ridge, particularly when the muscle is put into action by forced or resisted dorsiflexion with inversion at the ankle joint (**461**). It has the important function of maintaining normal dorsiflexion of the foot when raised from the ground and loss of the muscle or usually its nerve supply leads to the very disabling condition of foot drop when walking. The muscle is inserted into the medial cuneiform and the base of the first metatarsal and is supplied by the deep peroneal (anterior tibial) nerve L4 and L5.

Extensor hallucis longus arises from the middle two thirds of the fibula and the interosseous membrane deep to extensor digitorum longus (**461–462**). Its tendon becomes superficial in the approach to the ankle just lateral to tibialis anterior and becomes very obvious on the dorsum of the foot on forced extension of the great toe. (The muscle is supplied by the deep peroneal (anterior tibial) nerve L5 and S1.)

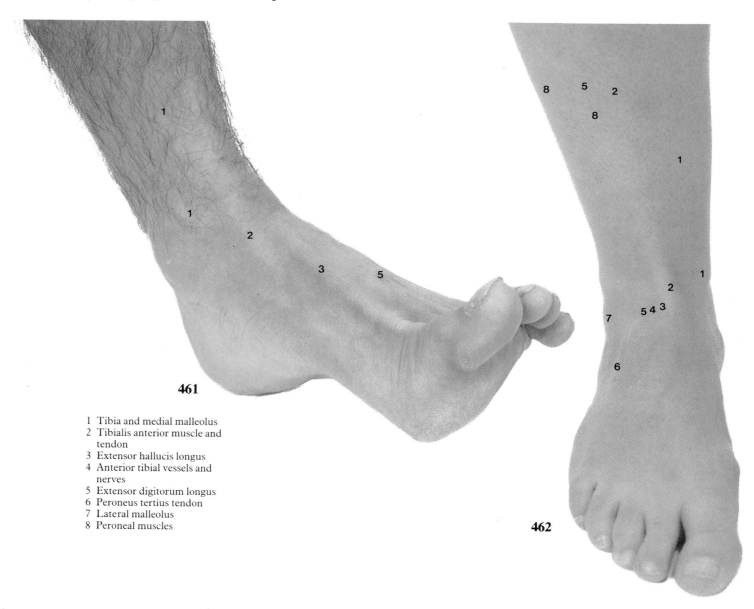

461

1 Tibia and medial malleolus
2 Tibialis anterior muscle and
   tendon
3 Extensor hallucis longus
4 Anterior tibial vessels and
   nerves
5 Extensor digitorum longus
6 Peroneus tertius tendon
7 Lateral malleolus
8 Peroneal muscles

462

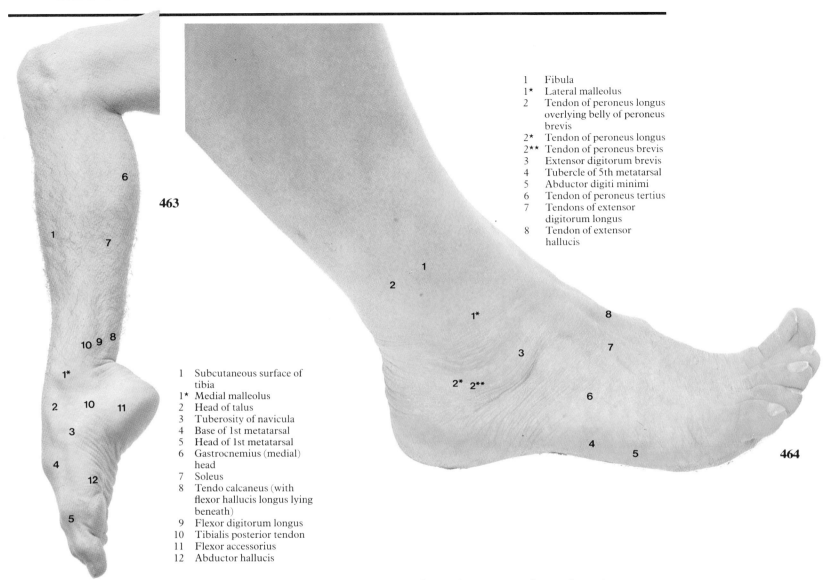

463

464

1 Subcutaneous surface of tibia
1* Medial malleolus
2 Head of talus
3 Tuberosity of navicula
4 Base of 1st metatarsal
5 Head of 1st metatarsal
6 Gastrocnemius (medial) head
7 Soleus
8 Tendo calcaneus (with flexor hallucis longus lying beneath)
9 Flexor digitorum longus
10 Tibialis posterior tendon
11 Flexor accessorius
12 Abductor hallucis

1 Fibula
1* Lateral malleolus
2 Tendon of peroneus longus overlying belly of peroneus brevis
2* Tendon of peroneus longus
2** Tendon of peroneus brevis
3 Extensor digitorum brevis
4 Tubercle of 5th metatarsal
5 Abductor digiti minimi
6 Tendon of peroneus tertius
7 Tendons of extensor digitorum longus
8 Tendon of extensor hallucis

Extensor digitorum longus arises from the upper two thirds of the fibula and thus immediately lateral to tibialis anterior where it can be felt in digital extension, most effectively in eversion at the ankle when tibialis anterior is relaxed (**464**). It divides into tendons for the lateral four toes which pass under the extensor retinaculum lateral to extensor hallucis longus with the vessels and nerve between them. (The muscle is supplied by the deep peroneal (anterior tibial) nerve L5 and S1.)

Peroneus tertius is a muscle which arises below extensor digitorum longus and runs down lateral to it to be inserted into the base of the fifth metatarsal. Although often neglected or simply considered as part of the above muscle it is usually quite a large muscle and an important extensor evertor of the foot (**464**). (The muscle is supplied by the deep peroneal (anterior tibial) nerve L5 and S1.)

Tibialis posterior arises from the tibia, interosseous membrane and fibula deep to soleus. It appears at the ankle medial to the tendo calcaneus and crosses close behind the medial malleolus where the tendon can be felt moving in firm or resisted inversion and plantar flexion (**463**). It does not stand out prominently as does its anterior counterpart. It is inserted into the navicular bone but slips go to all the tarsus bones except the talus. (Nerve supply, tibial nerve L4 and L5.)

MUSCLES ACTING OVER THE ANKLE AND FOOT

Flexor digitorum longus also arises from the tibia under cover of soleus and runs down across the ankle immediately behind tibialis posterior as the long flexor to the toes (**463**). (Nerve supply, tibial nerve L5 and S1.)

Flexor hallucis longus also arises deep to soleus from the fibula and runs down deep to the tendo calcaneus and lateral to flexor digitorum longus, which tendons it crosses in the sole of the foot to reach the great toe as its long flexor. (Nerve supply, tibial nerve L5, S1, S2 and S3.)

Peroneus longus arises from the lateral aspect of the upper two thirds of the fibula and the adjoining lateral condyle of the tibia and runs down behind the lateral malleolus and then below the peroneal tubercle and across the sole of the foot (**464–465**).

Peroneus brevis arises below peroneus longus and likewise runs behind the lateral malleolus but then above the peroneal tubercle to the base of the fifth metatarsal.

The peroneal muscles are both evertors of the foot and have some flexor activity. (Nerve supply, superficial nerve L5, S1 and S2.)

Short muscles of the foot. Although the long muscles are the major power source, the short muscles are most important for a functionally effective foot. The great toe has a short abductor, flexor and adductor, the latter playing an important part in maintaining the internal strength of the foot. The abductor runs along the medial border of the sole of the foot and ideally should be an abductor of the great toe; but its role in most feet is to give medial balance to the toe. In people who use their feet effectively, such as dancers and particularly female classical ballet dancers who have to dance on points, the muscle is vital for the axial control of the great toe. Failure of the muscle in many feet leads to hallux valgus and those with a tendency to this can usually prevent any further detereoration and even gain improvement by reactivating the muscle as an abductor (**466**).

At rest the great toe lay alongside the other toes. Abductor pollicis brevis (1) has been activated, pulling the great toe to a more normal position (2), so reducing the angle at the metatarsophalangeal joint where a bunion might eventually form if the toe was allowed to continue 'drifting'.

1   Lower end of fibula
1★ Lateral malleolus
2   Peroneus longus muscle (2★ tendon)
3   Peroneus brevis muscle (3★ tendon)
4   Superior peroneal retinaculum
5   Lateral belly of gastrocnemius
6   Soleus
7   Tendo calcaneus
7★ Position of bursa between tendon and calcaneum
8   Extensor digorium brevis
9   Peroneus tertius muscle (9★ tendon)
10 Tuberosity of 5th metatarsal
11 Abductor digiti minimi

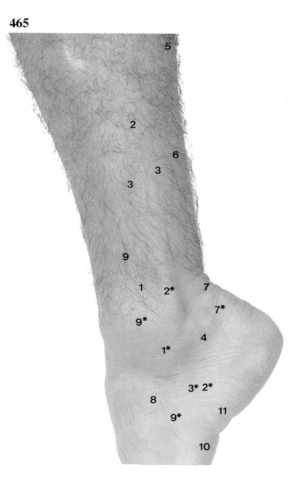

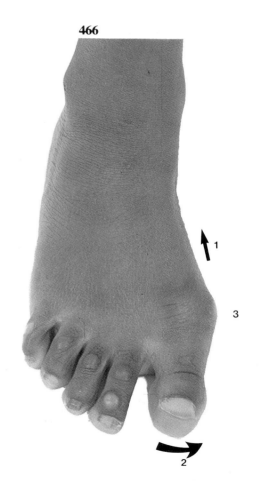

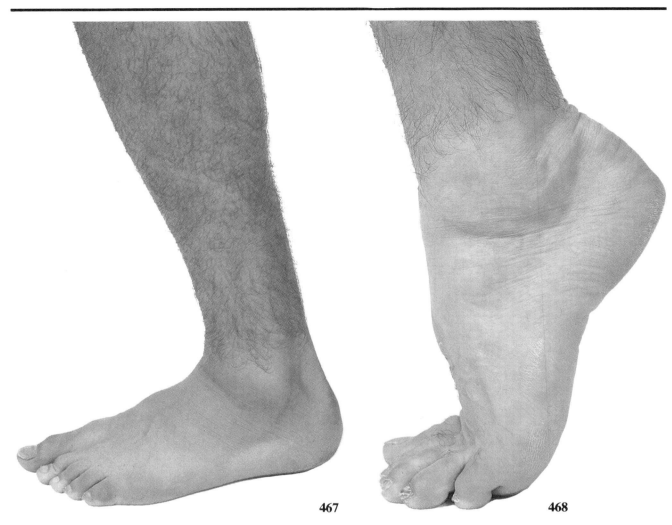

467

468

As the body is carried forwards in walking or running the long flexor muscles to the toes must relax to allow the dorsiflexion of the ankle. The short flexor muscles (including flexor accessorius on to the long flexor tendon) maintain digital flexion. Note how the pressure on the toes has led to blanching.

As the foot drives off, gastrocnemius and particularly soleus give the main plantar flexor power to the ankle. Additional power through to the tarsal joints is added by tibialis posterior (medially) and peroneus longus and brevis (laterally), which muscles also give collateral stability to the ankle and tarsal region. The long flexors of the toes then give the final drive though this is limited as pure toe movement in most footwear with a firm sole.

In addition to the great toe the other toes have a short flexor which has the same insertion as the long flexor digitorum superficialis in the hand. There is also a flexor digitorum accessorius. This muscle arises from the hollow on the medial side of the calcaneum below the medial malleolus where it can be felt contracting on digital flexion. It is inserted into the tendon of flexor digitorum longus and is often said to correct the line of pull of that muscle. This is hardly acceptable but what is important is that in the efficiently working foot the toes need to maintain flexor power even when the long flexor must relax during dorsiflexion of the ankle (**467**). Note how even in relaxation of the long flexors the toes are still maintaining enough flexor power to produce blanching from the pressure on the floor.

It is also important that the long extensors should have a comparable short support, vital to classical ballet dancers for point work. Extensors digitorum and hallucis brevis arise as a muscle mass mainly from the upper surface of the calcaneum and slips join the extensor mechanisms of the toes.

As the tendons of these muscles are of little general value they are often used for tendon grafts but care shold be taken before removing them in anyone for whom digital control in the feet is important.

In a strong foot this muscle mass has been mistaken for a bony lump, so hard can it become on contraction.

MUSCLES ACTING OVER THE ANKLE AND FOOT

The interossei are important muscles in the foot as they are in the hand. The long and short flexors operate primarily on the interphalangeal joints which acting alone will produce clawing of the toes much as occurs in the hand in ulnar nerve palsy. The interossei are the flexors at the metatarsophalangeal joints. They thus complete the full flexor control of the foot from the ankle, the midtarsal joints through to the toes. The need to maintain the strength of these muscles is well enough known and exercises are often prescribed for them. A totally unacceptable one is to pick up a pencil by the toes – this in fact only aggravates the clawing. Flexion must occur at the metatarsophalangeal joints for effective foot function.

When standing with the heels on the ground, the ankle is in a close-packed stable state.

On moving on to the toes soleus with gastrocnemius plantarflexes the ankle joint and give the main power to the movement. Tibialis posterior with the peroneals add flexion to the ankle and tarsal joints and also give lateral balance to the region, including the ankle joint, which otherwise would be free to rock, while the long and short flexors of the toes with the interossei give the necessary digital control. Regrettably many wearers of high heeled shoes have virtually none of this control and rely almost entirely on a tiny heel for safety.

Note also in **470** how the blood to the heel is driven out by this manoeuvre.

469

470

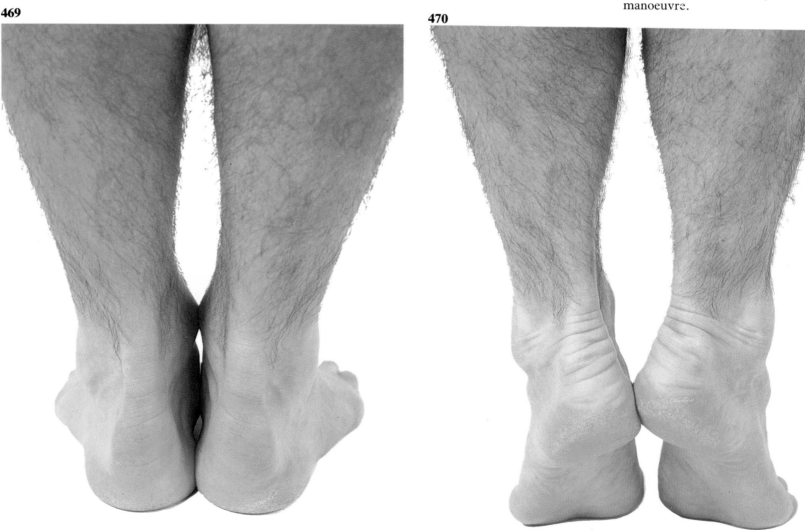

RETINACULA AND SYNOVIAL SHEATHS OF THE FOOT

The three groups of tendons passing the ankle are all controlled by retinacula, made of thickenings in the deep fascia, and lubricated as they pass by synovial sheaths (**471–472**).

The extensor tendons are bound down by two thickenings. The superior extensor retinaculum lies above the ankle joint and bridge across from the tibia to the fibula, binding down all the extensor tendons and peroneus tertius, together with the vessels and nerve. The inferior retinaculum is Y shaped. The single stem runs from the calcaneum and is continuous there as the inferior peroneal retinaculum, over the peroneal tendons. It then crosses the extensor digitorum longus and peroneus tertius before dividing into its upper and lower limbs. The upper limb has two strata; the deeper covers the anterior tibial vessels and the deep peroneal nerve with the more superficial covering the tendons of tibialis anterior and extensor hallucis longus. The lower limb covers all the tendons more distally as well as the nerve and the vessels, the latter now the dorsalis pedis.

The flexor retinaculum runs from the medial malleolus to the calcaneum but the lower part forms separate channels for the individual tendons, together with the posterior tibial vessels and nerve.

The peroneal tendons are covered by a superior retinaculum running from the lateral malleolus to the calcaneum while the lower is an extension of the inferior extensor retinaculum.

The synovial sheaths are individual for each tendon except for the extensor digitorum longus and peroneus tertius which is a combined one. The two peroneal tendons have their tendon sheaths joined proximally.

As in the case of the hand, the flexor tendons to the toes also have synovial sheaths through the fibrous flexor sheaths to each toe.

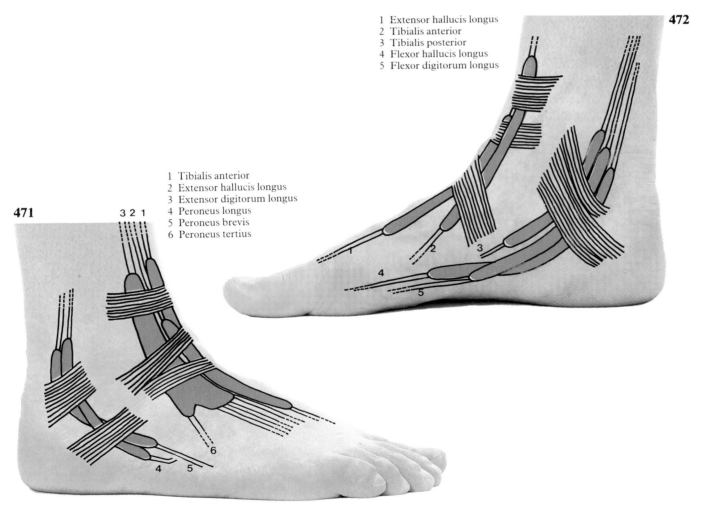

1 Extensor hallucis longus
2 Tibialis anterior
3 Tibialis posterior
4 Flexor hallucis longus
5 Flexor digitorum longus

472

1 Tibialis anterior
2 Extensor hallucis longus
3 Extensor digitorum longus
4 Peroneus longus
5 Peroneus brevis
6 Peroneus tertius

471

THE NERVES OF THE LEGS

In the arm the segmental innervation of the skin follows a relatively simple pattern. In the leg the simplicity has been disorganised by the embryonic rotation of the limb in order to bring the sole of the foot to the ground. Thus the posterior divisional nerves supply the front of the thigh and leg while the anterior division supplies the medial side of the thigh and the back of the leg and sole of the foot. The overall pattern of supply is shown in **473** and **475**.

The areas of supply expected of the individual cutaneous nerves are shown in **474** and **476**. *The genitofemoral nerve* (L1 & 2) runs down over psoas muscle to give two branches. The genital branch passes through the external inguinal ring to supply the cremaster muscle and skin of the scrotum and the adjacent thigh. The femoral branch runs down with the external iliac and femoral arteries to supply an area of skin below the inguinal crease.

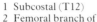

1 Subcostal (T12)
2 Femoral branch of genitofemoral
3 Ilio-inguinal (L1)
4 Lateral femoral cutaneous (L2,3)
5 Intermediate femoral cutaneous
6 Medial femoral cutaneous (L2,3)
7 Obturator (L2,3,4)
8 Infrapatellar branch of saphenous
9 Saphenous (L3,4)
10 Lateral cutaneous of calf (L5, S1)
11 Superficial peroneal (L4,5; S1)
12 Sural (L5; S1,2)
13 Femoral (L2,3,4)
14 Common peroneal (L4,5; S1,2)
15 Superficial peroneal
16 Deep peroneal

Nerve roots and areas of supply.

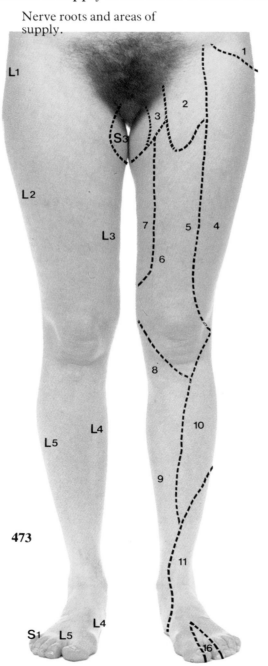

473

Positions of cutaneous and main nerve trunks.

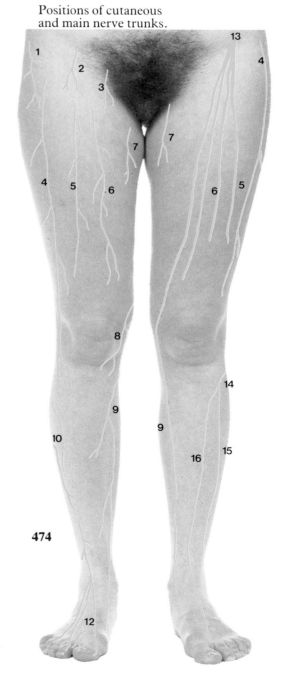

474

292

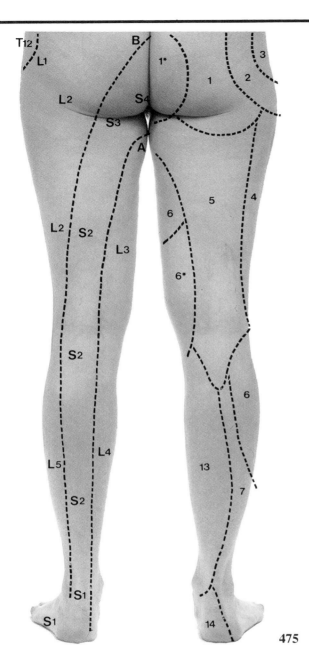

475

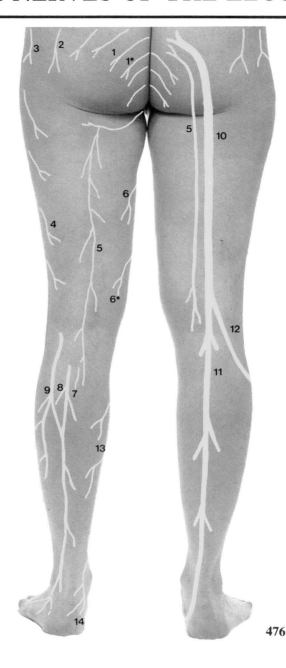

476

1 Posterior rami of lumbar nerves
1* Posterior rami of sacral nerves
2 Iliohypogastric (L1)
3 Subcostal (T12)
4 Lateral cutaneous of thigh
5 Posterior cutaneous of thigh
6 Obturator (L2,3,4)
6* Medial cutaneous of thigh (L2,3,4)
7 Sural (L5; S1,2)
8 Sural communication
9 Lateral cutaneous of calf (L5; S1)
10 Sciatic (L4,5; S1,2,3)
11 Tibial (medial popliteal, L4,5; S1,2,3)
12 Common peroneal (L4,5; S1,2)
13 Saphenous (L3,4)
14 Medial calcaneal branches of tibial (S1,2)

The cremasteric reflex is a useful test of the upper lumbar spinal segments. If the skin of the medial side of the upper thigh is scratched (in a male) reflex contraction of the cremaster muscle leads to retraction of the testis.

The lateral cutaneous nerve of the thigh (L2 & 3) runs over iliacus and enters the leg under the extreme lateral end of the inguinal ligament before piercing the deep fascia. It then divides into two branches, one the anterior supplies skin over the anterolateral aspect of the thigh and joins in the patellar plexus while the posterior branch runs through the fascia lata to supply the lateral aspect of the leg from the greater trochanter to the lower thigh.

The nerve can be blocked in the region of the origin of sartorius to give adequate anaesthesia to the lateral aspect of the thigh. However, more important clinically is the fact that the nerve often runs through the inguinal ligament

THE NERVES OF THE LEGS

where it may be subjected to compression, giving paraesthesia, particularly a burning sensation and numbness over the area of supply (meralgia paraesthetica). This can be relieved by surgical freeing of the nerve, dividing the deeper part of the ligament; sometimes the opening through the fascia lata may need to be widened.

The femoral nerve (L 2, 3 & 4 – posterior division) runs under the inguinal ligament, a finger's breadth lateral to the femoral artery i.e. lateral to the midinguinal point (**447**) where the artery should be palpable. It gives motor supply to the quadriceps group of muscles, sartorius and usually pectineus.

The cutaneous branches to the thigh are the intermediate and medial cutaneous nerves. The intermediate nerve(s) supplies the front of the thigh down to the knee and often arises as or with the branch to sartorius while the medial branch pierces the deep fascia a little lower down the line of sartorius to supply the medial side of the lower thigh and by a posterior branch the medial side of the leg below the knee. The saphenous nerve is the largest of the sensory branches and follows the long saphenous vein down the leg and behind the medial condyle of the knee to supply skin on the medial side of the leg, ankle and foot. Loss of the femoral nerve is unusual from injury but if so the loss of the quadriceps control of the knee is a serious problem; there would be sensory loss on the front of the thigh but there is usually adequate overlap below the knee.

The obturator nerve (L 2, 3 & 4 anterior division) passes as two branches through the obturator foramen to supply the adductor muscles and gives skin supply to the medial side of the upper thigh.

The sacral plexus is derived from the lower two lumbar nerves and the sacral. It supplies the major part of the leg other than that described above. The muscular branches to the quadratus femoris (L 4 5 S 1), obturator internus (L 5 S 1 & 2) pyriformis (S 1 & 2) superior gluteal nerve (L 4, 5 S 1) and the inferior gluteal nerve (L 5 S 1 & 2) have been noted with the muscles while S 4 gives vital innervation to the pelvic diaphragm including the anal sphincter. The major component to the leg is the sciatic nerve with sensory branches via the posterior cutaneous nerve to the back of the lower buttock and perineum and thigh as far as the knee.

477

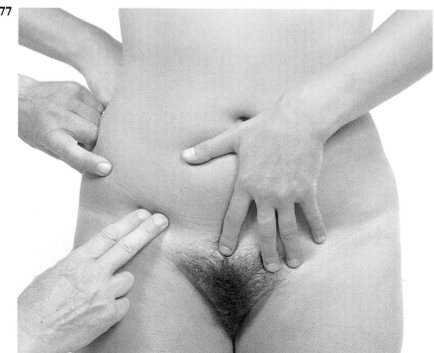

The femoral nerve can easily be found for local anaesthetic block for skin on the front of the thigh. The subject's index finger is pointing to the pubic sympysis and the examiner's to the anterior superior iliac spine. The examiner's middle finger overlies the femoral artery which can be felt pulsating at the mid-inguinal point, i.e. midway between symphysis and spine, while the index finger overlies the nerve.

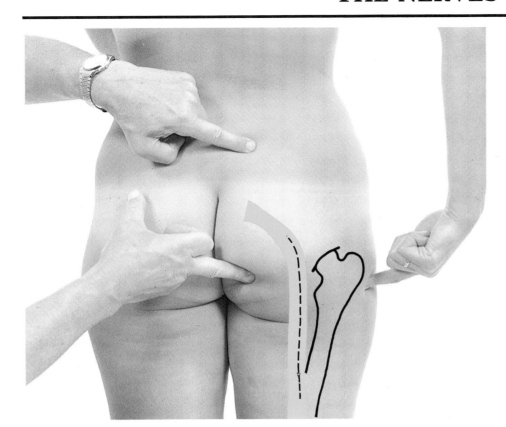

478

The fingers point to the posterior superior iliac spine, the ischial tuberosity and the greater trochanter. The positions of the femur and hip-joint, lying anterior to the nerve are indicated as also is the possible division of the sciatic nerve into medial and lateral components.

The sciatic nerve (L 4, 5 S 1, 2 & 3) leaves the pelvis through the greater sciatic foramen to enter the gluteal region (**478**). It is made up of medial and lateral components which usually divide in the back of the thigh to form the tibial (medial popliteal) nerve, the anterior division of all roots, and the common peroneal (lateral popliteal) nerve from the posterior divisions of all except S 3. It can however divide much earlier and may in fact run through the gluteal region already as separate nerves. In the gluteal region it enters about midway between the posterior superior iliac spine and the ischial tuberosity and then curves downwards to pass just medial to midway between the ischial tuberosity and the greater trochanter.

Of particular importance is the proximity of the lateral-common peroneal component to the acetabulum behind the hip joint. Damage to the nerve may occur in operations on the hip joint such as total hip replacement or in such injuries as posterior dislocation of the joint, with the resultant foot drop.

From the gluteal region the sciatic nerve passes down the middle of the back of the thigh. As it leaves the cover of gluteus maximus it comes to lie close under the deep fascia where it is vulnerable to injury but then runs deep again under biceps femoris. In the thigh it supplies all the hamstring muscles and the ischial component of adductor magnus. The medial component then continues through the centre of the popliteal fossa as the tibial (medial popliteal) nerve, to supply gastrocnemius and soleus, together with tibialis posterior, flexor hallucis longus and flexor digitorum longus before entering the foot behind the medial malleolus. Here it is tucked in under the medial side of the tendo calcaneus and can be palpated by pressure over the calcaneum just medial to the insertion of the tendon. Here it is also readily available for local nerve block. The nerve then runs into the sole of the foot where it divides into medial and lateral plantar nerves. These supply the short muscles of the foot, the medial giving cutaneous sensory supply to the medial part of the foot, leaving the lateral to supply the lateral part with the lateral one and a half toes.

THE NERVES OF THE LEGS

In the popliteal region the tibial nerve gives off the sural nerve (**479**) which runs down the back of the leg in company with the short saphenous vein, to supply (with the sural communicating nerve from the common peroneal nerve) the skin of the lower lateral part of the calf and the lateral side of the foot and little toe. It runs into the foot behind the lateral malleolus.

The common peroneal (lateral popliteal) nerve is the other smaller terminal branch of the sciatic nerve. It leaves the main nerve above or at the upper part of the popliteal fossa and runs downwards and laterally along the medial side of the tendon of biceps. It then winds forwards around the neck of the fibula before entering peroneus longus muscle where it divides into deep and superficial peroneal nerves. The former supplies the four extensor muscles and then continues over the front of the ankle, between the tendons of extensors hallucis and digitorum longus into the dorsum of the foot, with the dorsalis pedis artery, to supply the adjoining surfaces of the great and second toes.

The superficial peroneal (musculocutaneous) nerve runs downwards between extensor digitorum longus and the peroneal muscles, supplying the two peroneal muscles. It then goes on anterior to the lateral malleolus to supply most of the dorsum of the foot.

The lateral cutaneous nerve of the calf leaves the common peroneal nerve in the popliteal fossa to supply the lateral aspect of the calf. The common peroneal nerve is readily palpable by pressure over the neck of the fibula and can usually be felt rolling under the finger as it is moved up and down (**480**). Here it is very vulnerable to external trauma such as from the bumper bar of a car and not infrequently from pressure from plaster casts. It is also readily accessible for electrical stimulation or local anaesthetic block. Damage to the nerve, as to the lateral component of the sciatic nerve near the hip joint, leads to foot drop due to loss of the extensor muscles. When the foot is raised from the ground the toe drops and thus trails while being carried forwards in walking, with the need to throw the foot forwards by quick

1 Sciatic nerve
2 Tibial (medial popliteal) nerve
3 Common peroneal (lateral popliteal) nerve
4 Sural nerve
5 Sural communicating nerve
6 Tibial nerve running behind medial malleolus (The tibial nerve divides below the medial malleolus into the lateral and medial plantar nerves)

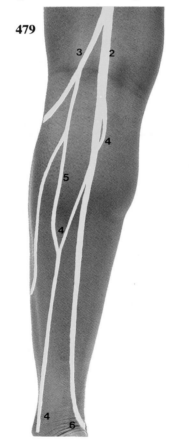

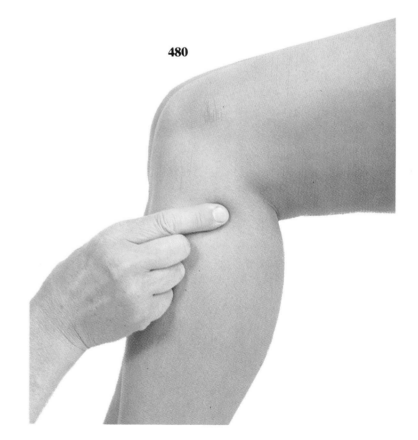

knee extension to place it on the ground. As the peroneal muscles are also likely to lose their nerve supply there will also be inversion of the foot. The front of the leg and upper surface of the foot will also be anaesthetic. Damage to part of the sciatic nerve is common from lower lumbar bone or disc lesions and these are likely to be root lesions. Total damage to the nerve is much more unusual, due to posterior wounds or posterior fractures and dislocations around the hip joint. This would lead to paralysis of the hamstrings and loss of all the muscles below the knee, together with a similar area of sensory loss, other than the medial side of the leg.

Injections are commonly given into the legs and the most usual sites are the buttock and outer thigh. The latter should present few problems as no major nerves are likely to be damaged in the region below the greater trochanter. This is a good site for personal injection, such as insulin for diabetics (**482**).

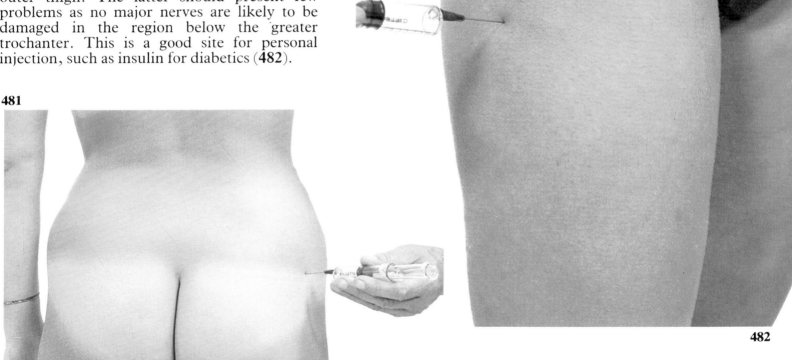

481

482

The region of the buttocks is less easy and in far too many cases the sciatic nerve has been damaged and even destroyed by such an injection. If care is taken to limit all injections to the upper and outer quadrant of the buttock this should be safe (**481**) but even with this knowledge damage has been done. Hence the best advice is to make it a little below the iliac crest and behind the anterior superior iliac spine or, above and anterior to a line joining the tip of the greater trochanter and the posterior superior iliac spine.

THE ARTERIES OF THE LEG

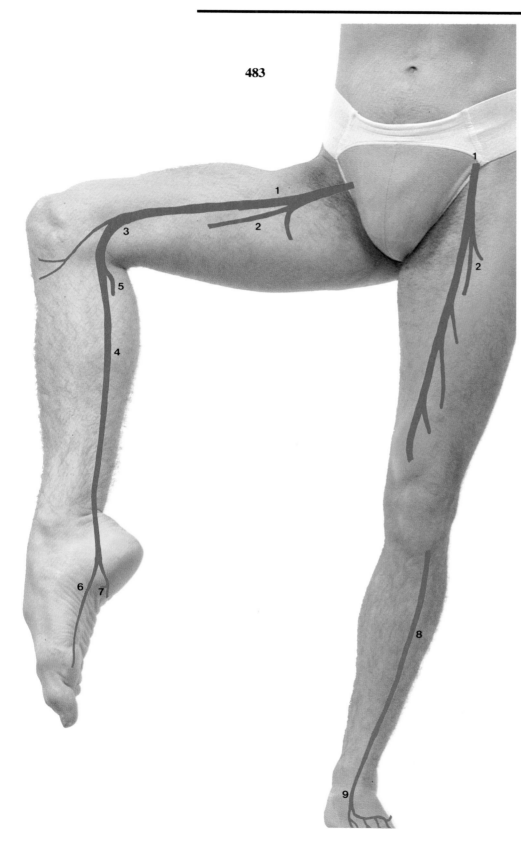

483

The *femoral artery* (**483**), the main axial artery of the leg is a continuation of the external iliac, which enters the leg beneath the inguinal ligament at the mid-inguinal point (i.e. midway between symphysis pubis and anterior superior iliac spine, **477**). Here it becomes superficial in the femoral triangle in the upper third of the thigh. In the groin it lies in front of the head of the femur, separated by the tendon of psoas. Being superficial it is, with the femoral nerve and vein on each side of it, vulnerable to injury. It is also readily available for canulation, if required, for a variety of clinical tests e.g. renal angiography etc. From the femoral triangle it runs down the leg under cover of sartorius in the subsartorial canal (of Hunter). It then winds around the medial side of the femur under the origin of adductor magnus, at the junction of the middle and lower thirds of the thigh, to enter the popliteal fossa. If the leg is flexed and rotated slightly laterally at the hip a line drawn from the mid-inguinal point to the adductor tubercle gives the surface projection in the upper two-thirds of the thigh.

In the popliteal fossa it changes its name to the popliteal artery, where it comes to lie deeply, closely related to the back of the femur, posterior capsule of the knee joint and then over popliteus muscle. If the knee is flexed the tension of the capsule of the popliteal fossa is relaxed and the artery can be felt pulsating against the back of the tibial table where it can also be compressed in arterial bleeding (**484**). The femoral artery can also be so compressed in the groin over the head of the femur or against the medial aspect of the femur in mid thigh.

1 Femoral
2 Profunda
3 Popliteal
4 Posterior tibial
5 Peroneal
6 Medial plantar
7 Lateral plantar
8 Anterior tibial
9 Dorsalis pedis

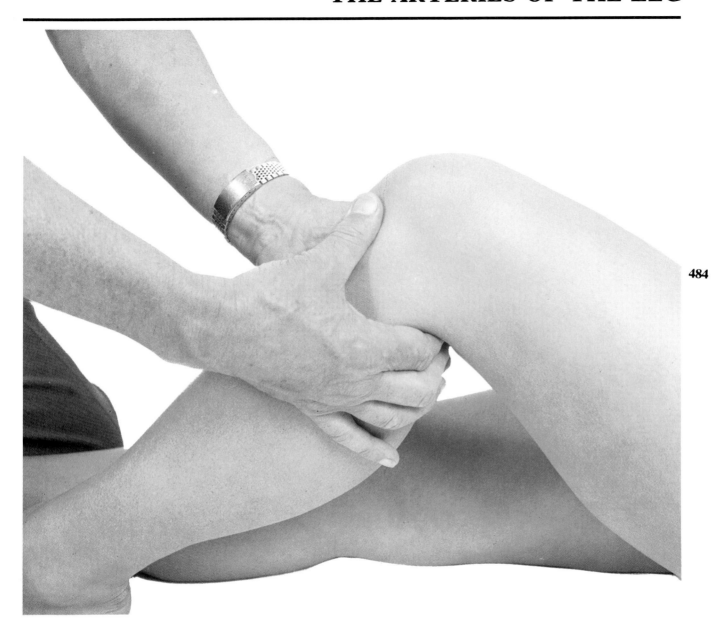

484

About 5 cm below the upper aspect of the tibia and about the level of the tibial tubercle the popliteal artery divides into posterior and anterior tibial arteries.

The *posterior tibial* artery runs down the leg with the tibial nerve, deep to gastrocnemius and soleus to appear more superficially behind the medial side of the tibia. At the medial malleolus it lies about mid-point between malleolus and the tendo calcaneus (with the nerve behind and lateral) before curving to the posterior part of the sustentaculum tali. Behind the malleolus the pulsations should be felt easily by light pressure against the lower part of the tibia, where here it is also available for compression in arterial bleeding (**485**). The order of structures from the malleolus laterally is tibialis posterior, flexor digitorum longus, posterior tibial artery (with its venae commitantes) tibial nerve and flexor hallucis longus, this last initially under the tendo calcaneus. From the ankle the posterior tibial artery runs into the sole of the foot, dividing into medial and lateral plantar arteries.

THE ARTERIES OF THE LEG

The *anterior tibial* artery passes through the upper part of the interosseous membrane to the front of the leg and then runs down on the membrane towards the ankle where it comes to lie on the front of the tibia. In the upper part of the leg it lies about midway between the tibial tubercle and the neck of the fibula while at the ankle it is midway between the two malleoli. Thus on the front of the ankle from medial to lateral the structures are tibialis anterior, extensor hallucis longus, anterior tibial artery with its venae commitantes, deep peroneal nerve and most laterally the tendons of extensor digitorum longus and peroneus tertius. Passing into the foot the artery runs on just lateral to the tendon of extensor hallucis longus as the *dorsalis pedis* artery, before passing through the space between the first and second metatarsal. The artery can be felt pulsating just lateral to the tendon of extensor hallucis longus over the cuneiform bones and lateral to the base of the first metatarsal (**486**).

Palpation of the arteries in the leg with their pulses is important clinically as it gives a ready assessment of their state; they are frequently involved in changes in their walls with subsequent reduced vascular flow.

Although for routine arterial canulation the radial artery is the most used, where there are problems, the dorsalis pedis is an excellent and safe alternative.

As the skin on the dorsum of the foot is of good quality with an axial vascular supply through the dorsalis pedis vessels, it makes an excellent free graft based on the anterior tibial vessels, to which the nerve can be incorporated where a suitable nerve is available in the recipient area.

485

If there is difficulty in feeling the artery in the natural position, it can be helped by dorsiflexing and everting the foot.

486

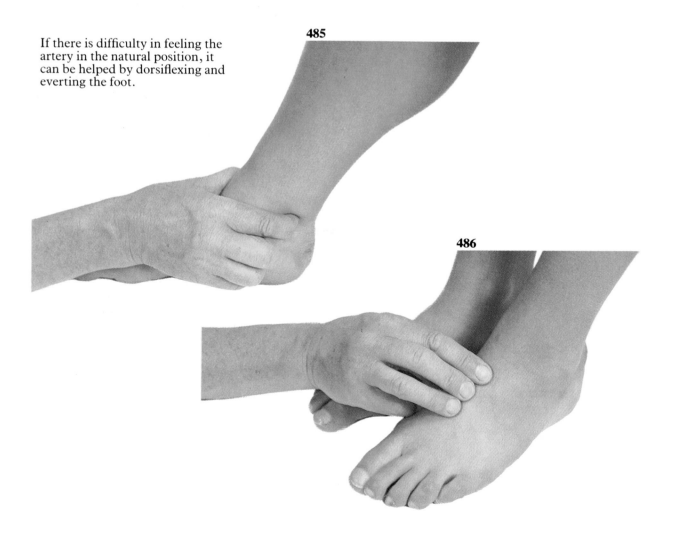

The veins of the leg are of particular importance for a variety of clinical reasons in addition to the problem of carrying the blood against gravity to the heart. Stasis in the deep veins from a variety of causes commonly leads to thrombosis which not only blocks the vein but may then lead to thrombi being sent into the circulation ending most commonly in the lungs. The superficial veins commonly become varicosed with the resultant deficiencies in superficial venous return.

487

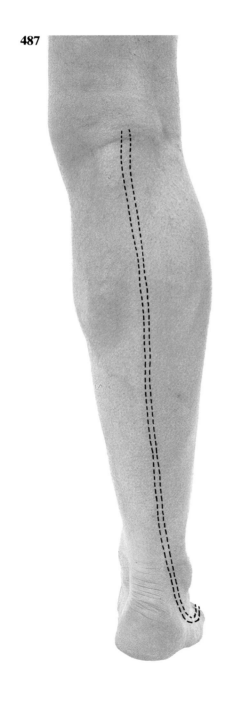

The superficial venous drainage from the toes develops on the dorsum and veins leave between the metatarsals to join a dorsal venous arch. The *small (short) saphenous vein* starts from the lateral aspect of the dorsal venous arch thus receiving blood mainly from the lateral toes and side of the foot. From here it runs behind the lateral malleolus up the back of the calf to the midline over the popliteal fossa. Here it pierces the deep fascia to join the popliteal vein (**487**). The *great (long) saphenous vein* begins on the medial side of the foot from the venous arch. It runs up in front of the medial malleolus and then behind the medial condyles of the tibia and femur before ascending still superficially along the posterior border of sartorius to the groin. It then passes through the deep fascia via the saphenous opening to join the femoral vein. The opening lies about 3-4 cms below the inguinal crease, to the medial side of the femoral artery. Before passing deep, the vein is joined by a 'cart-wheel' of veins of which the most important are the superficial external pudendal from the genital region, the superficial epigastric from the lower abdominal wall and the superficial circumflex iliac. Other veins join from the thigh while linkages between the two saphenous veins are common, particularly below the knee. Accessory saphenous veins may also run into the great saphenous vein.

Both saphenous veins are provided with valves to prevent the blood falling backwards. They are also severally connected by perforating and communicating veins with the deep veins, which are also supplied with valves to prevent the blood returning to the superficial system. Valve failure is a feature of and probably one cause of varicose veins, where there is poor venous return from the superficial regions with, in some cases, a tendency to ulceration.

The superficial veins in the foot offer an excellent site for infusions when they are readily visible and thus accessible. If however they are small, contracted or hidden in fat it may be necessary to cut down onto the great or, sometimes, the small saphenous vein at the ankle. Thus accurate knowledge of the positions of the veins is vital so that accurate placement of the incision is made. As the saphenous nerve runs with the great saphenous vein it is advisable to remember this in cutting down so as to avoid cutting the nerve with the consequent risk of the development of a painful neuroma.

THE VEINS OF THE LEG

As the main venous pump towards the heart comes from the muscles, and particularly soleus, acting upon the deep veins, the superficial veins can be discarded, and may have to be when they become severely varicosed and incompetent (**488**). They are also available as vascular grafts

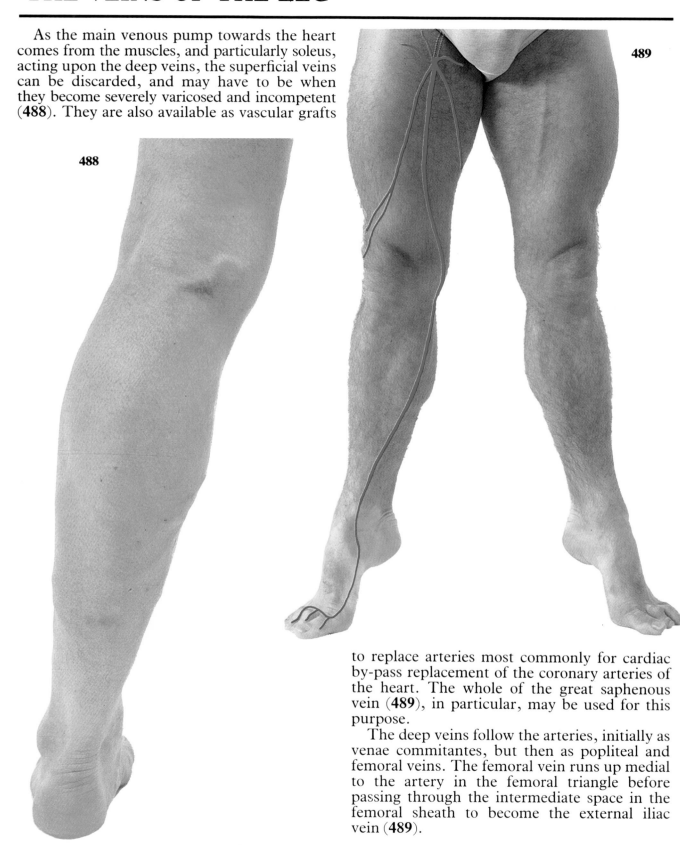

488

489

to replace arteries most commonly for cardiac by-pass replacement of the coronary arteries of the heart. The whole of the great saphenous vein (**489**), in particular, may be used for this purpose.

The deep veins follow the arteries, initially as venae commitantes, but then as popliteal and femoral veins. The femoral vein runs up medial to the artery in the femoral triangle before passing through the intermediate space in the femoral sheath to become the external iliac vein (**489**).

The lymphatics of the leg generally follow the standard pattern of the deep ones running with the arteries while the superficial ones follow the veins. The main drainage from the foot runs onto the dorsum and thence along the great saphenous vein, while those from the lateral side follow the small saphenous vein. The latter run up laterally towards the popliteal fossa where several lymph nodes are embedded in the popliteal fat. From here vessels run deep to follow the artery, ending in deep inguinal lymph nodes along the femoral vessels, although some lymphatics may also run superficially to join those following the great saphenous vein.

The lymphatics running with the great saphenous vein follow it to the inguinal region to end in superficial inguinal lymph nodes. The superficial inguinal nodes consist of a T-shaped group, giving lymph drainage to the area of vascular drainage of the great saphenous vein and its tributaries. The transversely running group lies parallel to and below the inguinal ligament. The more lateral ones receive drainage from the iliac region and the lower abdominal wall, mainly below the umbilicus; the more medial ones receive drainage from the external genital region and the anus. The vertical group, lying along the upper end of the saphenous vein receive the superficial drainage from the whole of the leg except for those which have gone through the popliteal nodes, and thence deep.

Infections etc from the lateral toes and side of the foot, together with the lateral part of the lower leg may be expected to produce a response in the popliteal nodes. Being embedded in fat these are far less easy to feel than are those in the inguinal region. The superficial inguinal lymph nodes not only drain a large area of the leg but also the lower abdomen and perineum and lie in the hollow of the groin where they can easily be felt (**490**). They are in fact commonly palpable even in a normal state. Pain and swelling in these nodes may well indicate infection or malignancy in any part of their drainage. As they drain the perineum and anus, the latter in particular being an infected region, it should be remembered that reaction in these nodes is more likely to come from that source than the leg.

From the superficial inguinal lymph nodes, vessels pass through the cribriform fascia to join the deep nodes along the femoral vessels. From here lymphatics pass through the femoral canal (the medial space in the femoral sheath) where another lymph node is also to be found. Other vessels run with the femoral artery and vein with all going to the iliac nodes. Although superficial drainage from the buttock follows the course of the leg or perineum, the deeper ones run with the arteries to the iliac nodes direct.

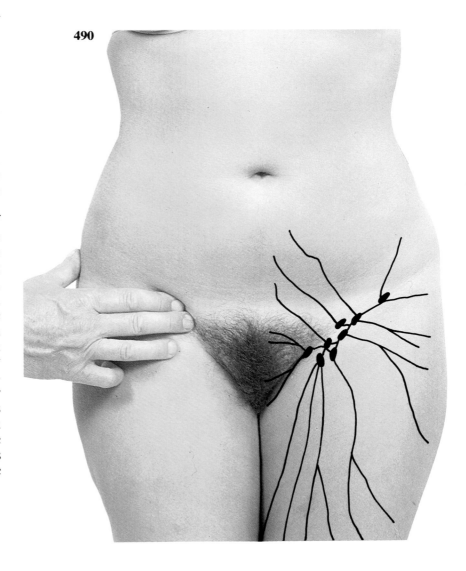

490